ENDOSCOPY IN INFERTILITY

System requirement:

- Windows XP or above
- Power DVD player (Software)
- Windows media player 10.0 version or above (Software)

Accompanying DVD ROM is playable only in Computer and not in DVD player.

DVD Content

Endoscopic Procedures in Infertility

ENDOSCOPY IN INFERTILITY

Editor

Kamini A Rao

DGO DORCP DCh FRCOG MCh FICOG PGDMLE (Law) FNAMS

President ISAR

Medical Director

Bangalore Assisted Conception Centre Pvt Ltd

6/7 Kumara Krupa Road, High Grounds

Bangalore

Co-editor

Christopher Chen

MBBS FAMS FRCOG FRACOG FRANCOG FACS FICS

CEO and Medical Director of

Christopher Chen Centre for Reproductive Medicine

Senior Consultant Obstetrician and

Gynaecologist and Infertility Specialist

Director of Gleneagles IVF Centre

Gleneagles Hospital

Singapore

JAYPEE BROTHERS

MEDICAL PUBLISHERS (P) LTD.

New Delhi

Anshan

Tunbridge Wells

UK

First published in the UK by

Anshan Ltd
in **2007**
6 Newlands Road
Tunbridge Wells
Kent TN4 9AT, UK

Tel: +44 (0)1892 557767
Fax: +44 (0)1892 530358
E-mail: info@anshan.co.uk
www.anshan.co.uk

ISBN 10 1-905740-62-X
ISBN 13 978-1-905740-62-8

British Library Cataloguing in Publication Data
A catalogue record for this book is available from the British Library

Printed in India by Ajanta Offset & Packagings Ltd., New Delhi

I dedicate this book to
my husband Dr AS Arvind and
my children Siddharth and Vyshnavi
for their unflinching support, love and encouragement

—Dr Kamini A Rao

Contributors

Aby K Koshy
Consultant Gynaecologist
Paul's Hospital and Cochin Gynaecological
Endoscopy Training Centre, Cochin, Kerala, India

Anil Chittake
Clinical Assistant
National Institute of Laser and
Endoscopic Surgery NILES – Mumbai
Aakar IVF – ICSI Centre, Mumbai, India

B Ramesh
Director
Dr Ramesh Hospital, Rajajinagar, Bangalore, India

Bimal Mathew John
Associate Director
Credence Hospital and Women's Health Institute
Near Ulsoor Bridge, Trivandrum, India

Chong Jin Long
Senior Consultant Anaesthetist
JL Anaesthesia Associates
Mount Alvernia Hospital, Singapore

Christopher Chen
CEO and Medical Director of Christopher
Chen Centre for Reproductive Medicine
Senior Consultant Obstetrician and
Gynaecologist and Infertility Specialist
Director of Gleneagles IVF Centre
Gleneagles Hospital, Singapore

Gautam N Allahbadia
Scientific Director
Aesculap Academy-Asia Pacific Center for
Minimally Invasive Surgery
Training and Research, Prince Aly Khan Hospital
Mazagaon, Mumbai, India

M Ramesh
Director,
BEST Institute and Research Centre
AV Hospital, Bangalore, India

Madhuri Patil
Director
Patil's Endoscopy and Fertility Center
5B, 2nd Floor, Priya Tower
1 Main, Ist Stage, BTM Layout
Bannerghatta Road, Bangalore, India

Manish Banker
Director
Advanced Fertility and Endoscopic Centre
Melbourne IVF Gujarat
Ahmedabad, India

Manish Shah
Consultant Gynecologist
Advanced Fertility and Endoscopic Centre
Melbourne IVF Gujarat
Ahmedabad, India

Meenakshi S
Consultant Gynecologist
Beams Hospital, 674, 16th Cross Road, Khar (W)
Mumbai, India

Nagendra Sardeshpande
Consultant Obstetrician and Gynecologist
Brahman Sabha and Dhanwantri Hospitals
Mumbai, India

Nikhil S Jani
Consultant Obstetrician and Gynecologist
Dr Danait Hospital, Andheri, Mumbai, India

Nozer Sheriar
Consultant Obstetrician and Gynecologist
Holy Family, Masina and Parsee General Hospitals
Gynecological Endoscopist
Bhatia and BARC Hospitals, Mumbai, India

Nutan Jain
Chief Endoscopic Surgeon and Infertility Specialist
Vardhman Infertility and Endoscopy Centre
A-36, Mahavir Chowk, Muzaffarnagar, (UP), India

PG Paul
Director
Paul's Hospital and Cochin Gynaecological
Endoscopy Training Centre, Cochin, Kerala, India

Prakash Trivedi
Chief Gynaecological Endoscopist and ART
Consultant, National Institute of Laser and
Endoscopic Surgery NILES – Mumbai

Jaslok, Wockhardt and BARC Hospital
Mumbai, India

Scientific Director
Akar IVF-ICSI Centre, Mumbai, India
Head of Dept. Obstetrics and Gynaecology
VC Gandhi, Rajawadi, Municipal Hospital
Hon. Prof. Pd. DY Patil Medical College
Mumbai, India

Pratap Kumar
Professor and Head
Dept. of Obstetrics and Gynaecology
Kasturba Medical College, Manipal, India

Pravin Patel
Director
Advanced Fertility and Endoscopic Centre
Melbourne IVF Gujarat, Ahmedabad, India

Rakesh Sinha
Gynecological Endoscopic Surgeon
Director
Beams Hospital
674, 16th Cross Road, Khar (W)
Mumbai, India

Ravi Kumar
Consultant Anaesthetist,
Bangalore Assisted Conception Centre
6/7, Kumara Krupa Road
Highgrounds, Bangalore, India

Sanjay Patel
Chief Endoscopic Surgeon
Mayflower Hospital, Ahmedabad, India

Sankar Das Mahapatra
Consultant Gynecologist
Vardhman Infertility and Endoscopy Centre
A-36, Mahavir Chowk, Muzaffarnagar, (UP), India

Shweta Raje
Consultant Gynecologist
Beams Hospital
674, 16th Cross Road, Khar (W), Mumbai, India

Shyam V Desai
Hon. Professor, Obstetrician and Gynecologist
N. Wadia Maternity Hospital, Mumbai, India

Sulbha Arora
Clinical Associate
Aesculap Academy – Asia Pacific Center for Minimally Invasive Surgery
Training and Research
Prince Aly Khan Hospital
Mazagoan, Mumbai, India

Sunita R Tandulwadkar
Chief IVF Consultant and Endoscopist
Ruby Hall Clinic
Pune, India

Tejas Dave
Consultant Gynecologist
Advanced Fertility and Endoscopic Centre
Melbourne IVF Gujarat, Ahmedabad, India

Tony Thomas
Consultant Gynaecologist
Paul's Hospital and Cochin Gynaecological Endoscopy Training Centre, Cochin, Kerala, India

Yogendra Jhala
Endoscopic Surgeon
Mayflower Hospital, Ahmedabad, India

Preface

New innovations in assisted reproductive technologies have opened up numerous options for treatment of infertility. The last 30 years has proven the value of and advantages of endoscopic access for gynecologic surgery which has had a great impact on the management of infertility. As a diagnostic tool, a combined laparoscopic and hysteroscopic examination is the gold standard for the evaluation of infertility. Gynecological endoscopic surgeries have changed and continue to evolve rapidly and several procedures considered difficult are now being successfully done laparoscopically. The advantages of shortened postoperative hospital stay, reduced postoperative discomfort, frequently lesser costs, and the opportunity to diagnose and treat at the same time has led to the immense popularity of endoscopic procedures. Advances in fiberoptic camera technology and improvement in technique and technology has revolutionized endoscopic procedures with great benefits to both the patient and the doctor.

This book presents an entire plethora of all possible surgical procedures in the treatment of infertility which can be carried out by endoscopy. Contributing authors have submitted high quality manuscripts which are of utmost practical application written in a simple, easy to understand style. The book is supported by a video DVD to teach and demonstrate the techniques described in the text.

Endoscopic diagnosis and surgery in the treatment of Infertility is here to stay. The future generation of gynecologists will have to learn only the laparoscopic technique for many of the common surgeries. We hope this book will be useful to those aspiring endoscopic surgeons and infertility specialists.

Kamini A Rao
Christopher Chen

Contents

SECTION ONE: GENERAL

1. **Prevention and Management of Complications at Laparoscopy** 3
   PG Paul, Aby K Koshy, Tony Thomas
2. **Fertiloscopy** 10
   Christopher Chen
3. **Tissue Harmonics in the Practice of Endoscopy in Infertility** 13
   Nutan Jain, Sankar Das Mahapatra
4. **Laparoscopic Management of Endometrioma** 25
   Rakesh Sinha, Meenakshi S
5. **Treatment of Peritoneal and Other Endometriosis** 36
   Pratap Kumar, Bimal Mathew John
6. **Endoscopy in Male Infertility due to Varicoceles** 40
   Christopher Chen
7. **Safety Aspects of Endoscopy** 45
   Madhuri Patil
8. **Endoscopic Instrumentation** 63
   Manish Banker, Pravin Patel, Manish Shah
9. **Anesthetic Management of Endoscopic Surgeries—Laparoscopy and Hysteroscopy** 72
   Ravi Kumar
10. **Anesthesia for Endoscopic Surgery in Infertility** 78
    Chong Jin Long

SECTION TWO: UTERUS

11. **Hysteroscopic Myomectomy** 87
    Christopher Chen
12. **Laparoscopic Myomectomy** 90
    Christopher Chen
13. **Laparoscopic Assisted Minilap Myomectomy** 95
    Nutan Jain

14. **Endoscopic Myomectomy in Infertility: Current Scenario and Our Experience** 107
Prakash Trivedi, Anil Chittake

15. **Hysteroscopic Management of Intrauterine Adhesions** 137
Nozer Sheriar, Nagendra Sardeshpande

16. **Role of Hysteroscopy in the Management of Infertility** 148
Rakesh Sinha, Shweta Raje

SECTION THREE: TUBES

17. **Laparoscopic Surgery for Distal Tubal Occlusion** 161
Pravin Patel, Manish Banker, Tejas Dave, Manish Shah

18. **Current Trends in the Management of Ectopic Pregnancy** 168
B Ramesh

19. **Hysteroscopic Cannulation for Proximal Tubal Block** 173
Sulbha Arora, Gautam N Allahbadia

20. **Falloposcopy and Salpingoscopy in Tubal Evaluation for Infertility** 180
Sunita R Tandulwadkar

21. **Role of Laparoscopic Tubal Recanalization in Modern Era of ART** 189
Sanjay Patel, Yogendra Jhala

SECTION FOUR: OVARIES

22. **Laparoscopic Electrocauterization of Ovarian Surface** 201
Shyam V Desai, Nikhil S Jani

23. **Laparoscopic Management of Benign Ovarian Mass** 207
Pravin Patel, Manish Banker, Manish Shah

24. **Laparoscopic Management of Adnexal Masses** 215
M Ramesh

Index *229*

Section One

GENERAL

1 Prevention and Management of Complications at Laparoscopy

PG Paul, Aby K Koshy, Tony Thomas

INTRODUCTION

Complications are inherent in any surgical procedure and laparoscopy is no exception. Since complications can occur even with a relatively easy procedure, it is imperative that all surgeons must learn to recognize the complications expeditiously and manage the events.

The risks increase exponentially with the complexity of procedures, the inexperience of the surgeon and with any deviation from the standard techniques.

The learning curve for laparoscopic procedures is lengthy and the risk of complications is greatest in the early period of the surgeon's learning. According to the ISGE survey, bowel injury occurred 5 times more frequently for surgeons who performed fewer than 100 laparoscopies per year.[1] The risk is higher when a new instrumentation or technique is utilized. The complication rates for diagnostic and minor laparoscopic procedures are less than 1 percent. Three national surveys conducted in the Netherlands, France and Finland included 25,764, 29,966 and 70,607 laparoscopic procedures respectively.[2-5] The total complication rates were 5.7, 4.6 and 3.6 per 1,000 procedures.

Complications can be divided into the following groups:

Anesthesia Related

An extreme Trendelenburg's position and increased intra-abdominal pressure during laparoscopy can compromise the patient. Prolonged ventilation with difficult intubation may fill the stomach with air and make it prone for injury with Veress needle or trocar. Ask the anesthetist to decompress the stomach with a nasogastric tube just prior to inserting the Veress needle through the left upper quadrant of the abdomen.

Patient Positioning and Nerve Injuries

Prolonged laparoscopic procedures under general anesthesia can lead to nerve injuries especially those involving the brachial plexus, ulnar, femoral and common peroneal nerves.

Any significant abduction, extension or external rotation of the arm can stretch the brachial plexus and cause nerve injury. An improperly placed shoulder rest can cause compression of the brachial plexus between the shoulder braces and first rib (Figure 1.1).The shoulder rest should be placed laterally on the acromioclavicular joint.

Placing the left arm extended at the elbow joint, pronated and tucked loosely by the side of the body (Figure 1.2) and the right arm flexed and kept on the chest as if on a sling can prevent both ulnar and brachial plexus injuries (Figure 1.3).

The patient's legs are then placed in the stirrups, with attention to the common peroneal nerve and femoral nerve. The common peroneal nerve is a branch of the sciatic nerve that passes very close to the head

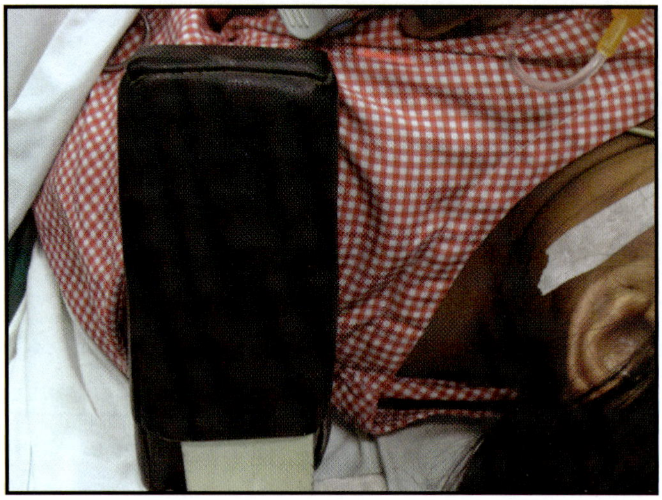

Figure 1.1. Shoulder rest should be placed laterally on the acromioclavicular joint

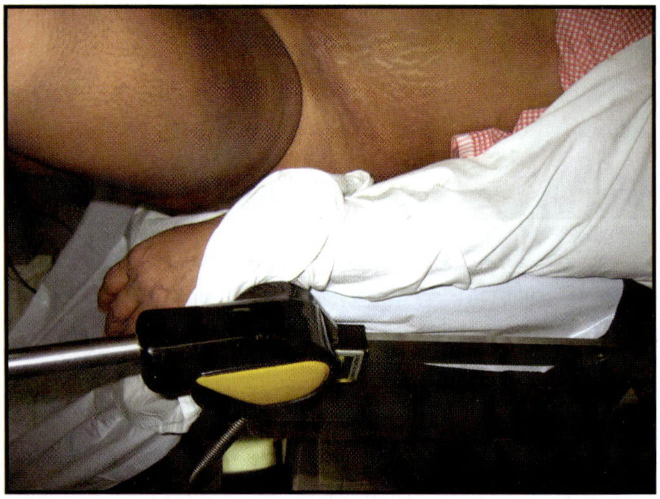

Figure 1.2. Positioning the extended left arm: Pronated and tucked loosely by the side of the body

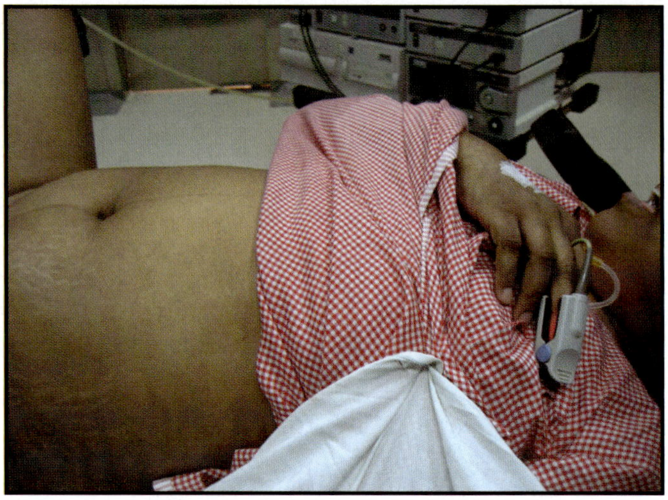

Figure 1.3. Positioning the flexed and adducted right arm

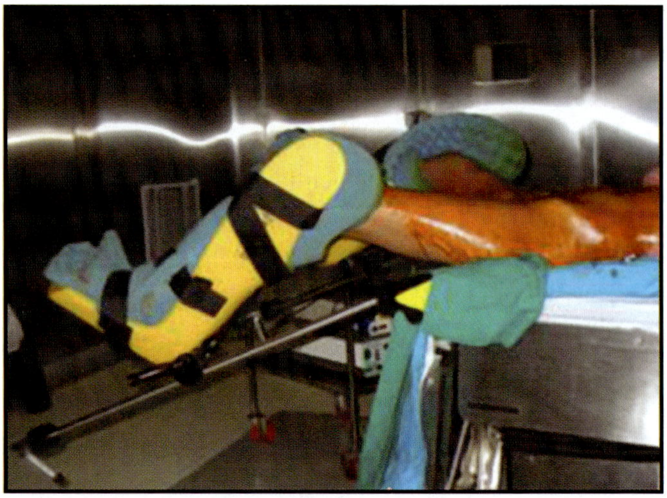

Figure 1.4. The leg placed in Allen stirrups

of fibula on its lateral aspect. Make sure that when the legs are placed in the stirrups and abducted there is a good cushion support to the common peroneal nerve (Figure 1.4).

The femoral nerve is also at risk of injury when the legs are placed at extreme flexion, external rotation and abduction. The femoral nerve can be stretched or compressed by the inguinal ligament especially when the legs are elevated for completing the vaginal part of a LAVH. It is important to deflex the knee when legs are elevated.

Postoperative numbness or tingling usually resolves by the fifth day and any symptom that persists beyond five days requires a neurological evaluation.

Trocar Related Injuries

It is the most common complication in laparoscopy. It is also the one of the most serious and potentially preventable complication in laparoscopic surgery. In a study of laparoscopic malpractice claims in the US, trocar injuries represented 31 percent of cases which was more than any other device. Trocars used in 24 out of 31 fatal cases were either shielded or optical trocars.[6] This finding is important because of the widespread use of trocars with these features and because laparoscopists may expect these features to reduce the risk of injury.

In an average patient the distance between anterior abdominal wall and retroperitoneal vessels is normally 3-4 cm. It can be increased to 8-14 cm by creating a pneumoperitoneum. We usually create a pneumoperitoneum with a Veress needle through an intra-umbilical vertical incision. Aspiration with a syringe is useful to avoid gas embolism before connecting it to the carbon dioxide source. We use a reusable trocar for primary entry. A Ternamian Endotip (Karl Storz, Tuttlingen, Germany) is used whenever bowel adhesions are suspected (Figure 1.5). It is important to get familiarized with the trocar and be very careful whenever a new trocar is used. Avoid the Trendelenburg's position before trocar insertion which can make the angle of insertion more perpendicular (Figure 1.6). A screwing motion of trocar gives better control while entering the abdomen than direct thrusting. The secondary trocars are placed under vision lateral to inferior epigastric vessels. The bladder should be emptied before introducing the suprapubic trocar.

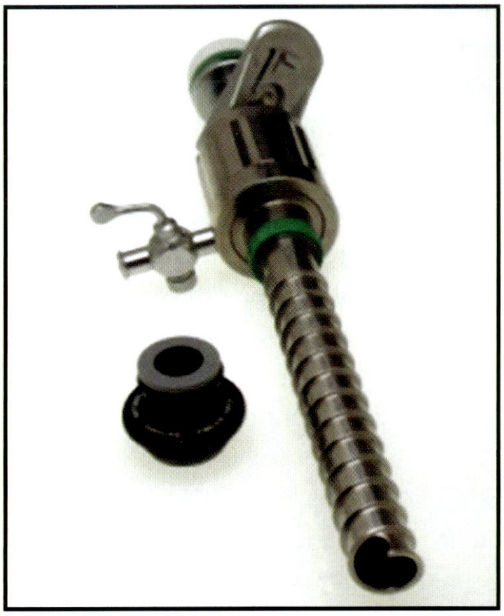

Figure 1.5. Ternamian endotip

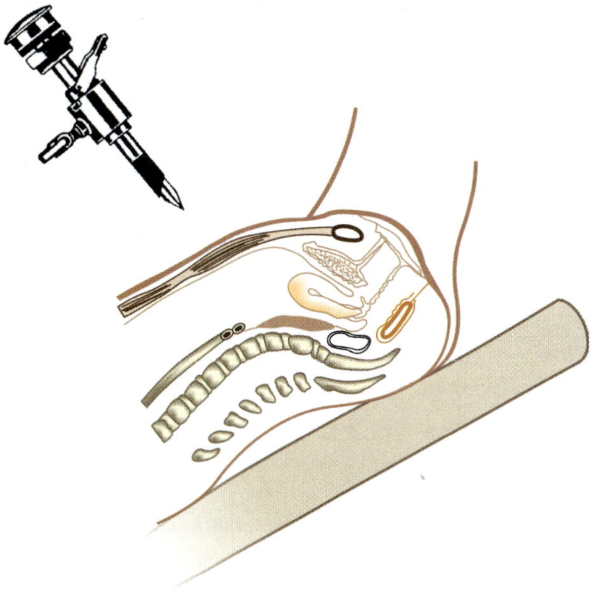

Figure 1.6. Trendelenburg's position: Avoid during primary trocar insertion

Intraoperative Complications

The three major areas of intraoperative complications include vascular, bowel and urological injuries. All intraoperative injuries can be life-threatening, especially if they go unrecognized.

Bladder and Ureteric Injuries

Serious complications are increasing as more and more major operative laparoscopy procedures are being performed. Urological complications can be either due to thermal or mechanical injuries.

The bladder is usually injured during dissection from the pubocervical fascia during laparoscopic hysterectomy. Patients with a previous cesarean section and those with endometriosis have a increased likelihood of this complication. The presence of gas and/or blood in the urinary drainage bag allows early recognition. Cystoscopy is confirmatory.

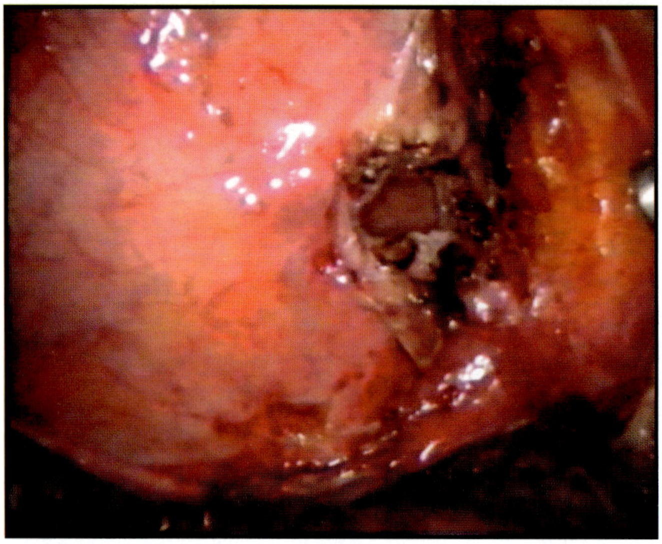

Figure 1.7. Intraoperative bladder injury

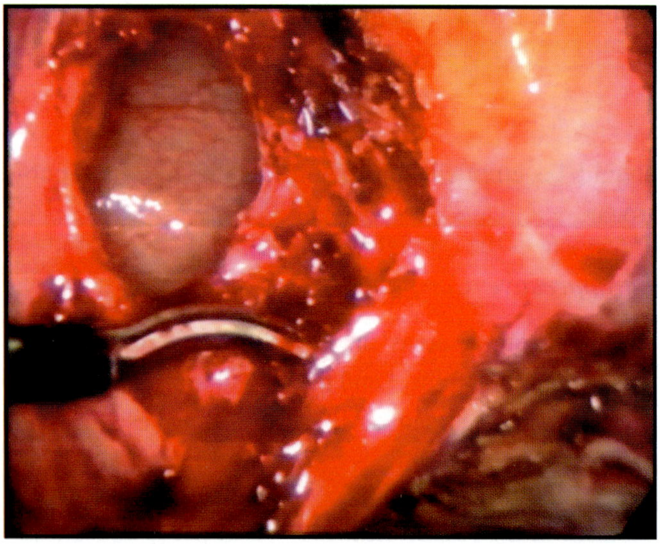

Figure 1.8. Intraoperative bladder injury: Coagulated area excised

Properly identifying the upper limit of the bladder is crucial in preventing injuries during laparoscopic hysterectomy. The bladder can be temporarily distended with saline to delineate the bladder outline. Bladder injuries can be repaired in one or two layers laparoscopically (Figures 1.7 to 1.9). Postoperative transurethral drainage for 7-10 days is sufficient.

The course of the ureters places it at extreme risk during major laparoscopic dissection. Thermal injuries and ischemic injuries can occur because of direct thermal application or loss of blood supply to the ureter. This may result in fistula formation that is unrecognized and presents 3-14 days postoperatively.

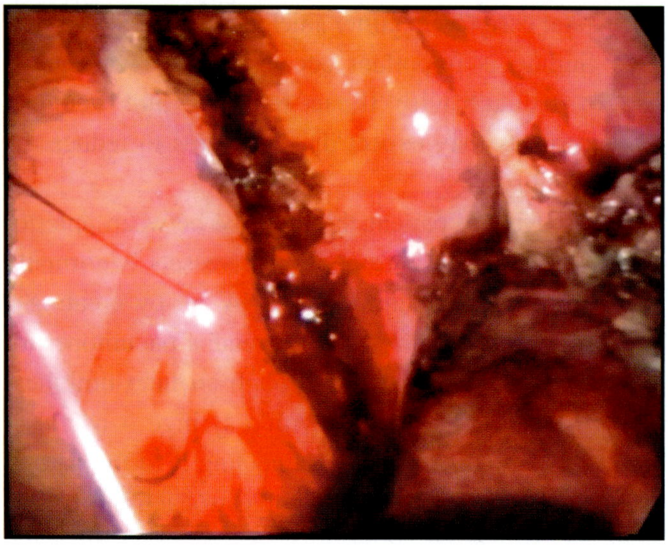

Figure 1.9. The bladder injury following laparoscopic repair

Endometriosis is a major factor for increasing the risk of serious urinary complications after operative laparoscopy.[7] Many ureteric injuries have been reported after laparoscopic hysterectomies.[8] Most occur in the distal portion of ureter, when the uterine vessels or cardinal ligaments are divided. Exposure, identification of anatomic landmarks and careful dissection will reduce the risk of injury. Illuminating ureteral catheters can be placed before performing difficult cases where the anatomy is markedly distorted. In suspected injuries, the integrity of ureter can be checked by performing a cystoscopy and looking for reflux of urine. If there is a suspicion of ischemic injury a stent can be placed with the help of a urologist.

The diagnosis of ureteric injury is usually made 48-72 hours postoperatively with pelvic pain and peritonitis. An IVP is indicated for a final diagnostic assessment. The therapeutic options are retrograde stenting, ureteroureterostomy and ureteroneocystostomy. Experienced laparoscopic surgeons may perform the anastomosis laparoscopically.

Gastrointestinal Injuries

The prevalence of bowel injuries in a combined survey of diagnostic and minor laparoscopic surgeries was 0.08 percent, whereas for operative laparoscopy the risk increases to 0.33 percent.[9]

The management of bowel complications varies according to the type and size of the injury, the segment of bowel involved and the general status of the patient. Although unintentional, operative injury to the bowel can occur and its occurrence can lead to significant consequences. Recognition and immediate attention to this problem is imperative. Delayed diagnosis of bowel injury is a major cause of sepsis and mortality. The combined Dutch and ISGE surveys reported 14 cases of delayed diagnosis (18%) with a mortality of 21 percent.[2]

Mechanical injury is usually caused by trocar insertion or as a result of operative trauma. The prevention of trocar related injuries to bowel include decompressing the stomach and a high index of suspicion for bowel abdominal wall adhesions. An enema will empty the bowel and make it easier to notice adhesions.

Injury to small bowel may occur during dissection of adhesions. Small bowel injuries should be left in place and the loop of bowel brought out through an extended incision and repaired. It can be repaired laparoscopically avoiding any stricture of small bowel (Figures 1.10 to 1.14).

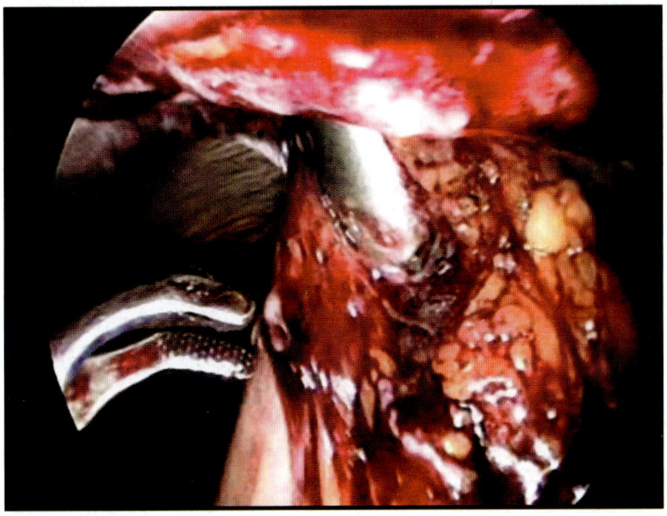

Figure 1.10. Bowel injury at primary trocar insertion

For small colonic injuries associated with minimal contamination, laparotomy with primary suture closure has been the accepted therapy. An experienced surgeon may close such an injury laparoscopically. Large injuries with contamination may require a diverting colostomy and repair at a later date.

Thermal injuries with monopolar or bipolar energy may be difficult to recognize at the time they occur. If identified, they generally require resection of the

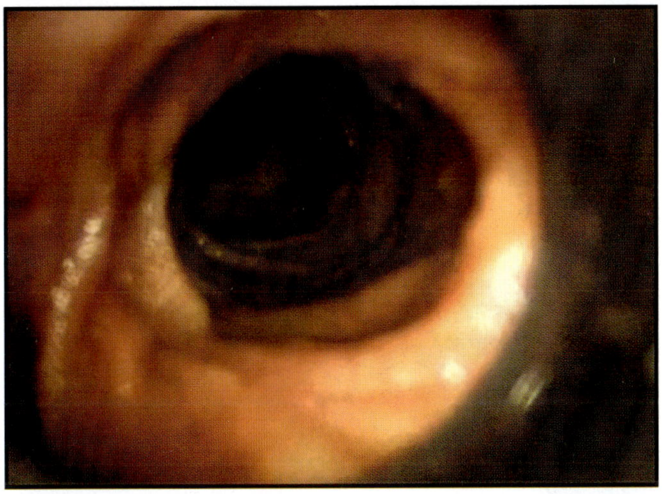

Figure 1.11. Visualizing the inner aspect of the bowel following intraoperative injury

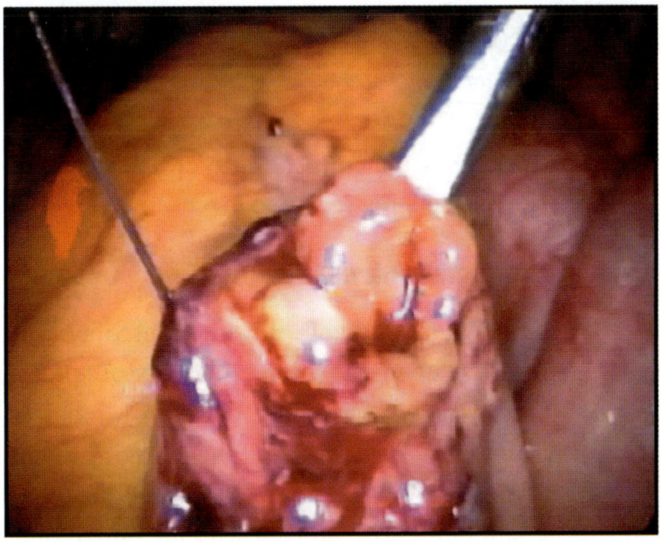

Figure 1.12. Laparoscopic repair of small bowel injury

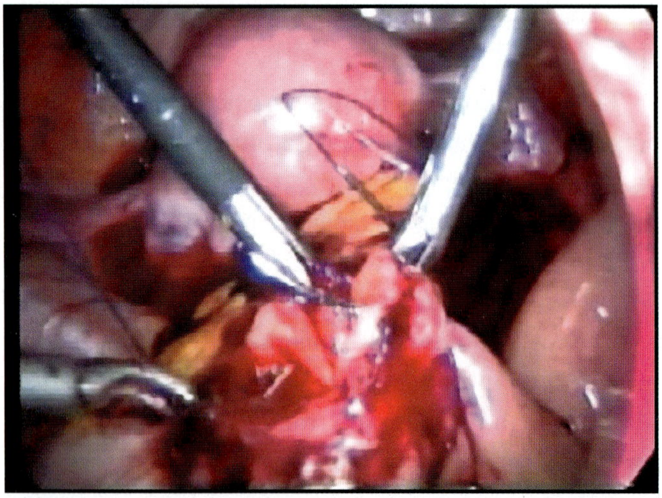

Figure 1.13. Laparoscopic repair of small bowel injury

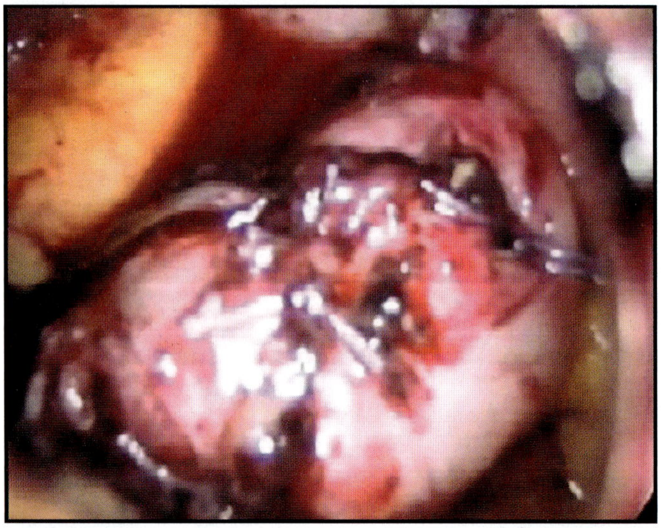

Figure 1.14. The bowel following laparoscopic repair

affected area with a 1-2 cm margin to ensure that only viable tissue is used for repair.

Morcellator Related Injuries

One of the most remarkable advances in operative laparoscopy has been the morcellator. Morcellator related injuries are not very rare. One study reported 14 cases of visceral injuries involving bowel, kidney, pancreas and vascular structures by morcellator.[10] The surgeon should familiarize himself with the functioning of the instrument before the actual use. The rotating blade of the morcellator should be visible throughout the procedure and it should be retracted when not in use. The specimen should be completely separated from surrounding structures and vessels before the morcellation.

Electrosurgical Injuries

Improper use of electrosurgery during a procedure, unfamiliarity with the equipment and the use of incompatible components contribute to many injuries. Electrical and thermal burns to the patient are usually predictable and more often than not preventable. Any break or breach in insulation of the instruments should be periodically checked. Direct coupling occurs when an active electrode makes an unintended contact with another electrode or instrument. The surgeon must be aware of the instruments in each port and he must see the tip of instruments when pressing on the pedal.

CONCLUSION

Although minimal access surgery has made tremendous advance in the field of gynecological surgery, it is not without its risks and complications. With careful attention to detail and a critical approach to patients who are at increased risk, complications can be anticipated in most circumstances and steps may be taken to minimize them. Careful postoperative observation of patients who are not recovering as expected will lead to early identification of those with complications.

REFERENCES

1. Brosens I, Gordon A. Bowel injuries during gynecological laparoscopy: A multinational survey. Gynaecol Endosc 2001;10:141-5.
2. Jansen FW, Kapiteyn K, Trimbos-Kemper T, Hermans J, Trimbos JB. Complications of laparoscopy: A prospective multicenter observational study. Br J Obstet Gynecol 1997;104:595-600.
3. Chapron C, Querleu D, Bruhat MA, Madelenat P, Fernandez H, Pierre F, Dubuisson JB. Surgical complications of diagnostic and operative gynecological laparoscopy: A series of 29,966 cases. Hum Reprod 1998; 13:867-72.

4. Harkki-Siren P, Kurki T. A nationwide analysis of laparoscopic complications. Obstet Gynecol 1997;89:108-12.
5. Harkki-Siren P, Sjoberg J, Kurki T. Major complications of laparoscopy: A follow-up Finnish study. Obstet Gynecol 1999;94:94-8.
6. Fuller J, Ashar BS, Carey-Corrado J. Trocar-associated injuries and fatalities: An analysis of 1399 reports to the FDA. J Minim Invasive Gynecol 2005;12:302-7.
7. Saidi MH, Sadler RK, Vancaillie TG, Akright BD, Farhart SA, White AJ. Diagnosis and management of serious urinary complications after major operative laparoscopy. Obstet Gynecol 1996;87:272-6.
8. Makinen J, Johansson J, Tomas C, Tomas E, Heinonen PK, Laatikainen T, et al. Morbidity of 10 110 hysterectomies by type of approach. Hum Reprod 2001;16(7):1473-8.
9. Brosens I, Gordon A, Campo R, Gordts S. Bowel injury in gynecological laparoscopy. J Am Assoc Gynecol Laparosc 2003;10(1):9-13.
10. Milad MP, Sokol E. Laparoscopic morcellator-related injuries. J Am Assoc Gynecol Laparosc 2003;10(3):383-5.

2 Fertiloscopy

Christopher Chen

INTRODUCTION

The reproductive system in the female, which includes both ovaries, fallopian tubes, and the uterus, as well as the rest of the pelvis, are regularly examined using the procedure called laparoscopy. This is often combined with an examination of the uterine cavity and cervical canal with the procedure called hysteroscopy. The combined operative procedures of laparoscopy and hysteroscopy require general anesthesia.

Before the advent of laparoscopy and hysteroscopy, a procedure called **culdoscopy** was employed by some gynecologists, back in the 1970s,[1-5] to examine the female pelvis. The operation required the use of neuroleptanalgesia and the patient was put in the knee-chest position so that gut could fall away cephalad, thereby exposing the posterior aspect of the female reproductive system for viewing through a telescope (like a laparoscope) called a culdoscope. The scope was introduced through a puncture hole via the posterior fornix. The limitation of this procedure was the restricted view of the pelvis, as the bladder and anterior aspect of the uterus could not be seen. Culdoscopy, because it was cumbersome and of limited usage failed to gain popularity and was superceded by laparoscopy when it was introduced into surgical practice.

In the late 1990s, Gordts et al[6,7] introduced a modification of the culdoscopy technique. Whilst still using the posterior fornix approach to the female pelvis, the patient was left lying on her back instead. To visualize the pelvic organs 200 ml or more of normal saline required to be instilled as a medium before visualization of the female pelvis was possible through a telescope. This technique was further pursued by Watrelot et al,[8,9] using local anesthesia.

CONCEPT OF FERTILOSCOPY

The term **Fertiloscopy** was introduced for the procedure. It was actually a trade name of one of the companies that developed the telescopic equipment for performing the above pelvic examination through the posterior fornix of the vagina after saline had been infused into the pelvic cavity. This step is also called **hydropelviscopy**. Dye can then be injected from the cervix to demonstrate tubal patency, the **dye test**. The fimbrial outer end of the fallopian tube can then be seen and assessed (**salpingo-scopy**), and the tubal mucosa magnified to be examined as well (**microsalpingoscopy**). The fertiloscopy procedure is concluded with **hysteroscopy**. The whole operation is minimally– invasive and is performed under local anesthesia.

INDICATIONS FOR FERTILOSCOPY

When can fertiloscopy be used? When infertility in the female is an issue. It can be used to examine the ovaries for cysts, endometriotic disease of the ovaries and pelvis, tubal infertility, and uterine fibroids. Cases of unexplained infertility can be identified, as well as decision-making with regards to enlisting cases for IVF therapy.

PROCEDURE OF FERTILOSCOPY

The operation of fertiloscopy can be done as an outpatient procedure with the patient on her back, in the lithotomy position. Asepsis of the vulva and vagina are obtained using povidone iodine, and a speculum then inserted to display the cervix and posterior vaginal fornix which should feel free. Local anesthesia is then injected, using 2 ml of lignocaine plus adrenaline, introduced about 1 cm below the cervix. Alternatively, neuroleptanalgesia may be used and the patient treated as a day surgery case.

A long Veress needle is next introduced through the posterior fornix into the pouch of Douglas and 200 ml of pre-warmed normal saline then instilled. The fornix is then punctured to allow a 2.9 mm hysteroscope into the pouch. A 3-chip video camera is clipped onto the scope for viewing of the pelvic organs on a TV monitor. Alternatively, a flexible hysteroscope can also be used.

The pelvic examination is performed systematically, observing the back of the uterus, the tubes and ovaries, and the rectum. Methylene blue dye hydrotubation then follows via the uterine cavity. The dye should flow out of the fimbrial openings demonstrating tubal patency. Salpingoscopy, or even microsalpingoscopy can then be performed. With salpingoscopy, the scope is directed at the fimbriae to assess their state of health. Where possible, the scope is inserted through the fimbrial opening and the ampulla observed as far up as possible. The state of the tubal mucosa is determined. Proceeding with microsalpingoscopy, the staining of the nuclei of the tubal cells by methylene blue dye determines the functional capacity of the tube. The greater the degree of staining, the lesser the functional state of the mucosa.

The examination is concluded with a hysteroscopy and endometrial biopsy. The scope is introduced through the cervical canal into the uterine cavity as a hysteroscope. Abnormalities of the uterine wall such as polyps and synechiae can be recognized and dealt with immediately. The entire procedure lasts about 15 minutes. The patient is discharged home 2 hours later, if the operation is performed under local anesthesia, or 6 hours if after neuroleptanalgesia.

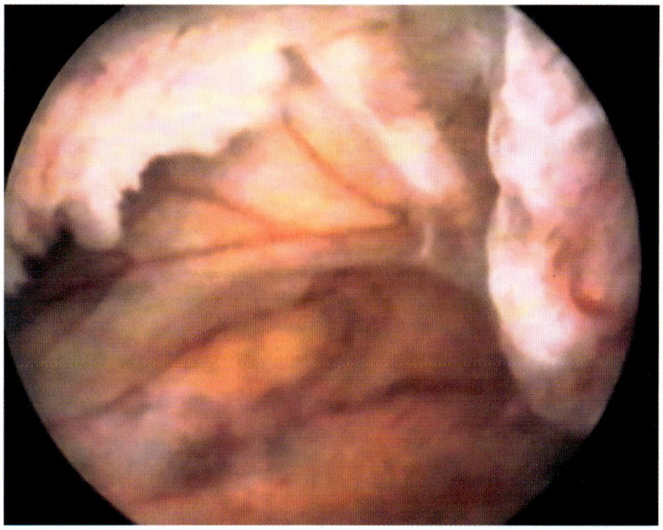

Figure 2.1. Normal tubal fimbriae and ovary during fertiloscopy

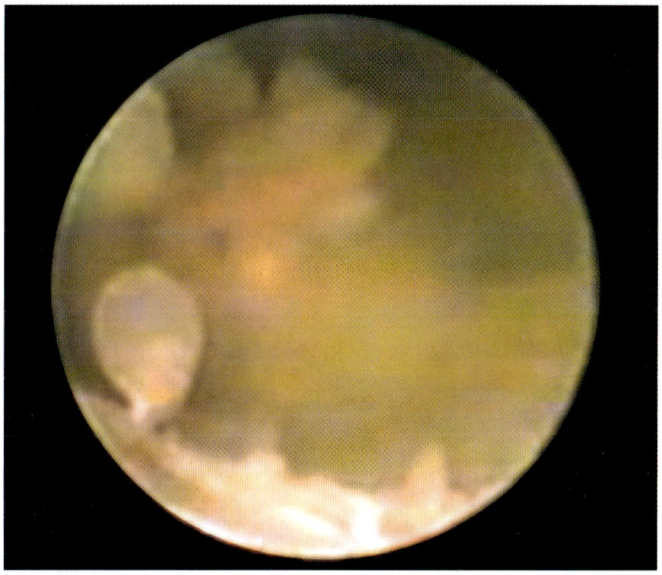

Figure 2.2. Tubal ampulla with fimbrial ends of the tube at fertiloscopy

Some illustrations of fertiloscopy are showed in Figures 2.1 and 2.2.

This book comes with an accompanying video recording demonstrating the appearances at fertiloscopy. The posterior aspect of the uterus, the tubes, and ovaries can be seen, with dye emerging from the fimbrial orifices.

Fertiloscopy is largely a diagnostic procedure, with obvious limitation over its usage.

CONTRAINDICATIONS TO FERTILOSCOPY

The conditions that are described below should be identified so that failure or complications of the procedure can be avoided. Scarring of the posterior fornix and of the recto-vaginal septum can cause rectal adhesions and result in rectal injury should the Veress needle or scope be introduced. A birectal and vaginal digital examination beforehand should alert the operator to this danger.

The pouch of Douglas may be filled and obliterated by large ovarian cysts (such as endometriotic cysts), bulky posteriorly situated myomas, or fixed retroversion of the uterus with obliteration of the pouch caused by endometriosis or old pelvic inflammation. Fertiloscopy should clearly not be performed.

SOME RESULTS OF FERTILOSCOPY

In a study of 160 women presenting with infertility,[10] the failure rate of the procedure was about 3 percent, principally due to severe adhesions in the pouch of Douglas. This failure rate could rise as the number of cases performed increase. Rectal injury occurred in 0.6 percent. Again, this figure could increase as more and more cases are done.

Normal findings occurred in 37 percent of patients, endometriosis in 13 percent, and old pelvic inflammatory disease in 36 percent. Tubo-ovarian adhesions were found in 17 percent and hydrosalpinges in 5 percent of cases.

COMMENTS

The justification for the use of fertiloscopy lies in its being able to being performed as an office procedure and under local anesthesia, or under neuroleptanalgesia. Like laparoscopy, individual surgical skills require to be developed.

Fertiloscopy has its limitations as being a largely diagnostic procedure. Operative procedures are not possible. Ultimately one has to resort to operative videolaparoscopy to resolve the conditions that require surgical treatment.

Whilst it appears to be cost-effective, in reality, if operative videolaparoscopy has to be done, costs will become cumulative. The patient will then have to undergo yet a further operative procedure.

At best, fertiloscopy and laparoscopy can be seen as complementary procedures.

REFERENCES

1. Chen C, Ratnam SS, Cheng M, Lim SM, Chew SC, Khew KS. Culdoscopic Sterilization: The Singapore Experience. 8th World Congress of Fertility and Sterility, Buenos Aires 1974;162.
2. Cheng MCE, Khew KS, Chen C, Ratnam SS. Culdoscopic Ligation as an Outpatient Procedure. American Journal of Obstetrics and Gynaecology 1975;122:109.
3. Chen C, Ratnam SS, Cheng M, Lim SM, Chew SC, Khew KS. Culdoscopic Sterilization: Our Experience with 1,000 Cases Performed as an Outpatient Procedure in Singapore. In: Campus da Paz A, Drill A, Hayashi M, Rodrigues W, Schally AV (Eds): Recent Advances in Human Reproduction, Excerpta Medica, 1975;220.
4. Chen C, Ratnam SS, Cheng M, Lim SM, Chew SC, Ng A, et al. The Feasibility of Outpatient Abortion Combined with Culdoscopic Sterilization. Proceedings, 10th Singapore-Malaysia Congress of Medicine, Stamford College Press 1975;10:340.
5. Litynski GS. Hans Frangenheim–culdoscopy vs. laparoscopy, the first book on gynecological endoscopy, and "cold light". JSLS 1997;1(4):357-61.
6. Gordts S, Campo R, Rombauts L, Brosens I, et al. Transvaginal hydro laparoscopy as an outpatient procedure for infertility investigation. Hum Reprod 1998a;13:99-103.
7. Gordts S, Campo R, Rombauts L, Brosens I, et al. Endoscopic visualization of the process of fimbrial ovum retrieval in the human. Hum Reprod 1998b;13:1425-8.
8. Watrelot A, Gordts S, Andine JP, Brosens I. Une nouvelle approche diagnostique: la Fertiloscopie. Endomag 1997; 21:7-8.
9. Watrelot A, Dreyfus JM, Andine JP. Fertiloscopie: la culdoscopie de l'an 2000. Indications et résultats. Endomag 1998;23:17-8.
10. Watrelot A, Dreyfus JM, Andine JP. Evaluation of the performance of fertiloscopy in 160 consecutive infertile patients with no obvious pathology. Hum Reprod 1999;14 (3):707-11.

3 Tissue Harmonics in the Practice of Endoscopy in Infertility

Nutan Jain, Sankar Das Mahapatra

INTRODUCTION

The search for an ideal energy source for laparoscopic surgery has been ongoing since the first laparoscopic surgeries were performed. Ideally the energy source should be effective safe, quick and cost efficient. Additionally it should not interfere with visualization as a result of smoke or aerosol production. The search of alternative methods has lead to development of the ultrasonic cutting technology which has found increasing use in open and endoscopic operations because of its safety in comparison to other energy sources. Ultrasonic energy for dissection and coagulation has now been used with advantage in many types of laparoscopic surgeries. Although the ultrasonic energy have been used in difficult gynecological laparoscopic surgery, it is necessary to evaluate the safety and applied value of the ultrasonic energy sources in gynecological operations with special references to infertility.

PRINCIPLES OF ACTION OF HARMONIC ENERGY SOURCES

The principles of harmonic cutting is based on conversion of electrical energy into mechanical energy by Piezoelectric crystal system during the time of excitation of hand piece. This mechanical energy is transferred to tissue though blade tips with maximum amplitude of 55, 500 cycles/ second. When blade comes in contact with the tissue, pressure causes coaptation of blood vessels followed by breaking of hydrogen bonds and denaturation of protein in cells that forms a sticky coagulum. This allows simultaneous cutting and coagulation to take place at a lower temperature than electrosurgery. Cutting and hemostasis can be achieved with minimal tissue damage and minimal risk. Electrical energy from the generators is converted to mechanical energy at the hand piece and no electricity passes through the patient. So low temperatures and less contact time first results in cavitations, a steam bubble in the tissue. There is an explosion of cells in the parenchyma and blistering in connective tissues resulting in dissection of anatomical planes, therefore surgical dissection is considerably reduced. By applying additional pressure on the tissues there is defragmentation of hydrogen bonds, which occurs at 63°C leads to coaptation. Coaptation is the sticking together of collagen tissues. At higher temperature protein denaturation occurs that leads to coagulation (Figures 3.1A to D).

In case of high frequency (electrical, laser) coagulation occurs by heating tissues to denature the protein. Ultrasonic energy provides less thermal spread than electricity. Cutting with ultrasonic energy are done by cavitational cutting and fragmentational cutting. Cavitational cutting is transient pressure changes that causes intracellular water to vaporize at lower temperature leading to very precise cutting and dissection. This cavitational effect does not destroy tissue and enhances

PRINCIPLE OF ULTRASONIC ENERGY

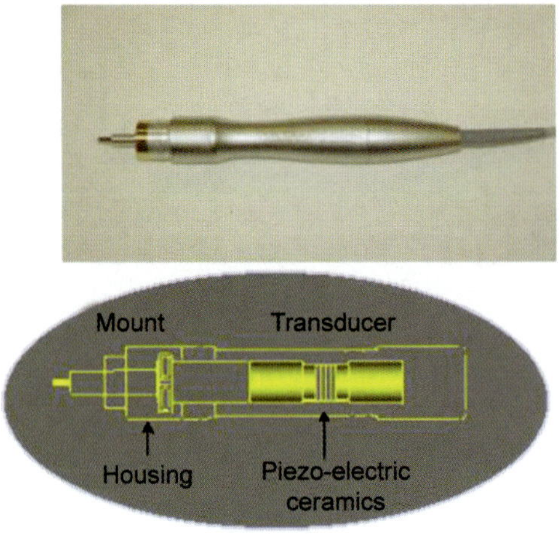

Figure 3.1A. Ultrasonic energy

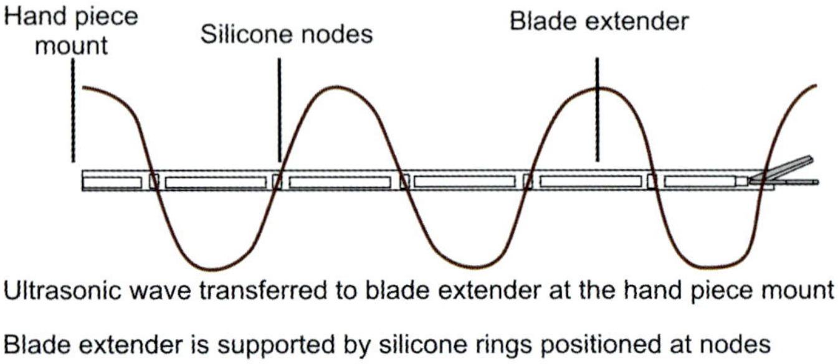

Figure 3.1B. Motion through blade extender

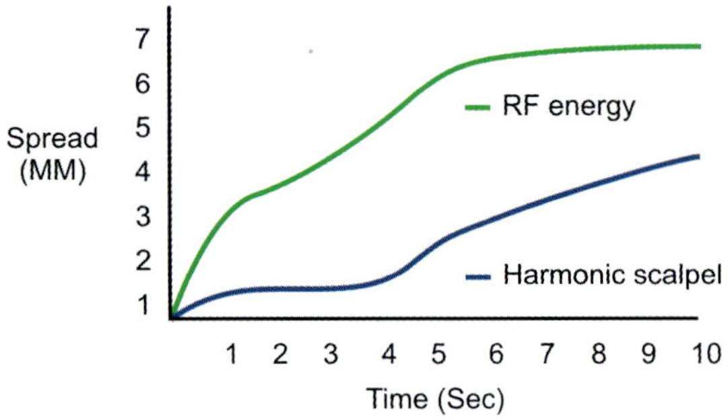

Figure 3.1C. Lateral thermal effect

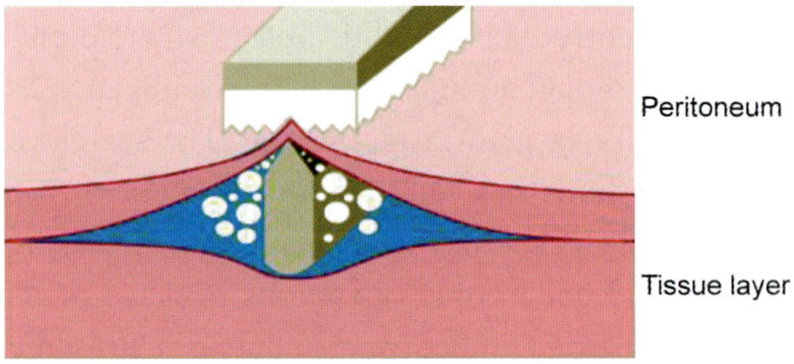

Figure 3.1D. Cavitational effect

visualization of the vascular plane. Power cutting is that the blade cuts the tissue by stretching it beyond it's elastic limit (breaking rubber band by stretching it too far). Mechanical cutting effect is most easily achieved in high protein density areas such as collagen or muscle rich tissues.

Following factors effect cutting and coagulation

1. Tissue tension
2. Blade sharpness
3. Exposure time
4. Power level
5. Grip force

More power is faster cutting but less hemostasis. Less power is slower cutting but more hemostasis. More tissue tension is faster cutting but less hemostasis. Less tissue tension is slow cutting but more hemostasis. Power and tension are the key controlling factors

Instruments

The basic instrument is an alternating current generator with foot switch (Figures 3.2A and B) and main cable as well as reusable hand pieces for different instruments.

The generator is a microprocessor controlled high frequency switching, power supply device that pulses the acoustic system in the hand piece with AC current. This results in vibration of the transducer at its natural harmonic frequency of 55.5 KHz. The microprocessor senses changes in the acoustic system to maximize power

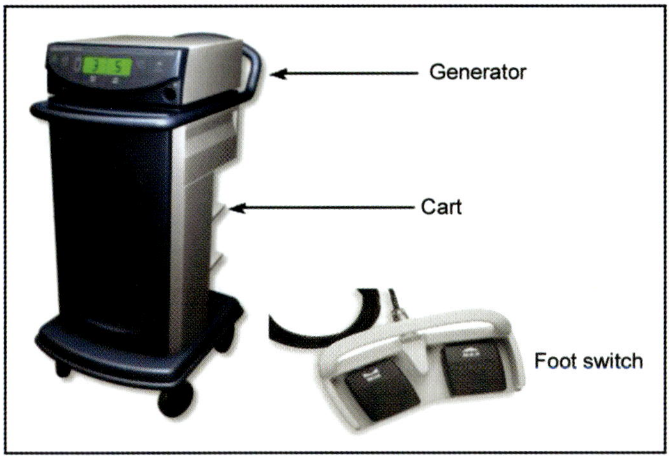

Figure 3.2A. Harmonic scalpel

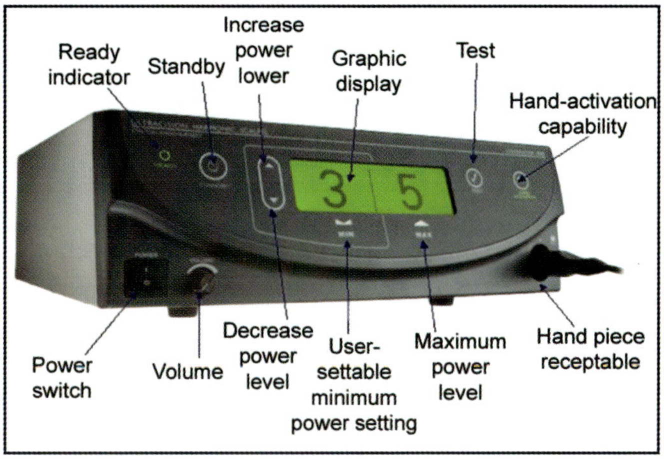

Figure 3.2B. Generator 300

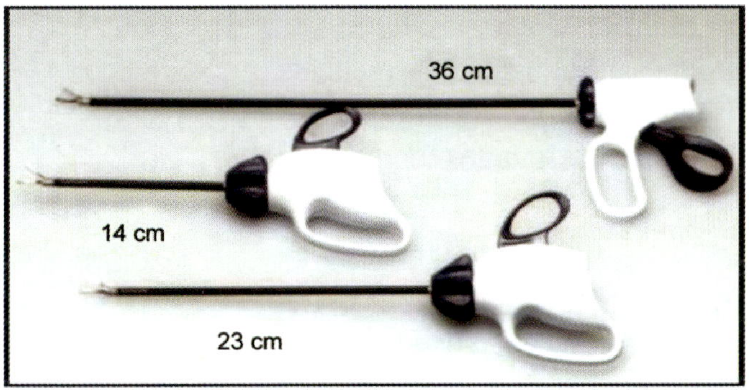

Figure 3.2C. 5 mm curved shears

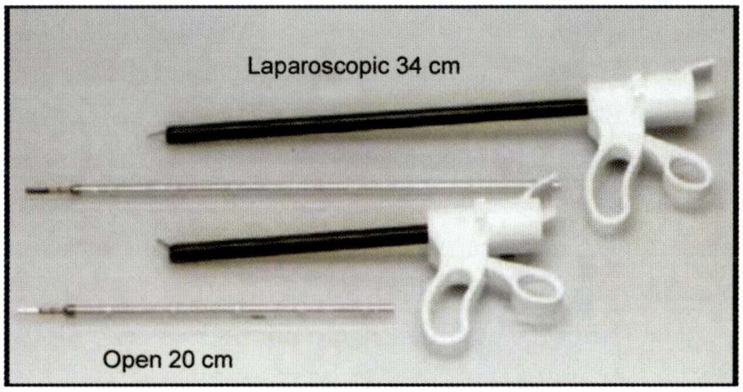

Figure 3.2D. 10 mm pistol grip shears

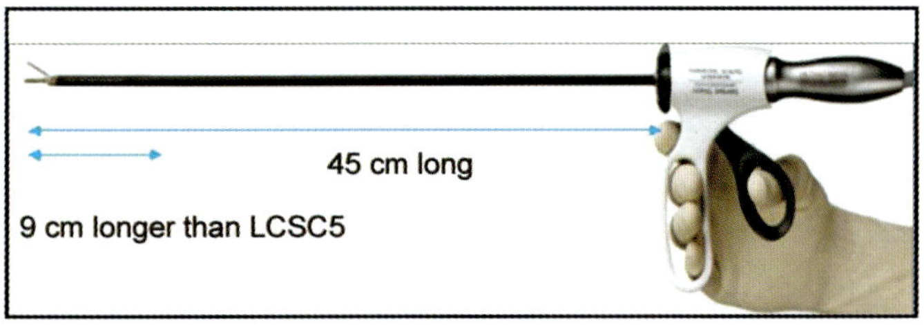

Figure 3.2E. Long shears

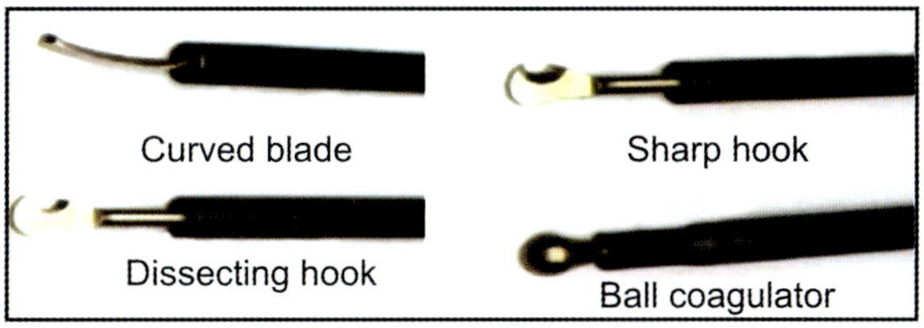

Figure 3.2F. 5 mm blades

and alerts the user of system faults. The mechanical vibration established in hand pieces is conducted to a blade via extending rod, which is necessary for laparoscopic use.

The foot switch consists of left pedal and right pedal. The right pedal is set at 3, left pedal is set at 5.

The hand piece with Piezo-electric crystal system is attached to the generators by a silicone tube. An integrated air duct cools the hand piece. The hand instruments are of 5 mm or 10 mm (Figures 3.2C to E). The rod is housed in a 10 mm hollow stainless steel tube or sheathed in Teflon to produce a 5mm diameter tube. The entire system vibrates ultrasonically at a frequency of 55000 cycles per second with maximum longitudinal displacement of 80 micro meter. Hand instruments are following types. Laparoscopic coagulating shears, hook tipped blades, sickle shaped blade and ballpoint coagulator (Figure 3.2F) The hand instruments possess multi-functions with three different sides (Sharp, Blunt, Flat) that can be used according to anatomical necessity. The sharp and blunt sides are designed for tissue cutting where relatively less coagulation is needed. The flat blade is used during coagulation but less cutting. Hook tipped blades and sickle shaped blades are used to give incision over the myoma and adhesiolysis.

The harmonic scalpel system consists of:

1. Generator with foot switch
2. Generator (2nd type) 200
3. LCS
4. Multifunctional blades—mechanical work.

Advantages

There is no electrical energy used at the point of delivery, there is no risk of electrical injury at the operative site or at some remote site out of the field of view because of depth of penetration of the energy lateral to the intended focus is minimal.

There is little risk of injury to adjacent structures. The superficial depth of penetration of the energy results in fewer complications. The technology reduces operating time because it requires few if any instrument changes during the dissection. This reduction in operating time along with the less use of other instruments such as scissors also significantly reduces cost. Finally since the temperature of the instruments never rises higher than 80°C there is little smoke production. A small spray of normal saline is seen but this falls out of the field of view without obscuring the view.

These advantages make the ultrasonic energy and laparoscopic coagulating shears valuable additions to our laparoscopic tools. Because of the above advantage, adhesiolysis and dissection near delicate organ like bladder, intestines or ureter is possible in complete safety. In a nutshell ultrasonic energy sources has definite advantage over electrosurgery following are the advantages:

1. No electricity to or through the patient.
2. Minimal thermal damage.
3. Minimal smoke.
4. Minimal char and desiccation
5. Multifunctional.
6. Precise cutting and coagulation.

Operative Techniques

Myomectomy

Application of harmonics in infertility related procedures is gaining popularity. Different data are available in doing myomectomy by using ultrasonic energy sources. Utilization of ultrasonic energy for laparoscopic myomectomy is first reported by Miller in the year 1993. Subsequently reported by Stringer and Mcarus. It would appears that myomectomy via this technique is safe in patients interested in achieving future pregnancy. While initially utilizing the 5 mm hook blade of the harmonic scalpel for myomectomy but currently the ultrasonic instrument of choice for myomectomy is the harmonic energy curved blade. It is a 5 mm diameter instrument, which enables rapid cutting and dissection.

Attention is now directed toward the uterus and the myomata. The major deterance to myomectomy is blood loss. In order to minimize this blood loss, the myometrium around the myoma is infiltrated with a dilute vasopressin solution (Figures 3.3A to F).

LAPAROSCOPIC MANAGEMENT OF MYOMECTOMY

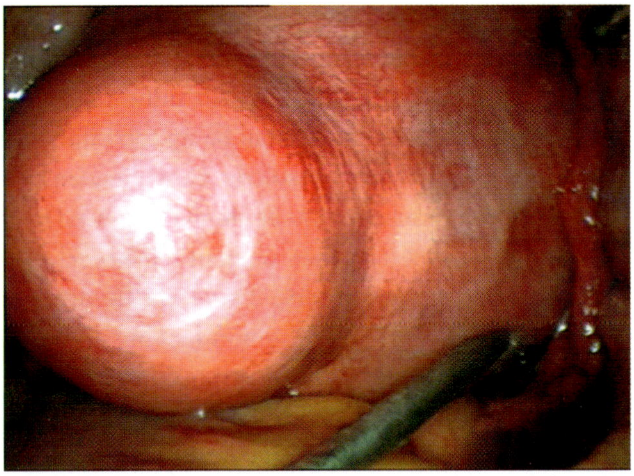

Figure 3.3A. Initial appearance of myomas

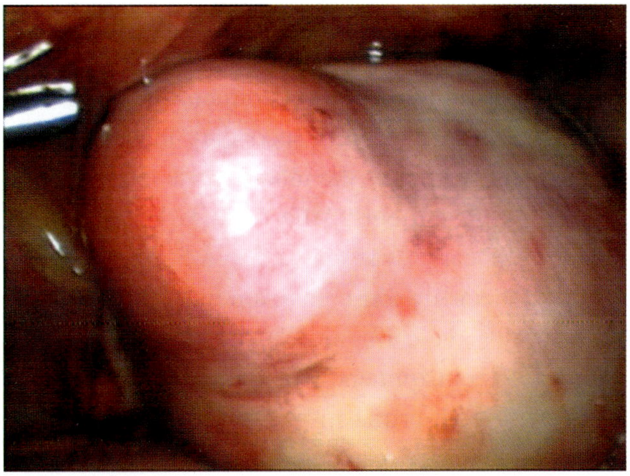

Figure 3.3B. Blanching of myoma after injecting pitressin

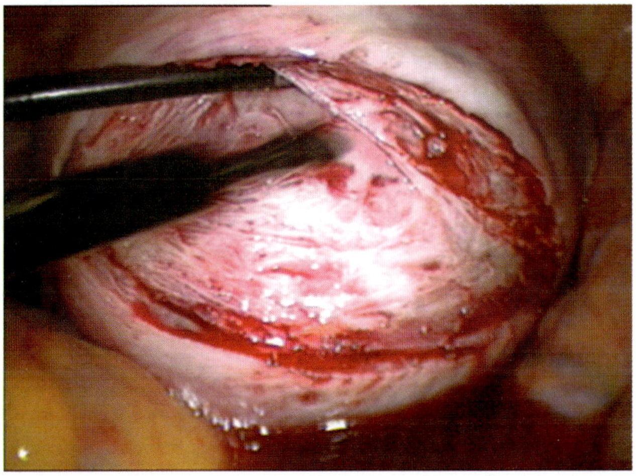

Figure 3.3C. Transverse incisions over the myoma by harmonic scalpel

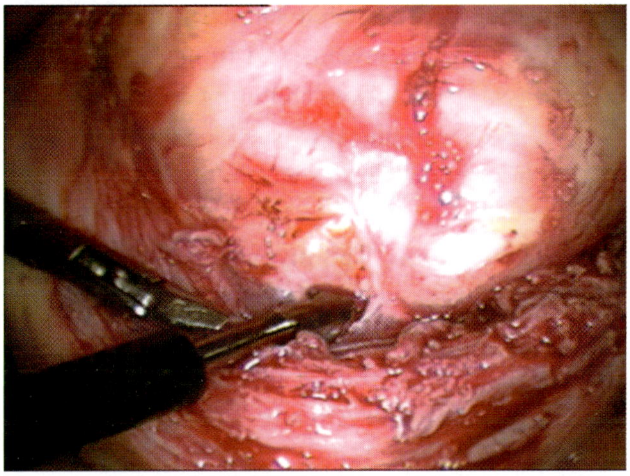

Figure 3.3D. Enucleation of myoma by harmonic scalpel

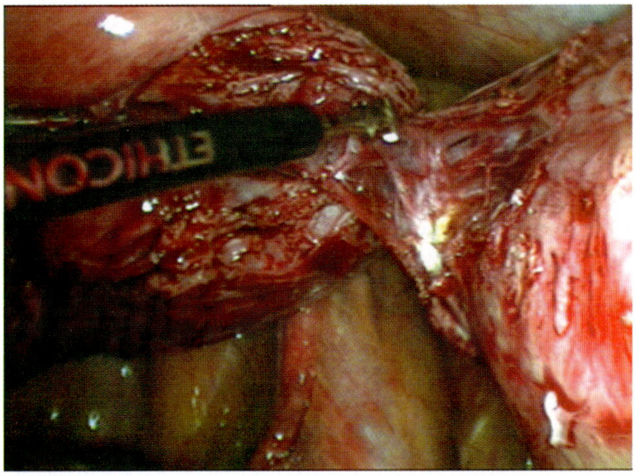

Figure 3.3E. Completed enucleation of myoma

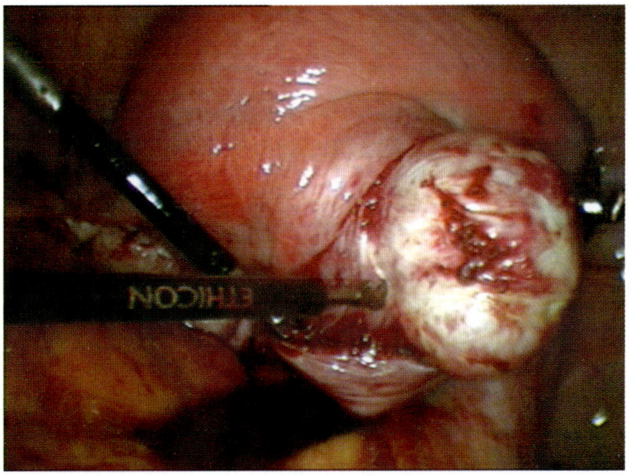

Figure 3.3F. Enucleation of other myoma

While initially utilizing the 5 mm hook blade of the Harmonic Scalpel® for myomectomy, the initial workers began to use the laparoscopic coagulating shears® (LCS®) when the ultrasonic instrument was released. Unfortunately, lateral 10 mm secondary incisions were required; along with this, the inherent risk of herniation was noted. Subsequently, the 10 mm LaparoSonic Coagulating Shears® was reduced to a 5 mm diameter. Currently, the ultrasonic instrument of choice for myomectomy is the harmonic scalpel curved blade. It is a 5 mm diameter instrument, which enables rapid cutting and dissection. All criticism of laparoscopic myomectomy regarding fear of scar, dehiscence during pregnancy or labor become non-existent Traditionally in open surgery myoma bed has been sutured in two or three layers obliterating the myoma bed from deeper planes to the more superficial ones. Suturing in two or three layer gives more anatomical closure and added strength to the myoma bed, which can endure the stress of pregnancy and labor. There is lesser risk of hematoma or a fistula formation. The myoma incision is given transversely over the most bulging part of the myoma. Prior injection of pitressin reduces the bleeding from incision site. Vicryl 1-0 on a taper cut needle is the preferred suture material. A suture about 45cm in length is loaded on a needle holder and introduced in the peritoneal cavity by the Clarke Reich technique of removing the smaller valve less apple trocars. The angle knot is taken by passing the suture on the upper and lower edges of the myoma bed. Intracorporeal knot is tied making a secure square surgeon's knot. From this point on continuous suturing is done passing the needle from the lower flap to the upper edge without locking. The assistant plays an important role in pulling the slack of the suture and keeping adequate tension on the suture when the surgeon passes the successive sutures. Needle holders in both hands give a much better grip and needle alignment becomes easier. The needle is gripped as it comes out of the upper flap and is realigned immediately without letting it fall. This adds a lot of speed and convenience to continuous curved needle suturing. It is extremely important to keep aligning the needle as soon as it exits from the upper flap of the myoma bed. The bites in the tissue are taken according to the thickness of the myometrial bed and keeping in mind that it gives good anatomical closure without being too bulky or too thin, both of which will result in either inadequate or bad tortuous suture line. Sutures should be placed evenly, bringing the tissue together without excessive tension or misalignment of layers. The first layer is thus completed by passing running non-locking suture from one end of the myoma bed to the other where it is anchored by a square knot (Figures 3.4A to F). If the myometrial defect is small and adequate suture length still remains, the same suture is used to stitch the superficial myometrium and serosa up to the starting point of the first layer at the angle. While suturing the superficial layer it is extremely important to pass the sutures at an even distance and take almost same amount of tissue in each bite to give a neat look to the finished suture site. At the end of the suture line a good anchoring square knot is used and can be tied to the tail end of the first knot tied at the start of the suturing. So, in this way, there is only one knot in the entire myoma bed. The amount of adhesions formed per suture line is directly proportional to the number of knots. Lesser the number of bulky knots, lesser the adhesion formation. Copious irrigation and lavage is done and complete hemostasis achieved. No adhesion barrier is used.

Dissection performed using ultrasonic energy results in decreased thermal damage. This may be of benefit in promoting healing and maintenance of uterine integrity by avoiding the extent of blanching and lateral char experienced with thermal modalities and adhesion potential for tissue necrosis and postoperative adhesions. Proper use of energy source to excise the myoma and provide hemostasis and subsequent repair of uterus in multiple layers are important. Optimal healing must be the goal not only to restore normal architecture and also to close the dead space in order to decrease the risk of bleeding in the myometrium.. This is very important in patients of infertility requiring myomectomy. So

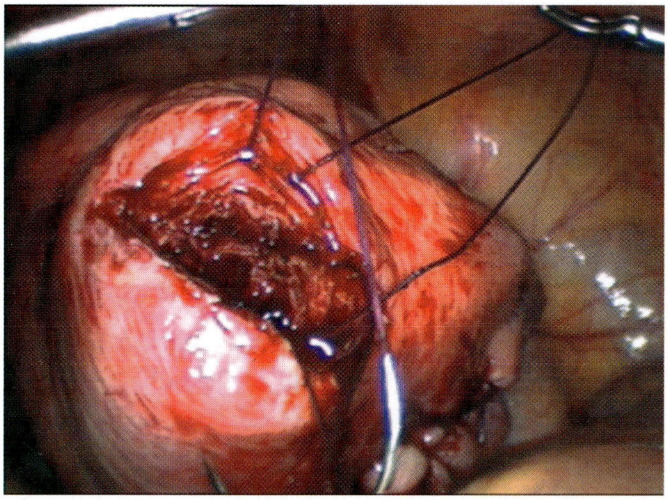

Figure 3.4A. Beginning of the first layer closure

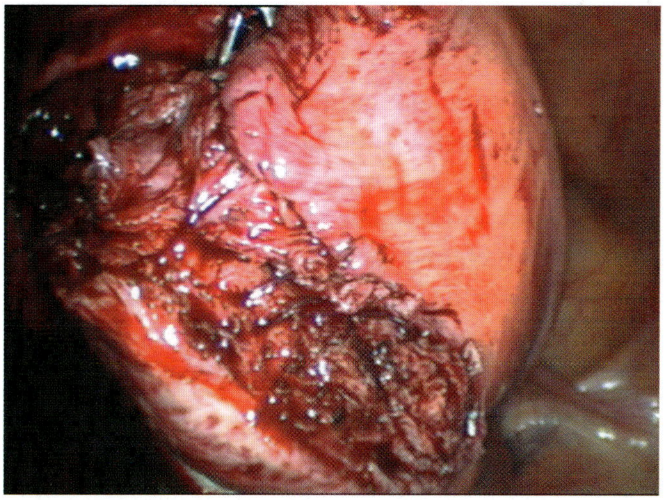

Figure 3.4B. First layer closure almost completed

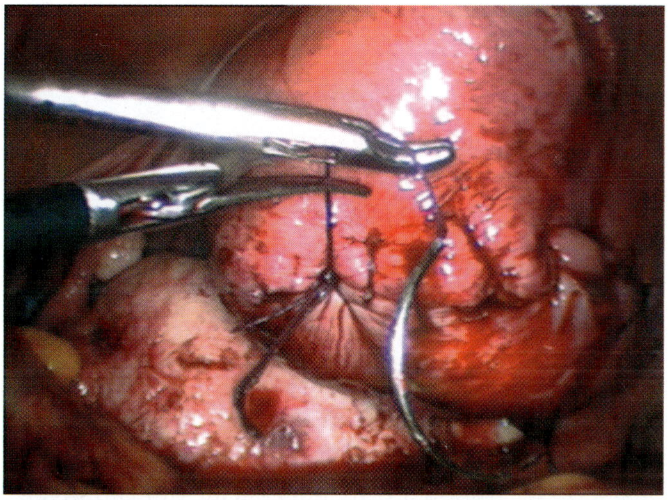

Figure 3.4C. Second layer closure completed

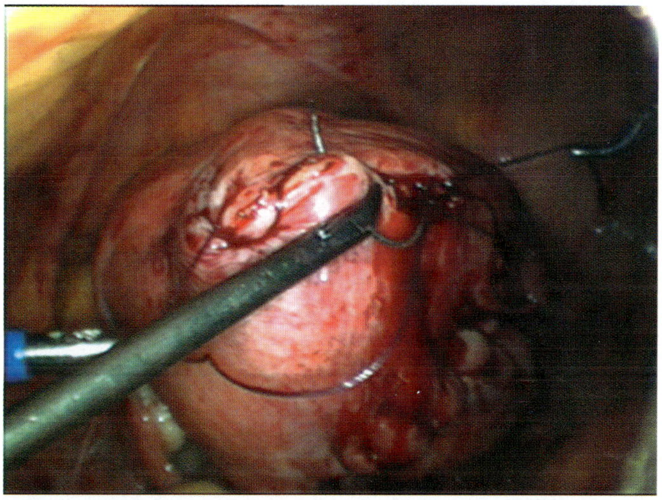

Figure 3.4D. Second layer closure of other myoma

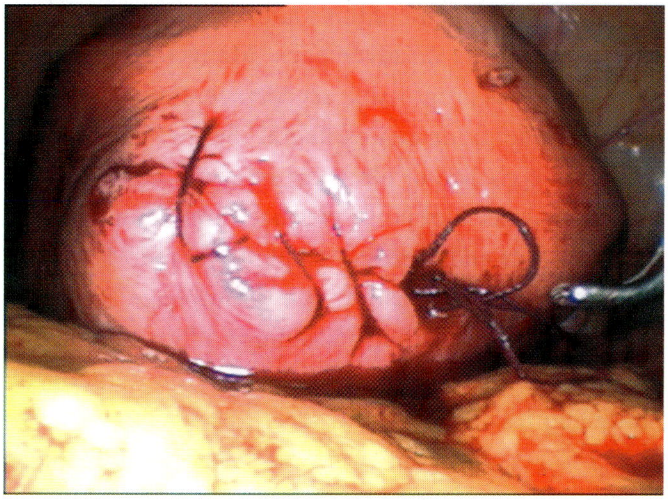

Figure 3.4E. Complete closure of other myoma

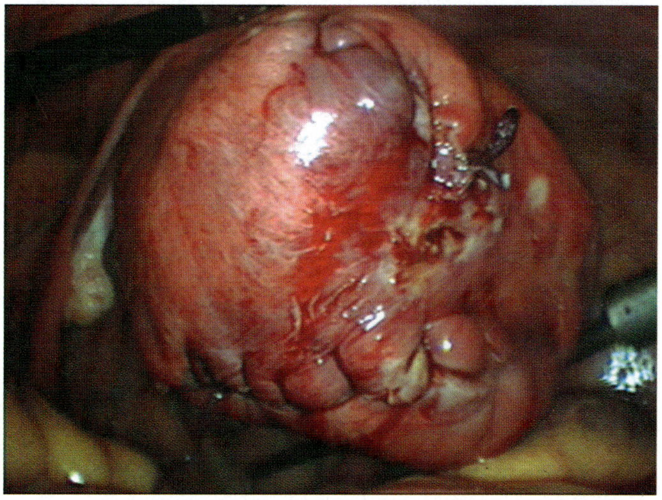

Figure 3.4F. Final appearance after completed myomectomy

ultrasonic energy source can play a great role in myomectomy specially in patients with infertility.

Adenomyomectomy or debulking of a large adenomatous uterus can also be easily performed by using harmonic energy (Figures 3.5A to F). The preferred instrument is an ultrasonic long hook. The incision is vertical, the preferred one as it helps in coring out large chunks of adenomyotic tissue. Thick, fibrotic tissue of adenomyosis cuts well with the ultrasonic hook without causing smoke or char. Gross debulking of uterus is carried out. If a localized adenomyoma is present then an adenomyomectomy similar to myomectomy is carried out. Though the plane of cleavage is not handy but coring out is carried out by harmonic shears or hook blade. Hemostasis is easily obtained. The uterine reconstruction is best obtained by interrupted vertical mattress sutures using 1-0 polygylactin suture material (Figures 3.6A to F). Attempts at meticulous closure like myoma in continuous fashion is not possible due to very firm tissue dealt for approximation. Postoperatively patient's benefit greatly in symptoms of dysmenorrhea, dyspareunia and infertility.

Adhesiolysis

Laparoscopic adhesiolysis for fertility procedure includes Salpingo-ovariolysis, fimbrioplasty, salpingostomy, and enterolysis. Laparoscopic adhesiolysis has proven its effectiveness. Several reasons explain the advantages of laparoscopy.

- Closed internal environment, which avoids the drying of the peritoneum and therefore the recurrence or de novo adhesion formation.
- The approach of certain pelvic adhesions, which is much easier via laparoscopy than via laparotomy, particularly for adhesions in the inferior and lateral sections of the pelvis, under the ovaries in particular,
- The positive pressure exerted by the pneumoperitoneum, which creates a "barohemostasis" and therefore limits generalized bleeding considerably.
- The reduced occurrence of postoperative infections.
- Furthermore, the length of the operation and the period of convalescence are much shorter.

Laparoscopic adhesiolysis is indicated in all cases of tubo-peritoneal infertility:

- If the adhesions are isolated, then the chances of pregnancy are high,
- If the tubes are blocked, to make a precise assessment of the lesions, - and if the tubes are very severely damaged, to help in preparing the patient for safe oocyte retrieval during IVF.

For pure adhesiolysis, the indication and the prognosis depend on the spread of the adhesions, best evaluated by the adhesions score. The laparoscopic adhesiolysis technique is not universal. The choice of the instrumentation and the approach angles can vary significantly from one surgeon to another.

There are four possibilities open to the laparoscopic surgeon:

- The technique utilizing ultrasonic energy.
- The technique with elective use of the CO_2 laser.
- The technique with the dissecting forceps, scissors and bipolar coagulation.
- The technique with elective use of unipolar coagulation.

The technique with effective use of ultrasonic energy for laparoscopic adhesiolysis is gaining popularity. The instrument uses ultrasonic mechanical energy for cutting and coagulating tissue instead of electrical energy. It denatures tissue protein allowing the instruments to both cut tissue and seal vessels up to 5 mm. Although it has its limitations, the benefit of this multifunctional instrument may outweigh its disadvantages. Many factors can be attributed to its progressive acceptance. First the lack of electrical energy decreases lateral thermal damage and reduces the chance of electrical injury to other viscera. Secondly ultrasonic energy produces minimum charring, carbonization and bleeding (Figures 3.7A to F) this is thought to possibly, lead to less macrophage activation and adhesion formation. In addition ultrasonic energy allowing for better visualization by the surgeon by producing less smoke. Ultrasonic instruments have the ability to grasp, cut and cauterize tissue simultaneously requiring fewer instrument changes through port site.

LAPAROSCOPIC MANAGEMENT OF ADENOMYOMECTOMY

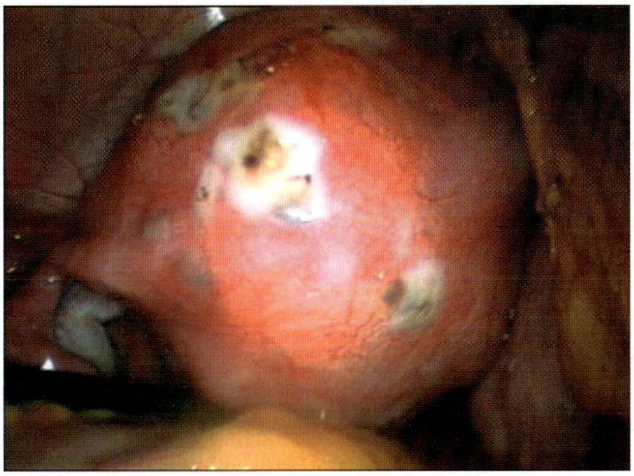

Figure 3.5A. Initial appearance of adenomyosis

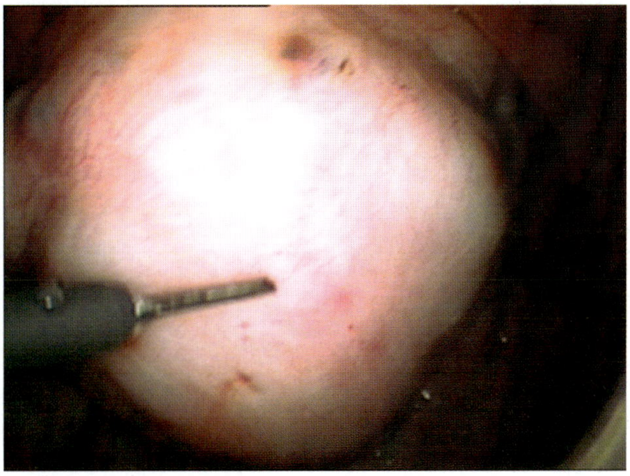

Figure 3.5B. Injecting petressin

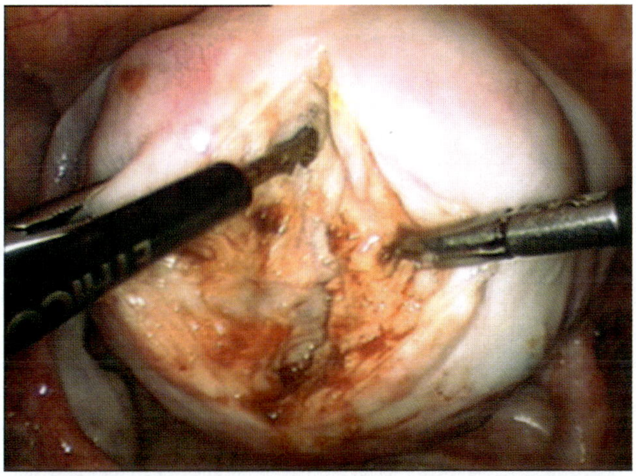

Figure 3.5C. Vertical incision with harmonic scalpel

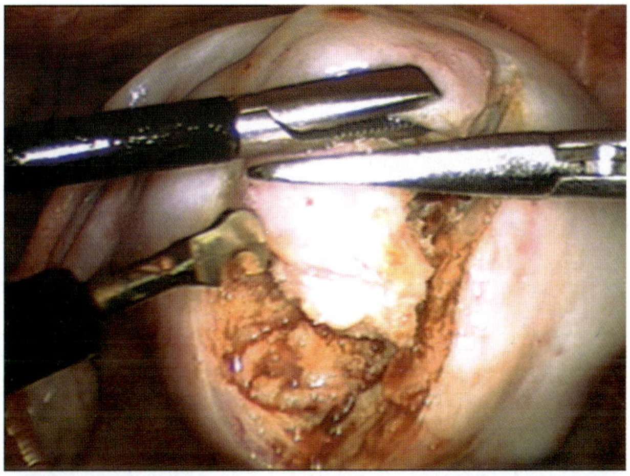

Figure 3.5D. Beginning cutting of adenomyoma

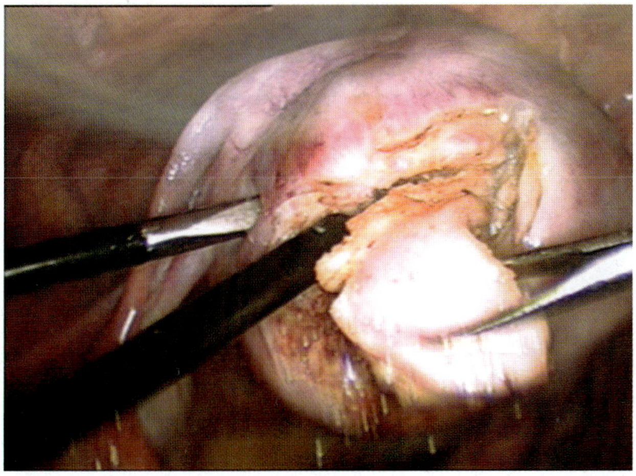

Figure 3.5E. Adenomyomectomy in progress

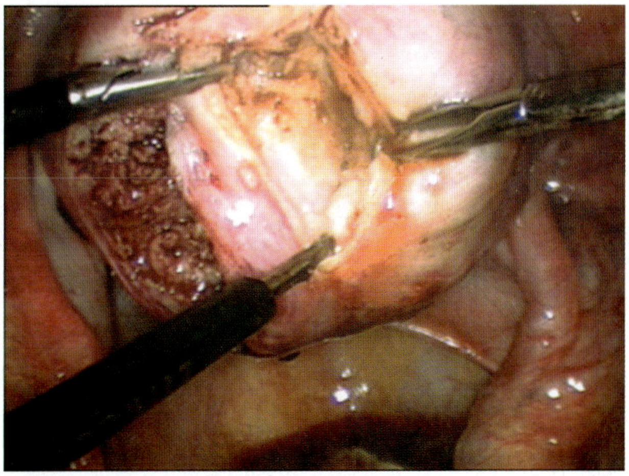

Figure 3.5F. Other side adenomyoma cutting by harmonic scalpel

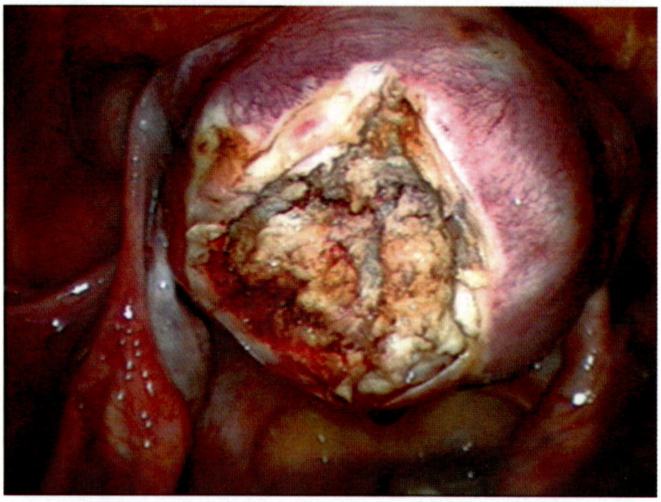

Figure 3.6A. Uterus after debulking of adenomyosis

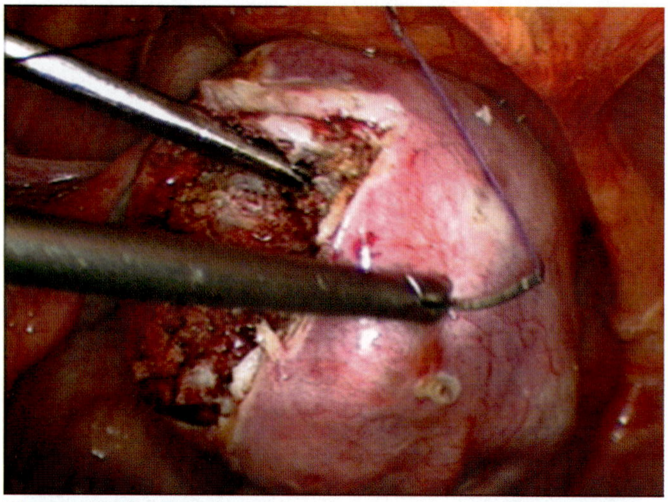

Figure 3.6B. Passing deep suture with 1.0 vicryl taper cut needle

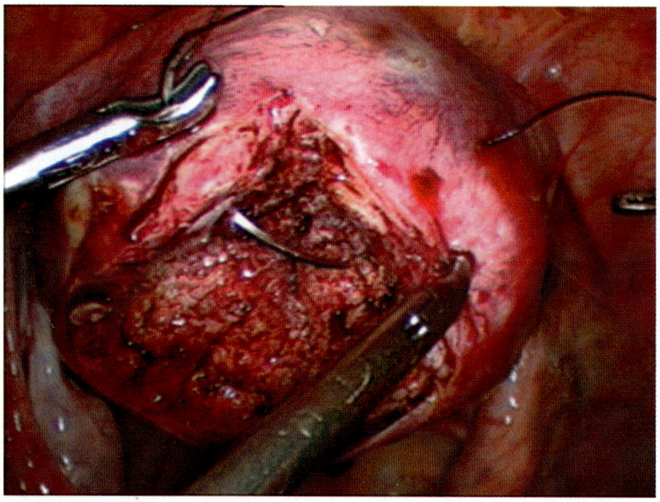

Figure 3.6C. Passing mattress suture

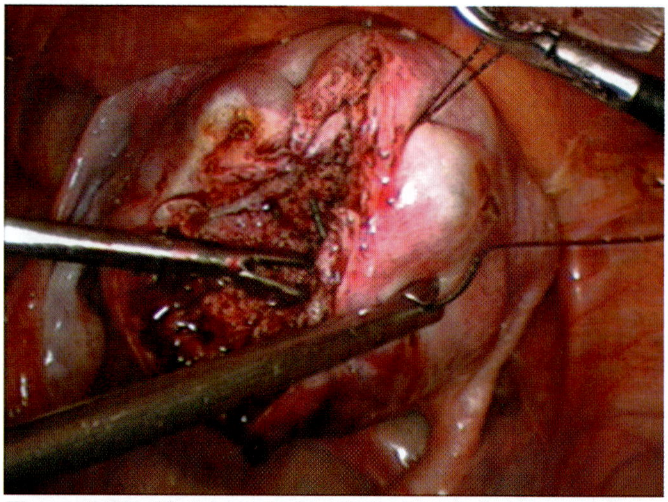

Figure 3.6D. First knot tied and starting IInd suture

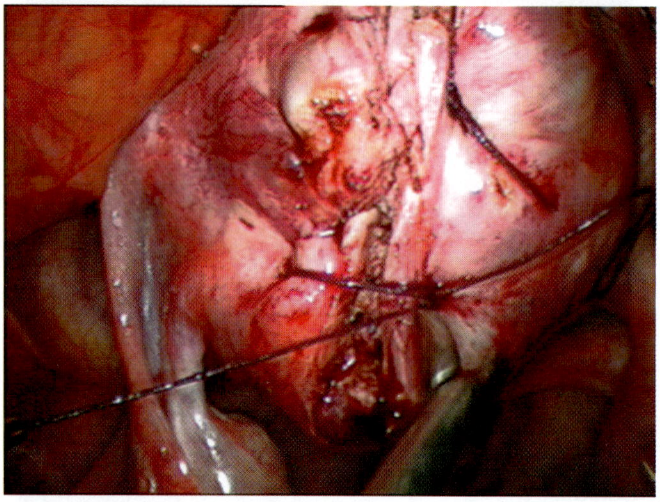

Figure 3.6E. Tying the knot

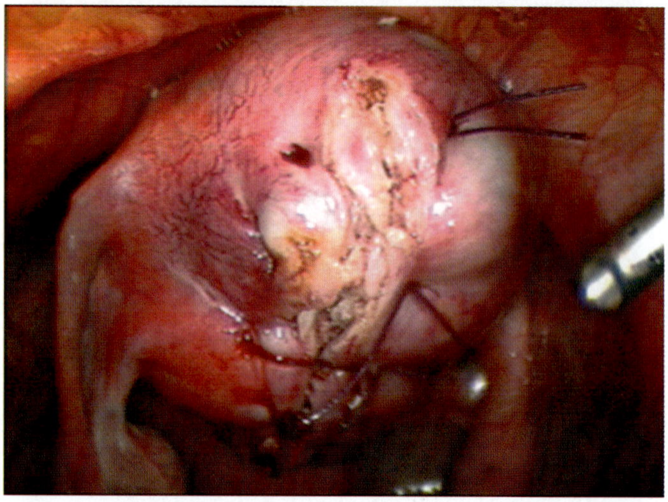

Figure 3.6F. Final appearance of adenomyomectomy

LAPAROSCOPIC MANAGEMENT OF ADHESIOLYSIS

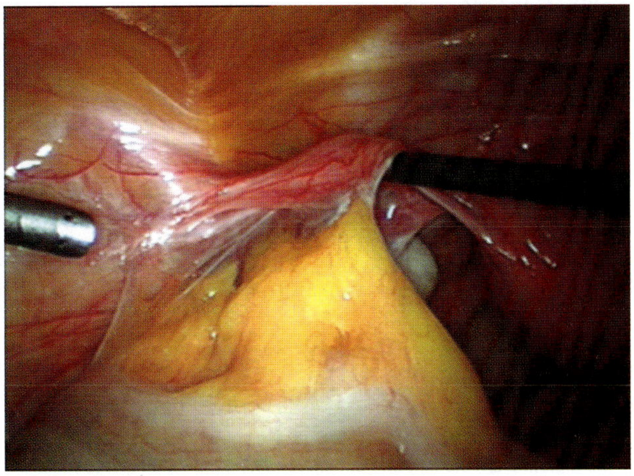

Figure 3.7A. Initial appearance of bowel adhesion

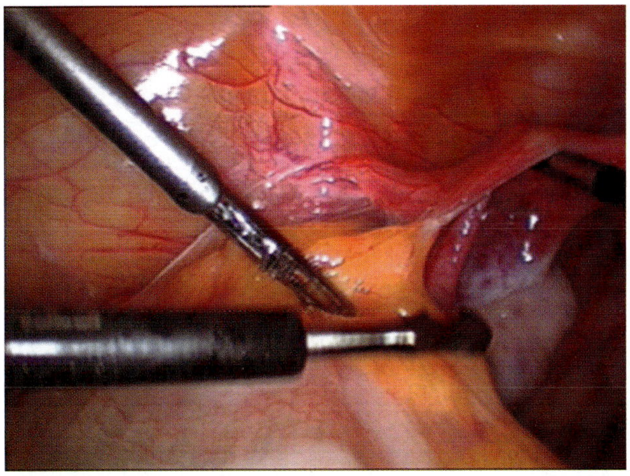

Figure 3.7B. Beginning the adhesiolysis by harmonic scalpel

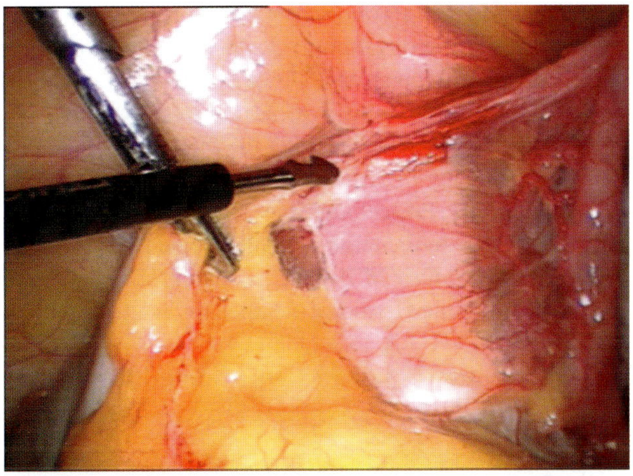

Figure 3.7C. Adhesiolysis done by harmonic scalpel

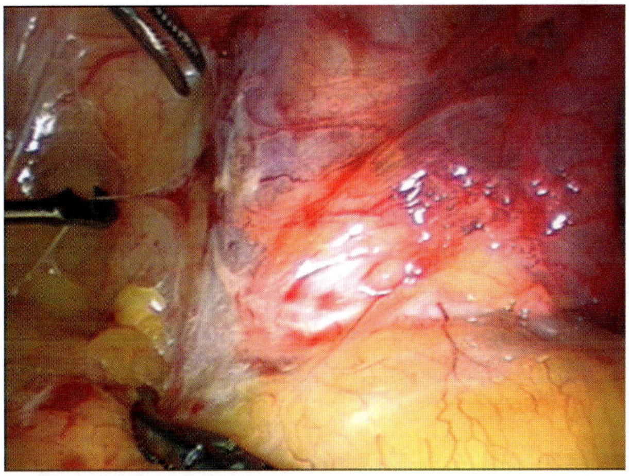

Figure 3.7D. Almost completed adhesiolysis

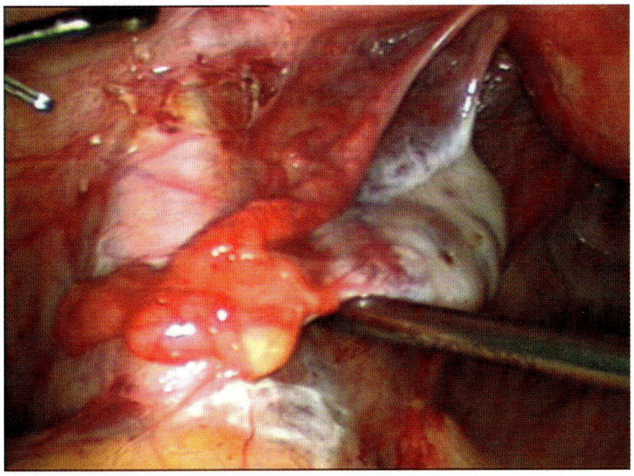

Figure 3.7E. Tube totally freed after adhesiolysis

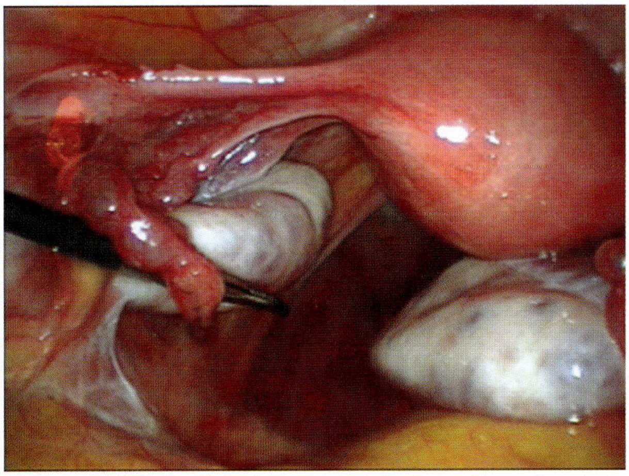

Figure 3.7F. Positive chromopertubation after adhesiolysis

Special Cases

Few special cases have to be dealt specifically. In these situations ultrasonic energy plays a great role.

Adhesiolysis between the intestines and another organ must be performed with special care. These are the adhesiolysis, which cause the worse accidents in laparoscopy, which is to say unrecognized intestinal wounds. No risk should be taken with thick adhesions, which do not interfere with the infertility. Ultrasonic energy has to play great role in this situation.

Results

The results of the pure adhesiolysis depend on the adhesion stage. In the case of slight or moderate adhesions, the pregnancy rate is around 60 percent as opposed to just 20 percent in severe cases. These figures are very similar to those obtained after microsurgery.

CONCLUSION

The ultrasonic cutting technique enables us to avoid the use of high frequency energy in endoscopic operative procedure. As advantages and disadvantages of various tools already at our disposal are scrutinized, we should see improvement in the quality of care afforded to our patients. The goal of operative laparoscopy is to reduce tissue damage, postoperative adhesions and to speed up recovery. Therefore the ultrasonic energy used in operative laparoscopy should not only reduce tissue injury but also decreases postoperative adhesion and inflammation. Ultrasonic energy used in gynecological operative laparoscopy is safe, effective and dependable. It is specially useful in adhesiolysis, salpingectomy, salpingostomy and myomectomy.

SUGGESTED READING

1. Application of ultrasonic in gynecologic operative laparoscopy. Chin Med J 2001;12:1283-5.
2. Marti L Robbins MD Shears. Excision of endometriosis with laparoscopic coagulating. The journal of the AAGL, 1999;6(2).
3. McCarus SD. Physiological Mechanism of the Ultrasonically Activated Harmonic Scalpel. J Am Assoc Gynecologic Laparoscopists #4:600-08:08/96.
4. Miller. Laparoscopic myomectomy for patients interested future fertility: Presented at the International Congress of Laparoscopy Endoscopy 23rd Annual meet.
5. Miller CD. Presented at the 22nd Annual Meeting of the American Association of Gynecologic Laparoscopist, San Francisco, CA. Miller CE. Laparoscopic Myomectomy Featuring the Harmonic Scalpel 1993.
6. Stringer NH. Laparoscopic myomectomy with harmonic. A review of 25 cases. J Gynecol Surg 1994;10:235-9.

4 Laparoscopic Management of Endometrioma

Rakesh Sinha, Meenakshi S

INTRODUCTION

Endometriosis is an enigmatic disorder characterized by the occurrence of endometrial glandular tissue outside the uterus; and is a challenging condition for clinicians, research scientists and patients alike. Endometriosis is commonly found in women of reproductive age group and affects 15 percent of fertile women and 40-50 percent of infertile women.[1] The most frequent site of endometriosis is the ovary. When the ovaries are involved, they become enlarged with cystic blood-filled spaces that on gross examination are termed as chocolate cysts or endometriomas (Figures 4.2 and 4.8). Ovarian endometriomas are among the most common ovarian cysts encountered during surgery.[2] The other frequent locations include the uterine ligaments, pouch of Douglas, pelvic peritoneum, fallopian tubes, rectosigmoid and bladder. WW Russel described the first case of ovarian endometriosis as early as 1899, in a woman of premenopausal age with a diagnosed cystic adenocarcinoma of the left ovary who had 'the right ovary enveloped in adhesions to the posterior face of the broad ligament'. Extensive research thereafter has added significantly to our knowledge of the disease spectrum. The treatment of ovarian endometriomas can be complex and difficult and varies with the presenting symptom complex. The aim of treating endometrioma is to alleviate symptoms, promote fertility and prevent disease progression.

PATHOGENESIS (FIGURE 4.1)

Sampson in1921 hypothesized that endometriomas might be formed by implantation of viable endometrial tissue on the ovarian surface from retrograde menstrual flow. This theory was supported by the fact that 90 percent of women demonstrated blood in the peritoneal fluid during the perimenstrual period. Ovarian endometriomas are more commonly found on the left side (Figure 4.10). The left sided predisposition of endometriosis and endometriomas is probably related to the decreased peritoneal fluid movement in the left side of the pelvis because of the presence of sigmoid colon.[3] These findings also support Sampson's retrograde menstrual theory. However, in 1957 Hughedson demonstrated that 90 percent

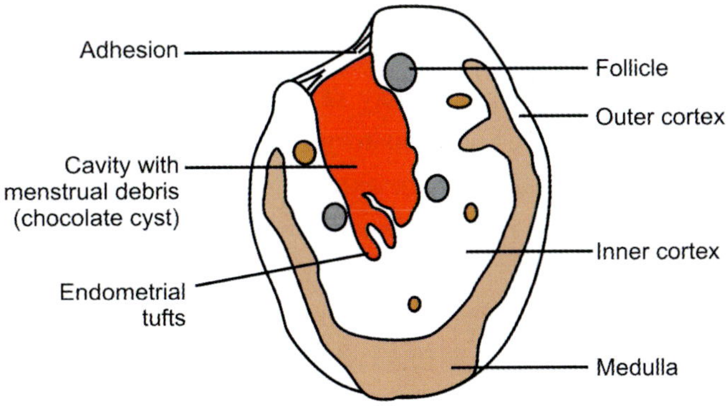

Figure 4.1. Section through the ovary with typical endometrioma

of endometriomas are formed by progressive invagination of the ovarian cortex due to accumulation of menstrual debris from the shedding and bleeding of active surface implants. The site of invagination is characterized by fibrosis and retraction of the ovarian cortex. Fibroreactive tissue progressively thickens the inverted cortex, and outgrowths of the endometrial epithelium extend over the surface or become embedded in the fibroreactive tissue covering the wall of the pseudocyst. However, other theories, such as its development from mullerian remnants in the ovary, implantation of endometrial tissue in functional cysts and metaplasia of coelomic epithelium in the ovary cannot be excluded.

Clinical Presentation and Diagnosis

The common clinical presentation of endometrioma is:

- Pelvic pain
- Infertility
- Dyspareunia, which may be a presenting feature if the endometrioma is adherent to the pouch of Douglas (Figures 4.9, 4.11 and 4.13).

The incidence of infertility directly attributable to endometriosis is difficult to assess. Some degree of infertility is found in 30-50 percent of women with endometriosis. Impaired folliculogenesis, ovulatory dysfunction and luteal phase defect are some of the postulated causes of infertility. Distortion of the tube due to peritubal adhesions can compromise motility as well as patency of the tube and can play an important role in advanced stages of endometriosis.

Pelvic examination may reveal the presence of an adnexal mass. Clinical history and examination alone may not correlate with the extent of disease. Sometimes endometriomas may be detected while investigating for infertility.

Biochemical tests do not contribute to the diagnosis of endometriosis. Ca 125 is of limited value in the diagnosis of mild disease. High levels may help to distinguish malignant lesions from benign conditions.

Imaging has become an important tool for the diagnosis of endometriomas. Transvaginal ultrasound is useful for diagnosis of endometrioma more than 2cm in size. Characteristic features are presence of diffuse attenuated internal echoes and hyperechoic foci in the cyst wall. Ultrasound may not differentiate endometriomas from hemorrhagic cysts, tubo-ovarian abscess and occasionally, cystadenomas. Features of malignancy like thick septae and solid areas can be detected on ultrasound.

The role of Doppler in the diagnosis of endometrioma is uncertain (Figure 4.12). A typical vascular pattern is described as "pericystic flow at the level of the ovarian hilus".[4] CT scan is not reliable for the diagnosis of endometriomas as their appearance on CT is nonspecific. MR imaging is useful to detect endometriomas larger than 1 cm; and this technique may be valuable for identifying endometriosis obscured by pelvic adhesions, particularly those involving the bowel.

Laparoscopy is the gold standard for the diagnosis of endometriomas. The visual diagnosis of a typical endometrioma demonstrates a sensitivity, specificity and accuracy of 97, 95, and 96 percent respectively.[5] Laparoscopy is highly sensitive as superficial peritoneal implants can be diagnosed only by direct visualization. The final diagnosis is confirmed by histopathology.

Staging of endometriosis depends on the size, extent and the complications of endometriotic implants. Based on laparoscopic findings endometriosis can be classified into four stages from mild (stage 1) to severe (stage 4). This staging, however, correlates poorly with symptoms of pain and dyspareunia, and does not predict the future fertility of the patient (Table 4.1).

MANAGEMENT OF ENDOMETRIOMAS

Endometriomas have a high chance of recurrence. No single therapeutic approach has emerged as the most effective modality for this condition. Management of endometrioma in the setting of infertility is challenging and their relationship has been debated for many years. The treatment of endometrioma depends on:

- Extent of disease
- Severity and range of symptoms

Table 4.1. Revised American Fertility Society classification of endometriosis-1985

Stage 1 (minimal) :		1-5		
Stage 2 (mild) :		6-15		
Stage 3 (moderate) :		16-40		
Stage 4 (severe) :		> 40		
Peritoneum				
Endometriosis		< 1 cm	1-3 cm	> 3 cm
Superficial		1	2	4
Deep		2	4	6
Ovary				
R	Superficial	1	2	4
	Deep	4	16	20
L	Superficial	1	2	4
	Deep	4	16	20
Posterior cul-de-sac obliteration			**Partial** 4	**Complete** 40
Ovary				
Adhesions		< 1/3 enclosure	1/3-2/3 enclosure	>2/3 enclosure
R	Filmy	1	2	4
	Dense	4	8	16
L	Filmy	1	2	4
	Dense	4	8	16
Tube				
R	Filmy	1	2	4
	Dense	4*	8*	16
L	Filmy	1	2	4
	Dense	4*	8*	16

* If the fimbriated end of the fallopian tube is completely enclosed, change the point assignment to 16

- Age of the patient and future childbearing
- Whether primary or recurrent disease.

Medical and surgical treatments with varying rates of success have been reported.

Medical Management (Table 4.2)

Endometrial implants regress in response to hormonal therapies as they have estrogen and progesterone receptors in them. Medical treatment alone is inadequate for the treatment of endometrioma. There may be a reduction in the size of the lesion but not a complete resolution.[6] Progestogens, Danazol or GnRH analogues are equally effective as all of them induce a hypo-estrogenic state and cause regression of active implants.

Table 4.2. Medical management of endometriosis

- Progestogens, Danazol or GnRH analogues inhibit ovulation and cause atrophy of endometriotic implants
- Choice of treatment depends on the symptoms and side effect profile
- Not very effective for treatment of endometrioma if used alone
- Not very suitable for patients with infertility
- Can be used preoperatively or postoperatively depending on the symptoms and disease pattern

Resolution can occur in 50-70 percent of cases and symptomatic improvement occurs in 80-90 percent of patients. Progestogens can cause spotting or break through bleeding. Other side effects are weight gain, breast tenderness and fluid retention. Danazol is associated with a multitude of side effects like weight gain, fluid retention, hirsutism, acne, hot flushes and mood changes.

GnRH analogues have become a standard means of therapy for pain relief in endometriosis. Many studies have analyzed the effect of preoperative use of GnRH analogues. Pretreatment with GnRH analogues may offer some advantage such as disease control at other peritoneal sites and slowing of disease progression.[7] Endometriomas >3 cm reduce marginally in diameter but recur rapidly and need surgical treatment. Donnez et al[8] in their study found that 82 percent of patients treated with buserelin subcutaneous implant had a 25 percent regression in size of endometrioma. Side effects include hot flushes, vaginal dryness, insomnia, mood changes and headaches. Long-term usage can cause osteoporosis; hence add-back therapy has been developed. But this may not be effective for endometriomas and not for patients who desire fertility. Other drugs like gestrinone, RU 486(Mifepristone) and tamoxifen have also been used for regression of endometriotic implants.

Aspiration of Endometriomas

Ultrasound guided aspiration of the endometriotic cyst is a simple technique, using the same set up as oocyte retrieval. The procedure may become cumbersome, difficult and is time consuming. Complete evacuation may not possible. Incidence of recurrence after aspiration is very high (30-98%).[9] To reduce the incidence of recurrence, injection of sclerosing agents like ethanol and tetracycline have been tried.[10] Recurrence, infection leading to abscess formation and adhesions are three potential complications of aspiration of endometriomas. Laparoscopic drainage is associated with a recurrence rate of 80-100 percent.

Surgical Management of Endometrioma (Table 4.3)

Surgery is the most appropriate approach for the treatment of endometriomata. Surgical therapy is warranted for women with pain symptoms who desire pregnancy as early as possible.

Certain principles are to be followed while treating ovarian endometrioma surgically. Malignancy should be ruled out as the incidence of carcinoma arising in endometriosis is 0.8 percent.[11] In addition, all active endometrial implants should be removed and damage to the ovarian tissue should be kept to a minimum in order to preserve ovarian follicles (Table 4.4).

Surgery can be either conservative or radical. Radical surgery implies. Total hysterectomy with bilateral oopherectomy. Hysterectomy does not imply cure, as recurrence can occur in 5-10 percent of women who have undergone this procedure.[12]

Table 4.3. Surgical management of endometriosis

- Laparoscopy is the gold standard for surgical management of endometriosis
- Treatment of choice for patients with endometrioma as medical therapy is often not very useful
- Effective treatment for pain and infertility
- Excision or ablation of endometriomas are two approaches with comparable results

Table 4.4. Principles of ovarian endometrioma treatment

- Rule out malignancy
- Surgical release of adhesions at the site of invagination
- Eversion of the invaginated cortex
- Remove all the ectopic endometrium
- Minimize the ovarian trauma in order to preserve ovarian follicles
- Minimize postoperative adhesion formation

Conservative surgery could be either through laparotomy or laparoscopic technique. Number of studies have compared laparoscopy and laparotomy for the management of endometriosis. The authors believed that laparotomy was performed due to lack of surgical skills for operative laparoscopy. Benefits of laparoscopy over laparotomy are reduced blood loss, a decrease in postoperative pain and hence the need for analgesics, shorter stay in the hospital and less postoperative adhesions; in addition to a magnified image of the lesion. The pregnancy rates, monthly fecundity and cyst recurrence are comparable in both modalities. A recent meta-analysis of all prospective randomized clinical trials comparing laparoscopic surgery and laparotomy showed that complications like bowel injuries, ureteric injuries and ovarian abscess formation were comparable in both.[13] The choice of surgical technique for laparoscopic management is still controversial.

Three different types of ovarian endometriosis can be classified as follows:

- Superficial lesions
- Endometriomas
- Deep infiltrating ovarian endometriosis (infrequent).

There are fundamentally two different laparoscopic techniques for the management of endometrioma

- Fenestration and ablation of the cyst wall
- Cystectomy or stripping of the cyst wall lining.

Numerous studies have debated the efficacy of cyst wall ablation and cystectomy. No definite conclusion has been made so far regarding the same.

We follow both the techniques depending on the size of the endometrioma, feasibility of excision and symptomatology of the patient taking into consideration the amount of normal ovarian tissue that would be preserved after the surgery.

With the patient in modified lithotomy position under general anesthesia, a 10 mm supraumbilical port and two ancillary 5 mm ports are introduced under vision. We use the 5 mm grasper, scissors and toothed needle holder for the procedure. Hemostasis is achieved using bipolar diathermy. Adhesions secondary to endometriosis can distort the pelvic anatomy, thereby reducing the fertility and increasing the associated pain. Adhesiolysis is performed by sharp dissection with scissors, bipolar diathermy or using the harmonic ultracision (Figure 4.3). Irrigation is performed with normal saline under pressure. All other areas with endometriotic implants are either fulgurated or excised (Figure 4.19). Studies have reported that the pregnancy rate after excision of the implants is similar to electro-diathermy.[14] Histological confirmation of the lesion is necessary in either procedure. The cyst wall is sent for histopathological examination after excision in toto or a biopsy is taken when ablation is performed. In small endometriomas, the endometrial lining can be easily identified by the presence of surface epithelium with stroma. Large endometriomas, however, are rarely completely lined by endometrial tissue. Biopsy should be taken from the area of maximum fibrosis, which could be the site of the implant. Other areas may show different lining like ovarian cortical tissue, fibro-reactive tissue with hemosiderin-laden macrophages.

For superficial endometriotic implants (<1cm diameter) electrocoagulation is done. Laser vaporization or excision can also be done.

Endometriotic cysts < 3 cm in size that can be easily removed without causing much damage to the normal ovarian stroma are excised completely. The inner lining of the cyst is dissected from the ovary by two grasping forceps or two toothed needle holders that are pulled in opposite directions (Figure 4.4) till the cyst wall is completely peeled off (Figures 4.5 and 4.6). This is then sent for histopathological examination. It is important to remember that unlike benign ovarian cyst that can be easily peeled off, chocolate cysts often rupture at the time of cystectomy. Peeling of the cyst wall may be difficult due to invagination and fibrosis of the cortex; the basic pathogenetic mechanism of endometrioma formation.

Endometriomas > 3 cm (Figure 4.14) in size that can be easily excised are managed by cystectomy as above. But most of the time the fibrosis is so dense that cystectomy may not be possible. In such instances we prefer to drain the cyst, irrigate the cyst and ablate the inner wall of the cyst (Figures 4.15, 4.16 and 4.18), so that no active endometrial lining is left behind. A portion of the cyst wall is sent for histopathology for confirmation of the diagnosis (Figure 4.17). We prefer to use GnRH analogues in cases of severe endometriosis for 3 months after surgery; wherein the active implants could not be completely excised or ablated due to extensive adhesions.

The remaining ovarian tissue is either left alone or reconstructed with the use of fine vicryl sutures (Figure 4.7). Number of sutures is kept at a minimum to prevent postoperative adhesions. Closure of the ovarian defect by endosuturing is suggested in order to decrease the risk of postoperative adhesions between the ablated areas and other pelvic structures.[15] Fibrin sealants have also been used for controlling microvascular or capillary bleeding from ruptured or surgically dissected tissues.[15]

Despite extensive studies, no definite conclusions can be drawn as to whether fenestration with ablation or cystectomy is the treatment of choice.

Donnez[16] et al reported a good pregnancy rate in a large series of patients who underwent laparoscopic internal wall vaporization. This procedure decreases the risk of ovarian damage. They also describe a three-step treatment, which involves laparoscopic drainage of the cyst, three months medical treatment with GnRH analogues and a second laparoscopic procedure to achieve laser vaporization of the remaining endometriotic implants. They achieved a 51 percent cumulative pregnancy rate, with an 8 percent recurrence rate.

Brosens et al[17] also reported that the endometriomas should be treated by laser vaporization after a preoperative medical treatment. Beretta et al, however, reported a high recurrence rate in endometriomas after fenestration and coagulation. Donnez et al believe that this could be due to insufficient coagulation of the cyst wall lining.

Many authors also believe that cystectomy will result in the removal of numerous oocytes thereby decreasing the follicular reserve during IVF cycles. Canis[18] in his study emphasized that the technique of cystectomy should be different from that used in the treatment of benign neoplasm. This is due to the fact that cyst wall is surrounded by fibrosis which makes the cleavage difficult.

Beretta[19] reported better pregnancy rates after laparoscopic ovarian cystectomy than after drainage and coagulation performed with bipolar. Alborzi[20] in his study concluded that laparoscopic cystectomy of endometriomas leads to a lower recurrence of signs and symptoms, a reduced rate of reoperation and a higher cumulative pregnancy rate than the latter. Advantage of cystectomy is that histopathological examination can be done and diagnosis can be confirmed.

A systematic review[21] from the Cochrane database concluded that excisional surgery for endometriomata provides a more favorable outcome than drainage and ablation, with regard to the recurrence of endometrioma, recurrence of symptoms and subsequent spontaneous pregnancy in women who were previously subfertile. However, they found no data to indicate the best surgical approach in women planning to undergo assisted reproductive techniques.

ROLE OF ADJUNCTIVE SURGICAL PROCEDURES

Endometriosis related pelvic pain could be managed by adjunctive surgical procedures done along with excision or ablation. Uterosacral nerve ablation and presacral neurectomy are two procedures that have shown to play a role in improving the efficacy of surgical treatment of women with pain.[22] Laparoscopic uterosacral nerve ablation is designed to destroy efferent nerve fibers in the uterosacral ligaments. Presacral neurectomy disrupts efferent sympathetic pathways from the uterus thereby relieving pain. Increased incidence of constipation and urinary urgency has been reported following presacral neurectomy.

ENDOMETRIOMA AND INFERTILITY

Pathogenesis

Endometriosis is thought to be one of the major causes for infertility. The cause and effect relationship between endometriosis and infertility is not clearly understood.

- Severe endometriosis can cause distortion of pelvic anatomy by adhesions and can lead to a mechanical disturbance in fertility.
- Periovarian adhesions can interfere with oocyte release.
- Tubal adhesions can impair transport into the uterine cavity.
- Presence of ectopic endometrial implants can lead to an autoimmune response resulting in implantation failure.
- Follicular defects like abnormal follicular growth, decreased follicular size and shortened follicular phase are observed in women with mild endometriosis.[23] Anovulatory cycles are found in 10 percent of infertile women with endometriosis.[24]
- Luteinized unruptured follicle has been considered an endocrine mechanism linking endometriosis and infertility. The dominant follicle in this condition fails to rupture after LH surge.

Treatment Outcome on Infertility

The question of expectant management, surgery only, surgery followed by IVF or IVF in the presence of endometriomas is controversial. In infertile women, ovarian endometriomas are treated surgically as medical therapy alone does not seem to be effective in enhancing fertility after treatment.

Takahiro et al[25] studied the impact of ovarian endometrioma on oocytes and pregnancy outcome in IVF. They concluded that endometriosis affects the oocyte number but not embryo quality or pregnancy outcome, irrespective of the presence of an ovarian endometrioma. The role of surgery in the management of ovarian endometriomas for infertility is not well defined. Tinkanen et al[26] studied the effects of operative treatment of recurrent ovarian endometriomas on the pregnancy rate with IVF. Patients with endometrioma had significantly more embryos to transfer as compared to women who underwent surgical therapy earlier. It was also reported that small subgroup of patients presented with dark

LAPAROSCOPIC RIGHT OVARIAN CYST EXCISION WITH OVARIAN RECONSTRUCTION

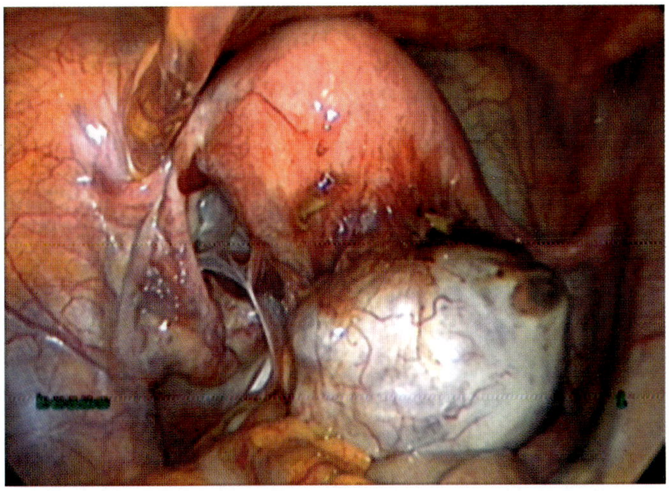

Figure 4.2. Uterus with right ovarian endometrioma

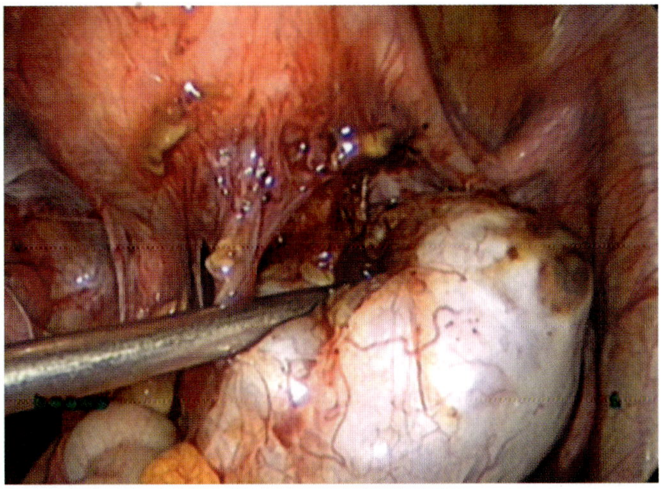

Figure 4.3. Adhesiolysis and aspiration of the endometrioma

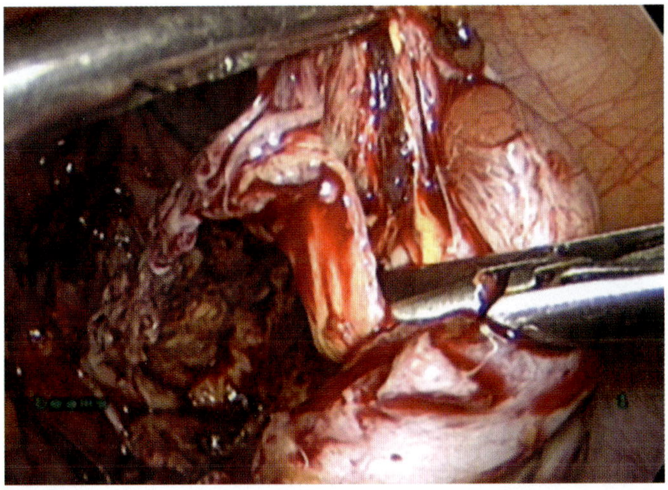

Figure 4.4. Separation of cyst wall from underlying ovarian tissue

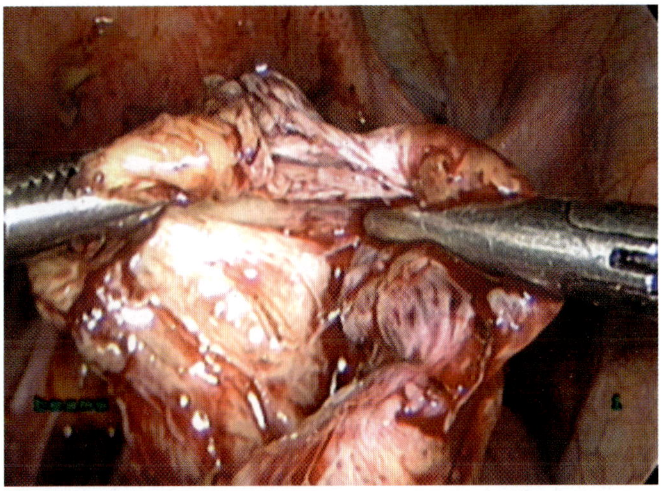

Figure 4.5. Peeling of the cyst wall

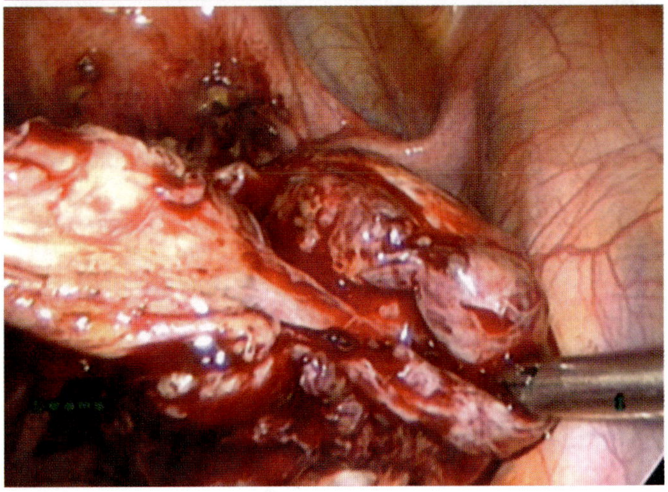

Figure 4.6. Complete excision

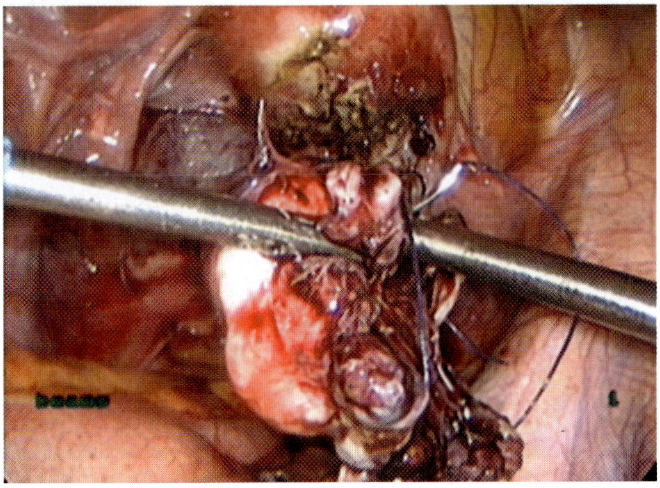

Figure 4.7. Ovarian reconstruction

OVARIAN ENDOMETRIOMAS

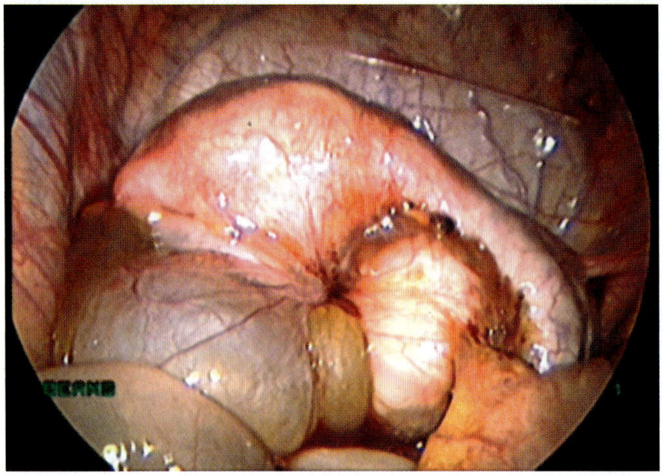

Figure 4.8. Bilateral ovarian endometrioma

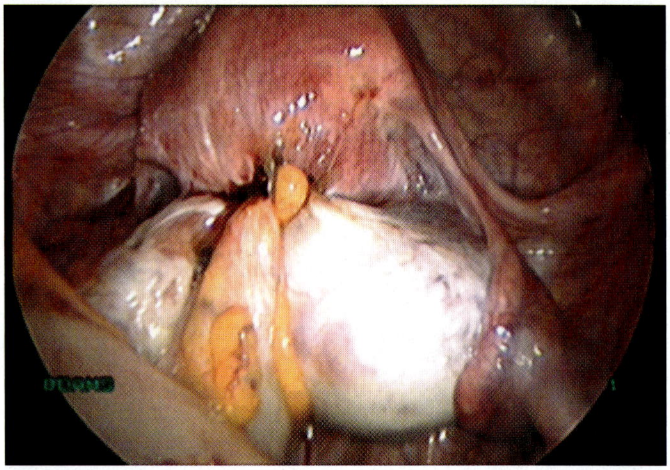

Figure 4.9. Bilateral ovarian endometrioma with severe rectosigmoid adhesions

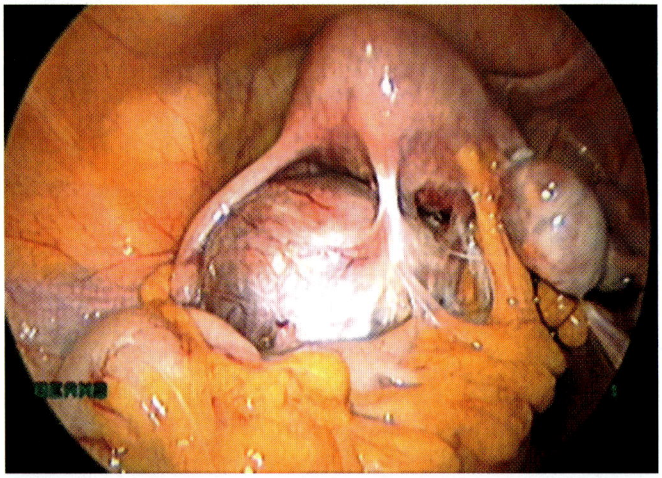

Figure 4.10. Left ovarian endometrioma

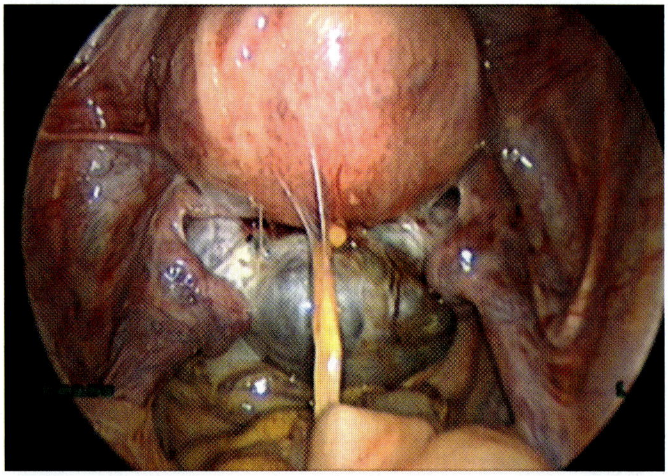

Figure 4.11. Right ovarian endometrioma

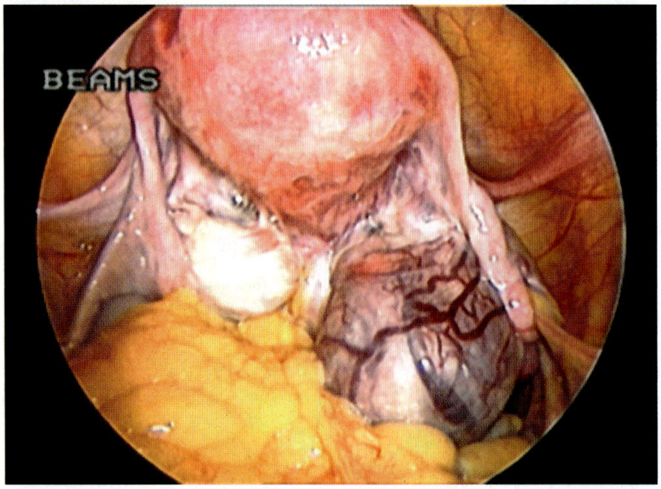

Figure 4.12. Right ovarian endometrioma with increased vascularity

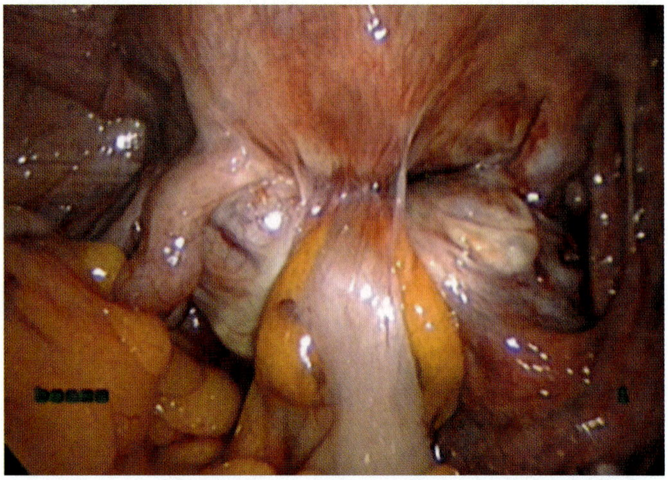

Figure 4.13. Bilateral endometrioma with rectal adhesions

LAPAROSCOPIC CYST WALL ABLATION WITH BIOPSY

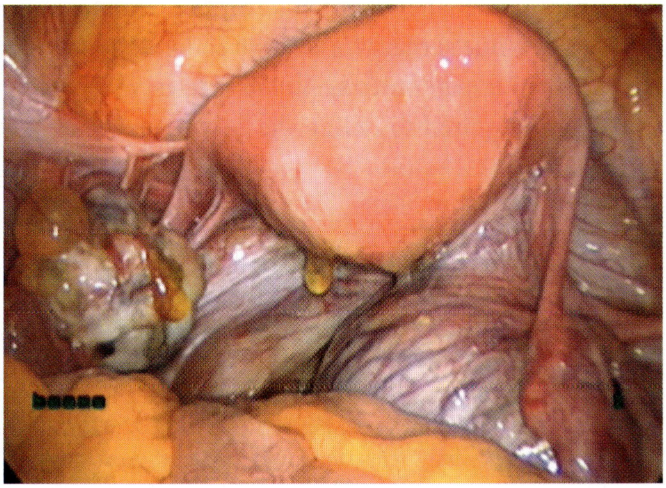

Figure 4.14. Uterus with bilateral ovarian endometrioma

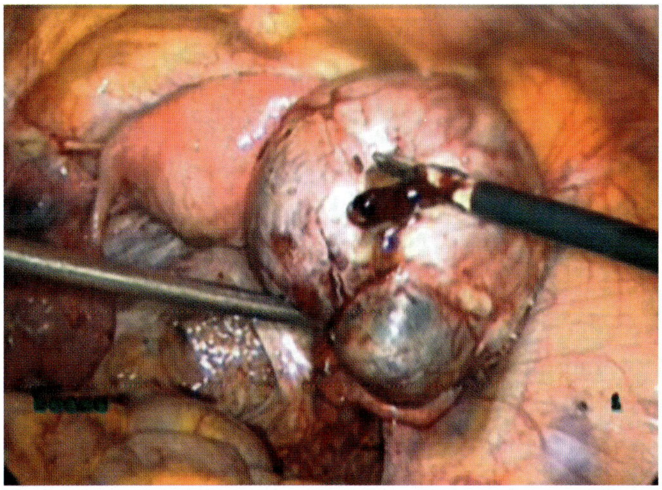

Figure 4.15. Right ovarian cyst incised

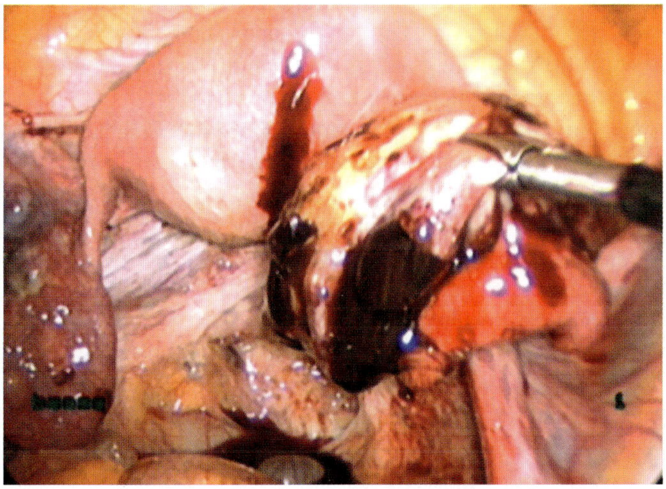

Figure 4.16. Cyst contents drained

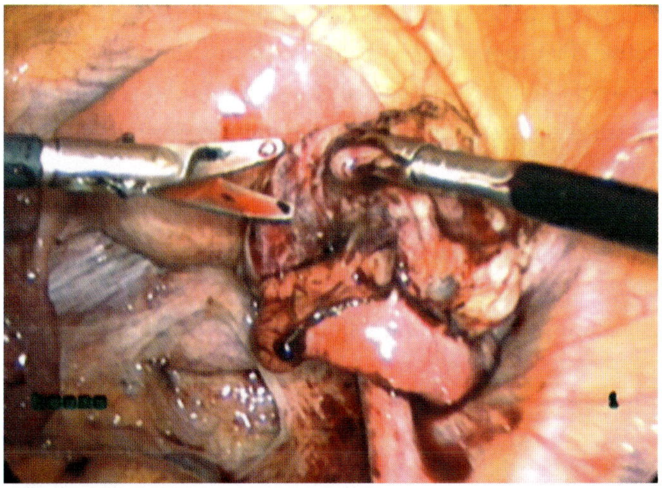

Figure 4.17. Ovarian biopsy taken

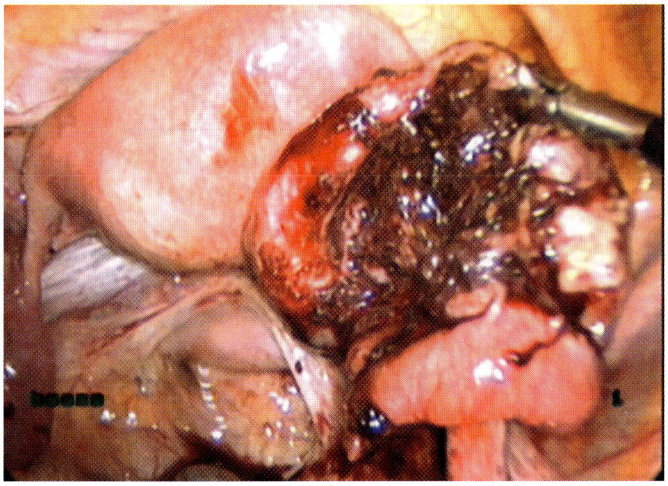

Figure 4.18. Ablation of cyst wall done

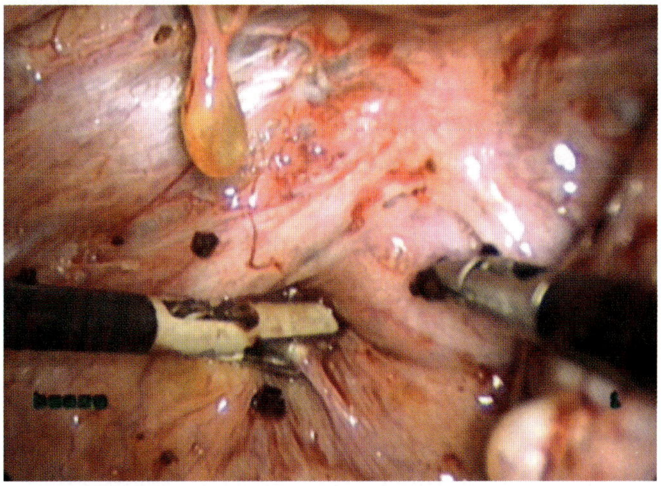

Figure 4.19. Fulguration of endometriotic spots

discharge coming out of the cervix which could probably be an endometriotic cyst draining the contents via the tube into the uterus. This may prevent the implantation of embryos in an IVF cycle.

Controversial data were reported after laparoscopic cystectomy on the ovarian response during ovarian stimulation for IVF. Garcia et al[27] investigated whether conservative surgery on ovarian endometriomas before an IVF cycle improves fertility outcomes. They concluded that laparoscopic cystectomy before IVF cycles does not improve fertility outcomes. Proceeding directly to controlled ovarian hyperstimulation in women with asymptomatic ovarian endometrioma might reduce the time to pregnancy and the costs of treatment. They also concluded that conservative surgical management in symptomatic women does not impair IVF or ICSI success rates. Damage to the ovarian tissue during surgery depends on the expertize of the surgeon and the number of surgeries done on the same patient before attempting IVF.[18]

Donnez et al evaluated the ovarian response to stimulation for IVF treatment in women who underwent cyst wall ablation. They concluded that cyst wall ablation does not impair IVF outcome.[16]

CONCLUSION

Endometriosis is an increasingly common condition in gynecological practice, the treatment of which remains controversial inspite of the vast body of literature available and the extensive research into it. Despite being described over a century ago, its pathogenesis remains elusive; and therein stems the cornucopia of treatments. Infertility and pelvic pain are the common presenting symptoms of endometrioma and surgical treatment offers the best results in both. Laparoscopic surgery has become the gold standard for management of endometrioma. Cyst wall ablation and cystectomy are the two treatment options and the optimal one should be decided based on the degree of ovarian damage that can occur with either procedure. Cystectomy is a valuable tool in experienced hands and is increasingly the preferred treatment option. Histopathological examination is important to rule out coincident malignancy and to aid further treatment and follow-up. While surgery for ovarian endometriomas has not shown to impair outcome in IVF cycles, prospective studies are required to define the best management of such patients.

REFERENCES

1. Drake TS, Grunnert GM. The unsuspected pelvic factor in the infertility investigations. Fertil Steril 1980;34:27-31.
2. Loh FH, Tan AI, Kumar J, Ng SC. Ovarian response after laparoscopic ovarian Cystectomy for endometriotic cysts in 132 monitored cycles. Fertil Steril 1999;72:316-21.
3. Haya Al-Fozan, Togas Tulandi. Left lateral predisposition of Endometriosis and Endometrioma. Obstet Gynecol 2003;101:164-6.
4. Alcazar JL, Laparte C, Jurado M, Lopez-Garcia G. The role of transvaginal ultrasonography combined with colour velocity imaging and pulsed Doppler in the diagnosis of Endometrioma.Fertil Steril 1997;67:487-91.
5. Vercellini P, Vendola N, Bocciolone L, et al. Reliability of the visual diagnosis of ovarian endometriosis. Fertil Steril 1990;53:1198-1200.
6. Rana N, Thomas S, Rotman C, Dmowski WP. Decrease in the size of ovarian endometriomas during ovarian suppression in stage IV endometriosis. Role of preoperative medical treatment. J Reprod Med 1996;41:384-92.
7. Robert Shaw, Ray Garry, Lindsay McMillan, et al. A prospective randomized open study comparing goserelin (Zoladex) plus surgery and surgery alone in the management of ovarian endometriomas.Gynaecological Endoscopy 2001;10:151-7.
8. Nisolle M, Clerckx F, Casanas-Roux F, Gillerot S, Bourgonjon D, Donnez J. Treatment of endometriosis. Evaluation of preoperative therapy with danazol, gestrinone and buserelin (nasal spray and implant)]. J Gynecol Obstet Biol Reprod (Paris) 1990;19(6):759-63.
9. Zanetta G, Lissoni A, Dalla valle C, Trio D, Pitelle M, Rangoni G. Ultrasound guided aspiration of endometriomas: Possible applications and limitations. Fertil Steril 1995;64:709-13.
10. Fisch JD, Sher G. Sclerotherapy with 5 percent tetracycline is a simple alternative to potentially complex surgical treatment of ovarian endometriomas before *in vitro* fertilization. Fertil Steril 2004;82(2):437-41.
11. Benoit L, Arnould L, Margarot A, Franceschini C, Collin F, Fraisse J, et al. Malignant tumours arising in extraovarian endometriosis: Three case reports and review of the literature. Ann Chir 2004;129(6-7):376-80.

12. Clayton RD, Hawe JA, Love JC, Wilkinson N, Garry R. Recurrent pain after hysterectomy and bilateral salpingo-oophorectomy for endometriosis: Evaluation of laparoscopic excision of residual endometriosis. Br J Obstet Gynaecol 1999;106(7):740-4.
13. Chapron C, Fauconnier A, Goffinet F, Breart G, Dubuisson JB. Laparoscopic surgery is not inherently dangerous for patients presenting benign gynaecological pathologies. Results of a meta-analysis. Human Reprod 2002;17:1334-42.
14. Tulandi T, Al-Took S. Reproductive outcome after treatment of mild endometriosis with laparoscopic excision and electrocoagulation. Fertil Steril 1998;69:229-31.
15. Donnez J, Nisolle M, Slatkine, Karaman Y, et al. CO_2 laser laparoscopy in peritoneal endometriosis and in ovarian cyst. J Gynecol Surgery 1990;5:391.
16. Donnez J, Wyns C, Nisolle M. Does ovarian surgery for endometriomas impair the ovarian response to gonadotropin? Fertil Steril 2001;76:662-5.
17. Brosens IA, Van Ballaer P, Puttemans P, Deprest J. Reconstruction of the ovary containing large endometriomas by an extraovarian endosurgical technique. Fertil Steril 1996;66(4):517-21.
18. Canis M, Pouly JL, Tamburro S, Mage G, Wattiez A, Bruhat MA. Ovarian response during IVF-embryo transfer cycles after laparoscopic ovarian cystectomy for endometriotic cysts of >3 cm in diameter. Hum Reprod 2001;16(12): 2583-6.
19. Beretta P, Franchi M, Ghezzi F, Busacca M, Zupi E, Bolis P. Randomized clinical trial of two laparoscopic treatments of endometriomas: Cystectomy versus drainage and coagulation. Fertil Steril 1998;70:1176-80.
20. Alborzi MD, Mozhdeh Momtahan, Mohammed Ebrahim Parsanezhad, Sedigheh Dehbashi, et al. A prospective, randomized study comparing laparoscopic ovarian Cystectomy versus fenestration and coagulation in patients with endometriomas. Fertil Steril 2004;82:1633-7.
21. Roger Hart, Martha Hickey, Panos Maouris, William Buckett, Ray Garry. Excisional surgery versus ablative surgery for ovarian endometriomata: A cochrane review. Human Reproduction 2005;20(11):3000-7.
22. Proctor ML, Farquhar CM, Sinclair OJ, Johnson NP. Surgical interruption of pelvic nerve pathways for primary and secondary Dysmenorrhoea (cochrane review). In The cochrane library, Issue 2003;2.
23. Ayers JWT, Birenbaum DL, Menon KML. Luteal phase dysfunction in endometriosis; elevated progesterone levels in peripheral and ovarian veins during follicular phase. Fertil Steril 1987;47:925-9.
24. Mahmood TA, Templeton A. Pathophysiology of mild endometriosis: Review of literature. Human Reprod 1990; 5:765-84.
25. Takahiro S, Shun-ichiro Izumi, Hidehiko, Matsubayashi, et al. Impact of Ovarian endometrioma on oocytes and pregnancy outcome in *in vitro* fertilization. Fertil Steril 2005;83:908-13.
26. Tinkanen H, Kujansuu E. *In vitro* fertilization in patients with ovarian endometriomas. Acta Obstet Gynecol Scand 2000;79(2):119-22.
27. Garcia-Velasco JA, Mahutte NG, Corona J, Zuniga V, Giles J, Arici A. Removal of endometriomas before *in vitro* fertilization does not improve fertility outcomes: A matched, case-control study. Fertil Steril 2004;81(5):1194-7.

5 Treatment of Peritoneal and Other Endometriosis

Pratap Kumar, Bimal Mathew John

INTRODUCTION

"If a man knows endometriosis, he knows Gynecology" was what Sir William Osler (1849-1919) said to describe the complexity and uncertainty of the disease. After years, the condition remains as enigmatic and we are still far away from consensus. While there are many controversies regarding treatment based on "Evidence Based Medicine" and complete resolution of endometriosis remains unlikely, the objectives for current treatment center around reducing pain, increasing the likelihood of pregnancy and delaying the recurrence of the condition.

CLASSIFICATION

Depending on the size and depth of the implant, bilaterality and the severity of adhesions, the American Society of Reproductive Medicine (1996) has classified endometriosis[1] as:

- Stage I–Minimal disease
- Stage II–Mild disease
- Stage III–Moderate disease
- Stage IV–Severe disease

Despite very poor correlation with severity of symptoms and very poor reproducibility, this remains the most accepted form of classification.

Currently, three different entities are recognized within the clinical condition of endometriosis:[2]

- Peritoneal endometriosis
- Ovarian endometriomas
- Rectovaginal endometriosis.

DIAGNOSIS

For women presenting with symptoms and signs suggestive of endometriosis, a definitive diagnosis still requires laparoscopic visual inspection, making it the "gold standard" investigation. Possible exception to this rule is when disease is visible in the vagina or elsewhere on examination. An elaborate history and thorough clinical examination remains vital to the diagnosis of endometriosis.

Immunoassays such as serum Ca-125, Placental Protein-14 and Antibodies to the endometrium are being studied, of which serum Ca-125 seems to be the most promising. However, there is overlap of positive assays with conditions such as Pelvic Inflammatory disease. 5-aminolevulinic acid fluorescence diagnosis and Aromatase P-450 messenger RNA expression are investigative modalities under research currently.

Imaging modalities have a limited role in the diagnosis of endometriosis, except transvaginal ultrasonography in the case of endometriomas[3] and MRI for deep infiltrating endometriosis.[4] Bowel barium enema, transrectal ultrasonography and intravenous pyelography are additional investigations that may help in the case of

Rectovaginal Endometriosis. Preoperative diagnosis of severe ureteral or rectal wall involvement of the disease is vital in surgical preparation, as well as in making available the assistance of competent urologists and surgeons during the procedure.

Endometriosis has multiple presentations and has been described as "protean" in appearance, making diagnosis even on visual inspection difficult. Histological confirmation of visually identified endometriosis has ranged from 9 to 90 percent. Various descriptions for the endometriotic lesions have been recognized such as red raspberries, purple raspberries, blueberries, blebs, peritoneal pockets, whitish scar tissue, stellate scar tissue, strawberry colored lesions, red vesicles, white vesicles, clear vesicles, powder-burns, yellow-brown patches, brown-black patches, adhesions, clear polypoid lesions, red polypoid lesions, red flame-like and gun shot lesions. Typically, the lesions are black, dark brown or bluish in color, while atypical presentations can be as red implants (red flame like, hemorrhagic or petechial lesions) or serous or clear vesicles. Thus diagnosing endometriosis solely on the basis of visual confirmation can lead to both misdiagnosis as well as over-diagnosis. 'Near-contact' laparoscopy, which results in up to an eight-fold magnification, can help to identify more atypical peritoneal lesions as small as 400 micrometers.[5] There is no consensus on whether histologic identification is required in the case of peritoneal endometriosis, but the current consensus is that visual inspection is adequate though positive histologic confirmation of atleast one lesion is ideal.

Treatment

Medical treatment for mild endometriosis generally provides effective pain relief, but the recurrence rate following cessation of therapy is high. NSAIDs may be effective for reducing endometriosis associated pain. Suppression of ovarian function for 6 months with COC, danazol, gestrinone, medroxyprogesterone acetate and GnRH agonists have been accepted and various studies show that all are equally effective. Depending on the patient, and considering drug side-effects and cost profiles, treatment should be tailor-made.[6]

In a meta-analysis that included seven studies comparing medical treatment to no treatment or placebo, the common odds ratio for pregnancy was 0.85 (95% CI 0.95, 1.22) indicating no cumulative increase in pregnancy rates following medical therapy for minimal and mild endometriosis.[7] These findings and other similar studies were analyzed and the present consensus is that hormonal treatment does not improve the fecundity of infertile women with stage I or II endometriosis.

Surgical treatment improves pregnancy rates and is the preferred initial treatment for infertility caused by endometriosis. Laparoscopic ablation of minimal-moderate endometriosis also appears to relieve pain associated with minimal to mild endometriosis. The Canadian Collaborative Group on Endometriosis recommended that laparoscopic destruction of endometriotic lesions should be the first line of therapy[8] while a later RCT by an Italian group suggested that surgical management of peritoneal endometriosis does not improve fertility.[9] Meta-analysis of the two randomized trials showed improvement in infertility associated with endometriosis with laparoscopic surgery. The Canadian trial clearly supported this outcome with an increased chance of conception (OR 2.03, 95% CI 1.28 to 3.24) and ongoing pregnancy rate after 20 weeks (OR 1.95, 95% CI 1.18 to 3.22). The smaller Italian trial did not show benefit in increasing the fertility rates (pregnancy OR 0.76, 95% CI 0.31 to 1.88; live birth OR 0.85, 95% CI 0.32 to 2.28). Combining the ongoing pregnancy and live birth rates there was a statistically significant increase in pregnancy rates with surgery (OR 1.64, 95% CI 1.05 to 2.57). Despite the lack of consensus, more studies are in favor of treating the lesions in the case of minimal and mild endometriosis, if and when laparoscopy is decided upon.[10]

With conservative surgery, the aim is to destroy visible endometriotic implants and lyse adhesions. The laparoscopic approach is the method of choice for treating endometriosis conservatively.[11] Ablation can be performed with YAG or carbon dioxide laser, Argon beam coagulator or electrodiathermy. Overall, the recurrence rate is 19 percent and is similar for all techniques.[12] For peritoneal endometriotic implants, carbon dioxide laser with a power setting of 40-50W in continuous firing mode is used. If a lesion is overlying a vital structure such as the ureter, urinary bladder, colon or large blood vessels, a retroperitoneal injection of fluid (aquaprotection) provides safer vaporization of the lesions. This allows a 100-200 mm depth of vaporization, thus substantially limiting the depth of penetration. After vaporization of an endometriotic implant, a curdy white material representing vaporization of the stromal layer is seen and the retroperitoneal fat is encountered which ensures complete removal of the lesion. There is no evidence that the outcome is affected by the method of ablation, by electrosurgery or laser delivery systems.[13]

The concept of adenomyosis of the retroperitoneal space should cover not only the rectovaginal space and the vesicovaginal space but also the area extending laterally in the direction of the cardinal ligaments. Deep fibrotic nodular adenomyosis involving the cul-de-sac requires excision of the nodular tissue from the posterior vagina, rectum, posterior cervix and uterosacral ligaments. There is lack of consensus on the extent of resection that is required in the case of rectovaginal endometriosis in particular. The concept that hysterectomy with bilateral salpingo-oophorectomy is a definitive treatment for endometriosis is proven incorrect now, especially in cases where there is infiltration of the rectovaginal, uterosacral and cardinal areas, leading to patches of endometriosis being left behind giving rise to persistence of symptoms. In cases where there is deep endometriotic infiltrates, referral to an expert laparoscopic surgeon is recommended for radical resection of the disease, which need not include hysterectomy or oophorectomy automatically. Laparoscopy allows radical microsurgery with its better magnification and easier access to the retroperitoneal regions compared to laparotomy.[14] But the decision for laparoscopy or laparotomy should depend primarily on the surgeon's expertise to remove the disease by either method.

As per the American Society of Reproductive Guidelines on Endometriosis in 2004, in women with stage III/IV endometriosis-associated infertility, conservative surgical therapy with laparoscopy or laparotomy is indicated. Analysis of several studies showed that there is improvement of fertility rates following surgery, with no evidence of benefit from medical therapy. For women with stage III/IV endometriosis who fail to conceive following conservative surgery or because of advancing reproductive age, IVF-ET is an effective alternative.

Presacral neurectomy is used be some surgeons to relieve severe dysmenorrhea. The nerve bundles are transected at the level of the third sacral vertebra, and the distal ends are ligated. Vascular injury to the middle sacral vessels is a potential complication, and prophylactic ligation may be done. Constipation is another common long-term adverse effect (94%) of this procedure and these complications should be considered and weighed against the benefits while deciding whether to perform this procedure.

Nodularity of the uterosacral ligaments may contribute to dyspareunia and low back pain with transmission of neural pathways via the Lee-Frankenhäuser plexus. Laparoscopic uterine nerve ablation (LUNA), performed to interrupt the pain fibers, had no advantage in terms of pain relief when compared to placebo in systematic reviews of various studies. However, when combined with laparoscopic ablation, LUNA significantly reduced pain attributed to endometriosis. Ablation of endometriotic lesions plus laparoscopic uterine nerve ablation (LUNA) in minimal–moderate disease reduces endometriosis-associated pain at 6 months compared to diagnostic laparoscopy; the smallest effect seen in patients with minimal disease. However, there is no evidence that LUNA is a necessary component, as LUNA by itself has no effect on dysmenorrhea associated with endometriosis.[15]

There is insufficient evidence to conclude that hormonal suppression (before or after or both) along with surgery for endometriosis is associated with a significant benefit in terms of improvement of fertility or reducing pain. There may be benefit of improvement in AFS scores with the pre-surgical use of medical therapy, but such benefits should be considered in the context of the adverse effects and costs involved with such therapies.[16]

CONCLUSIONS

- Laparoscopy remains the "gold standard" for the diagnosis of endometriosis
- Hormonal therapy does not by itself improve fecundity in women diagnosed to be infertile due to endometriosis
- Laparoscopic ablation of endometriotic lesions can improve fertility in the case of women with minimal and mild endometriosis, and may be safely recommended during laparoscopy
- In stage III or IV endometriosis, conservative surgery to excise or ablate all endometriotic lesions is recommended, and such surgery should not always be combined with hysterectomy or oophorectomy.

REFERENCES

1. American Society for Reproductive Medicine. Revised American Society for Reproductive Medicine classification of endometriosis: 1996. Fertil Steril 1997;67:817-21.
2. Nisolle M, Donnez J. Peritoneal endometriosis, ovarian endometriosis and adenomyotic nodules of the rectovaginal septum are three different entities. Fertility and Sterility 1997;68:585-96.
3. Moore J, Copley S, Morris J, Lindsell D, Golding S, Kennedy S. A systematic review of the accuracy of ultrasound in the diagnosis of endometriosis. Ultrasound Obstet Gynecol 2002;20:630-4.
4. Pratibha Arya, Robert Shaw. Current Obstetrics and Gynecology 2005;15:191-8.
5. Fred M Howard. The role of laparoscopy as a diagnostic tool in chronic pelvic pain. Bailliere's Clinical Obstetrics and Gynecology 2000;14(3):467-94.
6. Selak V, Farquhar C, Prentice A, Singla A. Danazol for pelvic pain associated with endometriosis (Cochrane Review). In The Cochrane Library, Issue 3. John Wiley and Sons Ltd, Chichester, UK 2004.
7. Hughes E, Fedorkow D, Collins J, Vandekerckhove P. Ovulation suppression for endometriosis (Cochrane Review). In The Cochrane Library, Issue 3. John Wiley and Sons Ltd, Chichester, UK 2004.
8. Marcoux S, Maheux R, Berube S. Laparoscopic surgery in infertile women with minimal or mild endometriosis. Canadian collaborative group on endometriosis. New England Journal of Medicine 1997;24:217-22.
9. Gruppo Italiano per lo Studio dell'Endometriosis, Ablation of lesions or no treatment in minimal-mild endometriosis in infertile women: A randomized trial. Human Reproduction 1999;14:32-4.
10. Jacobson TZ, Barlow DH, Koninckx PR, Olive D, Farquhar C. Laparoscopic surgery for subfertility associated with endometriosis (Cochrane Review). The Cochrane Library, Issue 3. John Wiley and Sons Ltd, Chichester, UK 2004b.
11. Saidi MH, et al. Complications of major operative laparoscopy. J Reprod Med 1996;4(17):471-6.
12. Revelli A, et al. Recurent endometriosis: A review of biological and clinical aspects. Obstet Gynecol Surv 1995;50(10):747-54.
13. Donnez J, et al. Surgical management of endometriosis. Best Practice and Research Clinical Obstetrics and Gynaecology 2004;18(2):329-48.
14. Charles Koh, et al. Laparoscopic microsurgery: Current and future status. Current Opinion in Obstetrics and Gynecology 1999;11(4):401-7.
15. Vercellini P, Aimi G, Busacca M, Apolone G, Uglietti A, Crosignani PG. Laparoscopic uterosacral ligament resection for dysmenorrhea associated with endometriosis: Results of a randomized, controlled trial. Fertil Steril 2003a;80: 310-9.
16. Yap C, et al. Pre- and postoperative medical therapy for endometriosis surgery. Cochrane Database Systematic Reviews. The Cochrane Library, Issue 3. John Wiley and Sons Ltd, Chichester, UK 2004.

6 Endoscopy in Male Infertility due to Varicoceles

Christopher Chen

VARICOCELE

The varicocele is a dilatation of the testicular veins within the spermatic cord due to retrograde blood flow arising from incompetency of their venous valves. Traditionally, the varicocele is considered to have a unilateral occurrence, more often on the left side. However, recent research has revealed a greater tendency to bilaterality of the condition.

The incidence of varicoceles among men being evaluated for infertility varies from 19 to 41 percent[1] and the latter figure is more reflective of the true incidence today.

The effect of the varicocele on male fertility is a reduction in sperm count, motility, and morphology.[2] It appears that renal blood refluxes into the testicle, causing damage as well as chromosomal breaks in the sex chromosomes. There is also consequential reduction of testicular male hormone production.[3]

DIAGNOSIS

Varicoceles are diagnosed by physical examination employing the Valsalva's maneuver in the standing position. The varicocele is subdivided into the following classes:[4]

Grade 3: Very large distension of the testicular veins causing bulging of the scrotal skin and visible on inspection.

Grade 2: Distension not visible but is palpable without Valsalva's maneuver.

Grade 1: Distension only palpable during Valsalva's maneuver.

Subclinical varicoceles are not palpable even during Valsalva's maneuver and require Doppler echography or color Doppler sonography for their detection.

All varicoceles, regardless, do decrease male reproductive function[5] and should be treated.

TREATMENT

The treatment of the varicocele is surgical, by occlusion of the testicular veins, the most common approach being through the inguinal route.[6] Scrotal varicocelectomy is not practised nowadays owing to its poor results. A high peritoneal approach is more thorough in its removal of varicoceles and is favored as a modality of treatment. Videolaparoscopic varicocelectomy is the latest in the treatment of the varicocele and employs the high peritoneal approach.[7,8]

CLINICAL STUDY

The author performed a study of 700 spouses of infertile couples, all of whom had varicoceles.[9] Their age ranges were between 26 and 68 years. Most were in the age group 30 to 34 years, with a 3 years history of infertility. All the men had semen analysis performed. Some showed single sperm defects, others double, and still others triple defects. The varicoceles were diagnosed by clinical examination of the external genitalia and the varicoceles confirmed by Doppler examination using a hand-held Doppler instrument. This machine produced a sound if there was retrograde venous flow from the varicocele. Videolaparoscopic varicocelectomy was performed on these men.

OPERATIVE TECHNIQUE OF LAPAROSCOPIC VARICOCELECTOMY

The technique of laparoscopic varicocelectomy as practised is described in detail as follows.

The patient is treated as a day surgery case, being admitted to the hospital in the morning and discharged the same day.[9] He is given a general anesthetic and lies in the supine position.

He is then shaved completely from the upper abdomen, above the umbilicus to the pubis and scrotum, to allow both laparoscopy and testicular biopsy to be performed. The skin of the abdomen and scrotum is scrubbed with an antiseptic wash followed by povidone iodine paint. Sterile drapes are then put on, exposing the abdomen and scrotum for the performance of surgery.

Microsurgical Testicular Biopsy

A Zeis operating microscope is positioned over the testis and a 0.5cm incision make into the scrotal median raphe, over either the left or right testis which is held firmly in the operator's left hand. The scrotum is opened in layers under the microscope until the tunica albuginea (fibrous covering of the testis) is exposed and the sharp point of the scalpel then incised into the tunica. The testis is squeezed so that the yellow-colored testicular tissue (seminiferous tubules) emerges and can then be cut, using a small pair of curved scissors (testicular biopsy). The biopsy is then immersed in Bouins solution and sent for histological examination. The testicular wound is very carefully closed with 2(O) vicryl, avoiding the risk of bleeding and testicular hematoma formation. The scrotal wound is similarly carefully closed with 2 (O) catgut. Povidone iodine is finally applied to the wound.

Pneumoperitoneum Creation

A Veress needle is then inserted into the umbilicus after ensuring the umbilical orifice has been thoroughly cleansed off dirt and povidone iodine applied earlier on. The needle must be sharp and as the needle is passed, 2 clicks should be obtained. This can be an extremely difficult step as the needle must be within the peritoneal cavity before CO_2 gas insufflation can occur and successful pneumoperitoneum achieved.

Various Difficulties

Various difficulties may be encountered at this stage. (1) The needle point may be extraperitoneal, not having penetrated deeply enough. This can occur with obesity or men with very muscular abdominal walls, making it difficult to lift up the abdomen during the needle puncture. Another situation can be experienced as the needle plunges into either of 2 abdominal columns of tissue that run between the pubis and the umbilicus on each side of the midline, giving the impression of extensive intra-abdominal adhesions beneath the umbilicus when there are actually none. The lack of free flow of CO_2 as shown by the insufflator gauge and failure to demonstrate loss of liver dullness are signs indicative of this problem. The difficulty is resolved by repeated attempts, making fresh punctures of the Veress needle at different sites within the umbilicus, until the pneumoperitoneum is successfully achieved. (2) The needle appears to be in the peritoneal cavity but the CO_2 gas passes intermittently and then stops completely. The cause of this is needle tip entrapment in the omentum. Gas collects and appears as a swelling beneath the apron of omentum. Total withdrawal and reinsertion of the needle should overcome this problem. The needle tip can also cause a small bleed from trauma to the omental vessels. A more worrisome complication is hematoma of the mesentery due to the needle puncture. Hematoma can also occur from accidental damage to blood vessels in the posterior abdominal wall. All these complications must be looked out for once the laparoscope is successfully introduced, and hemostasis ensured by cautery or simply application of pressure over the hematoma. (3) When gut adhesions to the abdominal wall, especially over the umbilicus, are suspected, e.g. past abdominal incisions or old scars, it is better not to even use the Veress needle in the first instance but to probe with a hypodermic needle attached to a syringe containing saline. If fecal material is withdrawn, then the operation must be abandoned. The patient is given intra- and post-operative antibiotics and admitted to hospital for observation. The outcome is uneventful.

Laparoscopic Procedure

In the usual operation, before passing CO_2 into the Veress needle, a 20 ml syringe containing saline is injected to test that the needle is intraperitoneal. The saline should flow freely on injecting the syringe and no blood or fecal contents should be withdrawn. The supply of CO_2 is then attached to the Veress needle and the gas should flow freely, resulting in abdominal distention, with subsequent loss of liver and splenic dullness. When gas flow is ceased, it indicates that the abdomen is ready for laparoscopy. A 5 mm trocar is inserted slowly and cautiously through the umbilicus. As it enters the abdominal cavity, gas escapes through the side port which is kept open during the start of the procedure. A 5 mm laparoscope is inserted and a 3-chip video camera attached, to view the abdomen through the TV monitor. Having ascertained this, then the CO_2 supply is connected to the trocar to keep the abdomen distended. In any patient where danger to gut may expect to occur during transumbilical trocar puncture, a 2 mm trocar is used instead, thereby minimising any trauma to the gut should this occur. A 2 mm laparoscope is then inserted into the trocar to view the abdomen for any damage. This is a useful procedure to adopt when faced with these circumstances.

The gut is already displaced by the CO_2 by this time and is further pushed cephalad by assuming the Trendelenburg's position. The theater is now dimmed so that the sides of the abdominal wall at the umbilical level can be transilluminated for the 2 lateral abdominal wall incisions of 0.5 cm to be made, thereby avoiding puncturing any blood vessels in their path.

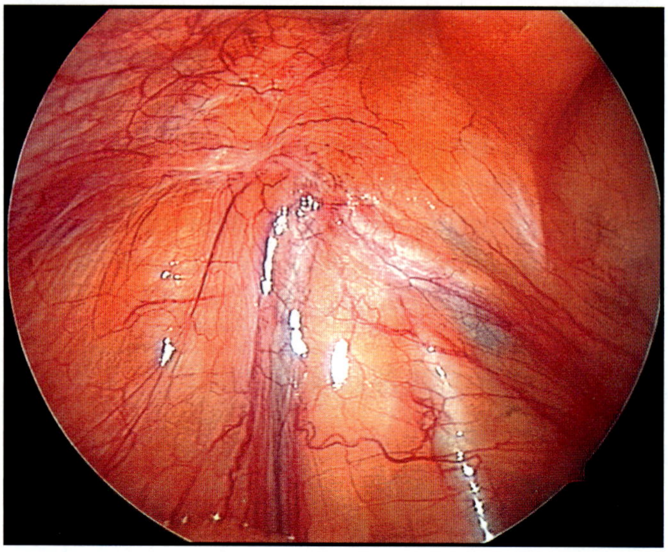

Figure 6.1. Left testicular vascular bundle entering internal ring with vas deferens of the right

Laparoscopic Varicocelectomy

After the 2 lateral trocars are inserted through the 0.5 cm abdominal incisions, both testicular vascular bundles on each right and left sides are identified.

The right bundle is operated on first (Figure 6.1). The vascular bundle is traced down to its entry into the internal ring and the vas deferens is also noted to emerge from the ring medially and running into the pelvis. These landmarks are always observed before proceeding further with the surgery. About a third of the distance up from the internal ring, the parietal peritoneum over the bundle is lifted up with pointed forceps and a 1cm transverse incision made. A pair of right-angled pointed hooks are then introduced through the lateral portals and the connective tissue between the vessels separated by teasing them apart.

The testicular artery must be identified and isolated first (Figure 6.2). It is seen as a pinkish vessel with varying degrees of prominence of pulsation. Unless the

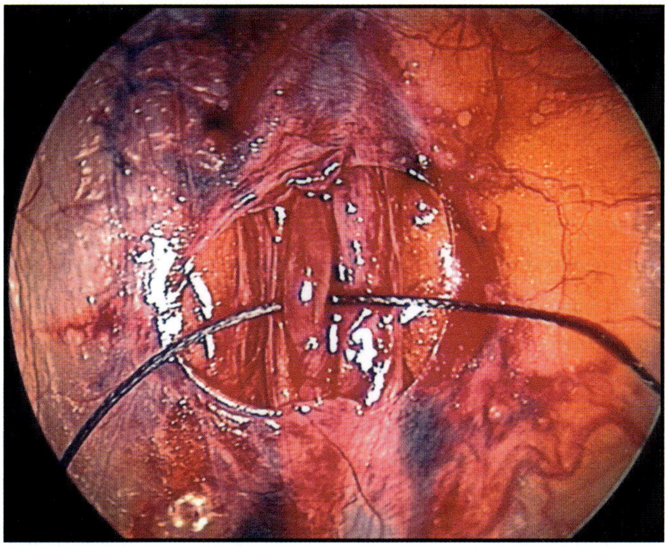

Figure 6.2. Left testicular artery dissected free with piece of marking suture beneath

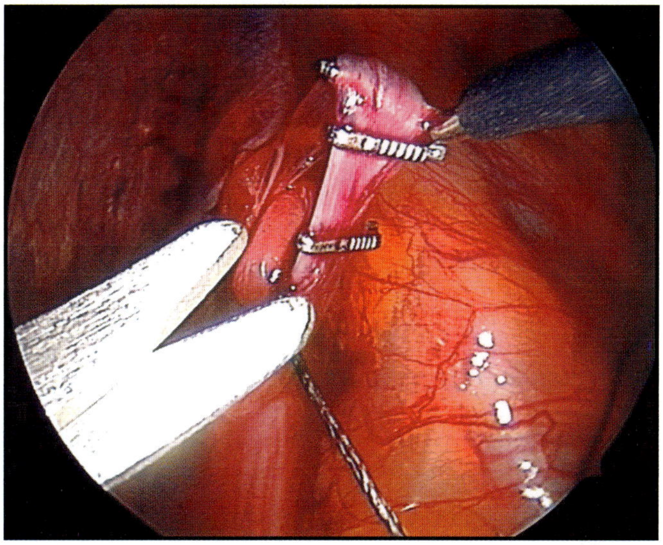

Figure 6.3. Bundle of left testicular veins clamped with 2 places and ready to be cut

artery is isolated and recognized with certainty, the operation cannot proceed. The artery is marked with a suture thread underneath it in order not to be mistaken for the testicular veins and be ligated inadvertently. More than one artery maybe encountered. There may be as many as 3 on each side.

Difficulty can be encountered with arterial bleeding due to tiny branches arising from the main arterial trunk. The bleeding can be quite substantial and pulsatile. This can be arrested by firm pressure with the forceps or with the use of a sponge plug which creates coagulation and occlusion of the bleeding vessel.

The testicular veins are exposed and clipped in 2 places with very small titanium clips and then cut in between (Figure 6.3). This ensures against recanalization. Bundles of veins are occluded in this fashion until all are eliminated. Where possible, lymphatic vessels are preserved to reduce the chances of hydrocele formation. The operation having been completed, the small peritoneal incision is sutured.

The operation then proceeds with the left side in the same manner as with the right, commencing with the peritoneal incision, isolation of the testicular artery or arteries, identification and occlusion of all the veins, and closure of the peritoneum.

Difficulties are often encountered on the left side because of adhesions of the descending colon over the testicular bundle, preventing access to the vessels until the adhesions are divided, the colon freed, and the vascular bundle then exposed. Thereafter, the varicocelectomy proceeds in the usual manner. The severity of the colon adhesions can vary from minor adhesions which are easily divided and freed, to very extensive ones, along a long length of the colon. The surgery having been completed, the abdomen is decompressed and then gas refilled to see if there is bleeding from the operated area. If this is detected, hemostatic sponges are inserted into the wound which provide the remedy by arresting the ooze.

At the conclusion of the operation, CO_2 is expelled completely from the abdomen and the lateral abdominal incisions sutured. The umbilical puncture usually does not require suturing unless the umbilicus is very shallow. (A video recording of the entire operation accompanies this book and may be viewed).

The patient recovers in 4 to 6 hours and is discharged from the day surgical ward.

He usually recovers well and returns to work in 2 days.

Sexual intercourse resumes in 1 to 2 weeks and he can play sport in 2 to 3 weeks.

The first response to the varicocelectomy is assessed by semen analysis 4 weeks later. During this period of time, the patient is given mesterolone, zinc and vitamin E. In the more severe cases of sperm defects, hormonal injections of FSH 150 iu, twice weekly alternating with hCG 5000 iu weekly are given for 3 months or longer, until improvement occurs, as monitored by semen analyses.

RESULTS OF THE CLINICAL STUDY

Among the 700 patients treated, the duration of the surgery varied between 1 to 2 hours and the patients returned home within 4 to 6 hours after the surgery. They were back at work within 2 to 3 days and felt well.

Testicular biopsies performed showed that the extent of damage of the seminiferous tubular elements by the varicoceles varied from 1 to 30 percent damage or greater. The damage was permanent.

The surgery was very well accepted by the patients. Many reported an increase in testicular size, improved sexual performance, increased libido, and erection was sustained for longer periods. They felt their ejaculation was strong, and some even had wet dreams. Some of the patient who experienced backache were relieved of their symptoms.

The semen profiles of the men preoperatively showed single defects in 53 percent, double defects in 28 percent, and triple defects in 19 percent before surgery. After surgery the semen parameters in terms of sperm count, grade of motility, and normal morphology improved among 80 percent.

An overall pregnancy rate of 43 percent occurred with their wives. The time it took the couples to conceive after surgery varied between 2 to 7 months.

CONCLUSION

The study demonstrates the feasibility of treating the varicocele using the videolaparoscopic approach. However, the technique requires familiarity and skill which need to be acquired over time. The distinct advantages of the approach are much recommended. It is a day surgery procedure, resulting in rapid recovery, saving on cost, and is well accepted by the patients. An important feature of the surgery is the degree of magnification obtained through the videolaparoscope, enabling a complete and thorough bilateral high ligation of the testicular veins, without risk of injury to the testicular artery. There is little likehood of recurrence of the condition, and no morbidity or mortality was encountered in the study.

The resultant improvement in the semen profile and the achievement of pregnancies favor its role for the treatment of the varicocele causing male factor infertility.

REFERENCES

1. Howards SS. Varicocele. Infertil Reprod Med Clin North Am 1992;3:429-41.
2. World Health Organisation. The influence of varicocele on parameters of fertility in a large group of men presenting to infertility clinics. Fertil Steril 1992;57:1289-93.
3. Ando S, Giachetto C, Beraldi E, et al. The influence of age on Leydig cell function in patients with varicocele. Int J Androl 1984;7:104-18.
4. Nagler HM, Zippe CD. Varicocele: Current concepts and treatment. In: Lipshultz LI, Howards SS (Eds): Infertility in the male. St. Louis: Mosby Year Book; 1991:313-36.
5. Dubin L, Amelar RD. Varicocele size and results of varicocelectomy in selected subfertile men with varicocele. Fertil Steril 1970;21(8):606-9.
6. Comhaire FH, Gerris J. Varicocele In: Comhaire FH (Ed): Male Infertility, London: Chapman and Hall Medical; 1996;231-49.
7. Hagood PG, Parra RO. Laparoscopic varicocelectomy. Urologic Laparoscopy, Philadelphia: WB Saunders Company; 1994:119-26.
8. Donovan JF Jr, Winfield HN. Laparoscopic varix ligation. Laparoscpic Urologic Surgery, New York, Raven Press; 1994;137-49.
9. Chen C, Chua BL. Laparoscopic varicocelectomy and male infertility. XXXIII World Congress of the International College of Surgeons. 2002, Taipei, Taiwan, Monduzzi Editore; 2002;277-80.

7 Safety Aspects of Endoscopy

Madhuri Patil

INTRODUCTION

As the indications for endoscopic surgery become wider safety protocols become more important in the prevention of complications. This is particularly important since most complications tend to occur in the hands of inexperienced surgeons.

SAFETY ASPECTS OF LAPAROSCOPY

Basic and advanced laparoscopic surgery is safe but not risk free. Complications tend to occur during the procedure or in the postoperative period, they may be either minor or major which are life-threatening. Safety at laparoscopy is a really underestimated problem. Complications of laparoscopy are often not reported, and we have a false impression of the safety of laparoscopy but if we use good surgical techniques and some new technology that's available to us, we can really serve our patients better and make the whole procedure safer for them. Laparoscopy is certainly advantageous as a way of operating, and we have to be sure that by giving the patients particular advantages, we're not causing them more complications. The vast majority of complications with laparoscopy are on entry, and most of the malpractice cases are concerning bowel and major vascular injuries, and about 80 percent of these happen on entry techniques. Another particular area of concern is the use of electrosurgery, which most laparoscopists utilize to coagulate, cut, and dissect. The third thing is one that is really a little more subtle and is the gentle treating of tissue. The other insult of laparoscopic surgery is the distension of the abdominal wall with carbon dioxide, which is moderately harsh on the tissue but if we can warm that gas as it comes in and humidify it, it's being clearly shown that this is advantageous.

Proper preoperative preparation and assessment and application of basic principles of good surgical techniques will help in preventing these complications. Adequate training including understanding the principles of electrosurgery and laser, knowledge of instruments available, and experience in recognizing the normal as well as abnormal is essential.

PREOPERATIVE WORK UP

Preoperative work up minimizes the intra and post-operative complications. The cardiac system is significantly affected by laparoscopy with the mechanical effect of pneumoperitoneum and the hemodynamic effect of absorbed CO_2 and the volume shift caused by patient positioning. Therefore it makes evaluation of cardiac and respiratory systems mandatory for a safe surgery.

Preoperative Checklist

- History and physical examination
- Evaluation of other medical problems

- Evaluation of cardiac and respiratory systems
- Normalization of fluids and electrolytes
- Antibiotics
- Deep vein thrombosis prophylaxis
- Complete evaluation of genitourinary tract
- Appropriate laboratory and radiologic studies
- Informed consent for laparotomy if necessity arises.

SELECTION OF PATIENT FOR LAPAROSCOPIC PROCEDURE

Proper selection is very important to avoid major complications on the table. Selection of patient for laparoscopy should be considered depending on the individual patient risk, disease process and expertise of the surgeon dealing with them. There are certain risk factors, which make the patient absolutely, or relatively contraindicated for laparoscopy, these should be identified and laparoscopy avoided in such patients.

CONTRAINDICATIONS TO LAPAROSCOPY

Absolute

- Hypovolemic shock
- Massive bleeding
- Hemodynamic instability
- Severe cardiac disease.

Relative

- Peritonitis
- Abdominal wall hernia
- Uncorrected coagulopathies
- Cirrhosis of liver
- Portal hypertension
- Multiple previous surgical procedures.

Laparoscopic surgery has provided the surgeon a technique, which will reduce the hospital stay, decrease postoperative pain and hasten recovery time for several diagnostic and therapeutic procedures. To have a safe laparoscopy the surgeon must be aware of the complications of laparoscopy, and at which step they can occur, so that he is careful at every stage of the procedure.

COMPLICATIONS OF LAPAROSCOPY

1. Complications of anesthesia.
2. Complications of pneumoperitoneum.
   - Pneumothorax, pneumomediastinum
   - Gas embolism – air or CO_2
   - Hypercarbia with acidosis
   - Effects of distention medium
   - Extraperitoneal gas insufflation.
3. Patient positioning.
4. Trocar or Veress needle related injuries - at entry into the peritoneal cavity.
   - Bowel injuries
   - Vascular injuries—vessels in abdominal wall, omental or mesenteric vessels, great vessels, bleeding from surgical site during dissection
   - Incisional site hernia
   - Bladder injury.
5. Injuries from energy sources - skin burns, bowel burns.
6. Injuries from operative instruments – injuries to ureter and bladder, bowel.
7. Postoperative wound infections or pelvic inflammatory disease.

PREVENTION OF ANESTHESIA COMPLICATIONS

The complication rate of anesthesia for laparoscopic surgery is approximately 0.05 percent. The risk of anesthetic complication is compounded by the steep Trendelenburg's position and the influence of pneumoperitoneum on cardiac function. An endotracheal tube and positive pressure respiration are essential for all laparoscopies. This helps in preventing regurgitation and inhalation of gastric contents and allows elimination of CO_2 from the circulation. These patients should be monitored continuously by an ECG record, NIBP and pulse oximetry. Potential complications are hypoventilation, esophageal intubation, gastroesophageal reflux, brochospasm, hypotension, narcotic overdose, cardiac arrhythmias and cardiac arrest. Laparoscopy when performed with CO_2 insufflation induces changes in several parameters of cardiopulmonary function; such has reduced pO_2, O_2 saturation, tidal volume and minute ventilation and increased respiratory rate.

SAFETY AT CREATING PNEUMOPERITONEUM

Creating a pneumoperitoneum with CO_2 and placing the patient into a head-down position for prolonged periods of time result in profound hemodynamic and respiratory changes during laparoscopy. The effects of pneumoperitoneum and postural changes depend largely on how much abdominal pressure increases. Pressure more than 12-15 mmHg may result in higher blood pressure initially followed by fall in cardiac output as the vena cava gets compressed at higher intra-abdominal pressure, which impairs the venous return. Inadequate muscle relaxation may further contribute to rise in abdominal pressure.

Both pneumoperitoneum and Trendelenburg's position produce cephalad pressure on the diaphragm resulting in its elevation and excursions being restricted leading to impaired volumetric expansion of lungs and overall lung collapse. Lung compliance is further compromised by increase in pulmonary blood volume that results from redistribution of blood from the abdomen to the thorax as abdominal pressure rises and the patient is tilted head down. Use of higher ventilation pressure overcomes this decrease in lung compliance.

The use of intraperitoneal CO_2 is also associated with increase in pCO_2 and decrease in pH. This rise in pCO_2 causes respiratory acidosis and catecholamine release. Mean blood pressure increases, with positive inotropic effect on the heart, with increase in stroke volume, heart rate and cardiac output. There is also a propensity to cardiac arrhythmias, which is compounded by halothane because it sensitizes the myocardium to catecholamine-induced ventricular ectopy.

Moreover constant flow of unheated CO_2 and irrigation of peritoneal cavity with clod fluids lower the body temperature. This hypothermia may contribute to a decrease in cardiac output by increasing systemic vascular resistance. It predisposes patients to cardiac arrhythmias and also increases myocardial oxygen demand by causing shivering. One could use CO_2 at 37°C by using a thermo-pneumo insufflators and also humidify gas at entry.

The key to minimizing these effects of pneumoperitoneum is to keep the increase in pCO_2 and intra-abdominal pressure to minimum. Good muscle relaxation, avoidance of lithotomy, and tilting of the patient excessively will help in decreasing the incidence of complications.

The other common problem is subcutaneous emphysema as a result of preperitoneal placement of an insufflation needle or leakage of CO_2 around the cannula sites due to excessive intraperitoneal pressure. When mild it is limited to the abdominal wall, but when extensive it involves the extremities, the neck and the mediastinum.

Gas may be introduced into the mesenteric or retroperitoneal spaces, resulting in pneumomediastinum, pneumopericardium or pneumothorax.

Proper positioning of an insufflation needle reduces the risk of subcutaneous emphysema. No one test absolutely predicts intraperitoneal placement. A variety of test that can be used are aspiration, demonstration of preinstillation negative pressure by placing drop of water on the pen end of insufflation needle followed by elevation of anterior abdominal wall, and maintenance of low insufflation pressure. Only after the peritoneal cavity has been adequately insufflated, should the trocar be introduced. Subcutaneous emphysema despite intraperitoneal placement of trocars can be avoided by low intraperitoneal pressure below 10-12 mm Hg.

Most CO_2 micro-emboli are absorbed, usually by the splanchnic vascular system, quickly and without any complication. However, severe cardiorespiratory compromise may result if large amount of CO_2 gains access to the central venous circulation by inadvertent intravascular placement of insufflation needle and unrecognized intravascular insufflation of gas, which may result in death. There is sudden unexplained hypotension, cardiac arrhythmia, cyanosis and development of heart murmur. Other clinical sequelae include increased tidal CO_2, due to pulmonary edema and pulmonary hypertension, resulting in right-sided heart failure. Routine use of aspiration test, and use of intra-abdominal pressure of less 15 mm Hg should prevent this life-threatening complication.

PATIENT POSITIONING

Patient positioning on operation table is critical to the success of laparoscopic procedures, but is not without potential problems. The lithotomy position may cause femoral or peroneal neuropathy or contribute to lower extremity ischemia or deep vein thrombosis. The Trendelenburg's position may reduce pulmonary reserve, increase airway pressure and cause gastroesophageal reflux. Abduction of arm may produce a brachial plexus injury.

Therefore it is critical to see that the patient is given a proper position taking care that there is no prolonged compression to any part.

It is also very vital to check that no part of the patient is in contact with the metallic parts of the table when electrical energy is being used.

SAFETY INVOLVING TROCAR OR VERESS NEEDLE RELATED INJURIES - AT ENTRY INTO THE PERITONEAL CAVITY

Maximum injuries occur at entry into the peritoneal cavity either by Veress needle or trocar. There is risk of bowel injuries, vascular injuries – vessels in abdominal wall, omental or mesenteric vessels, great vessels, bladder injury. At times due to trocar site facial defects there may be incisional site hernia.

Bowel Injury

Bowel trauma is probably the most serious complication in gynecologic laparoscopic surgery, when the incidence is combined with the likelihood of severe or even fatal consequences. Injury to the bowel frequently goes unnoticed during the procedure, leading to a delayed and insidious presentation with the infectious sequelae of perforation. The true incidence of injury to the bowel is difficult to calculate and depends upon factors such as the expertise of the operators whose practice is being assessed and the complexity of the procedures attempted. Factors that ultimately lead to bowel injury can be identified at all stages in the operative process, including.

- Selection of the patient and the procedure.
- Preoperative preparation and anesthesia.
- Gaining entry to the abdomen.
- The operative procedure itself.
- Leaving the abdomen.

Inadequate postoperative surveillance and inappropriate subsequent management of bowel trauma contribute enormously to the impact of the complications encountered. A vital prerequisite for safe surgery is the selection of an appropriate procedure for the patient's condition and state of health. Situations such as obesity, scarring from previous surgery, sepsis in the abdominal wall or peritoneal cavity, and ileus do not necessarily constitute absolute contraindications to laparoscopy, but are likely to involve an increased risk of complications. If a problem that cannot be corrected is encountered, consideration should be given to abandoning the procedure, as operating with a poor view invites a high risk of doing harm. Specific safety aspects to prevent bowel injury are:

- During insertion of a Veress needle, be sure that the valve is open. This permits room air to enter the abdominal cavity immediately on entry into the peritoneum, thereby allowing the bowel and its mesentery to fall away from the needle tip.
- The greatest dispute centers around whether to insufflate the peritoneal cavity before insertion of the primary trocar. One school of thought is to insufflate the peritoneal cavity before insertion of the primary trocar (Figure 7.1), to reduce the incidence of injury to bowel. For a trocar of given sharpness, the greater the tension of the abdominal wall, the less it will be indented by the tip before entry is gained (Figure 7.2). The alternative approach is to insert the primary trocar

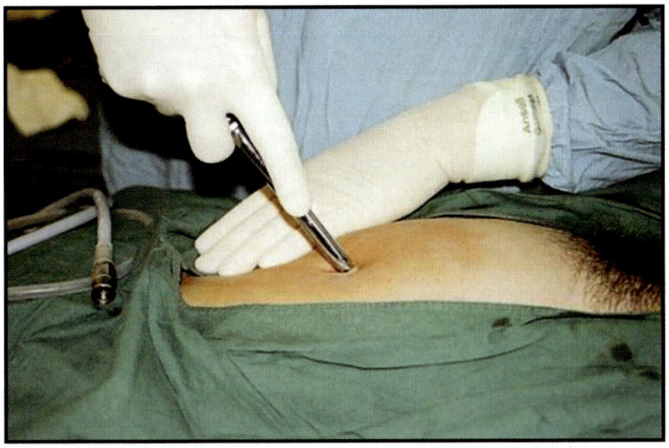

Figure 7.1. Primary trocar insertion after insufflations of abdominal cavity

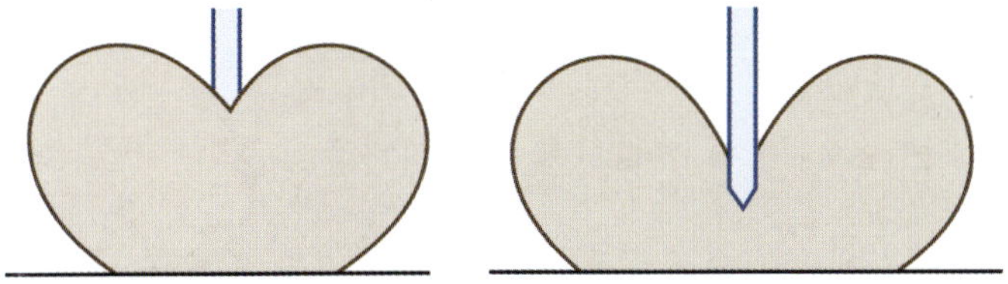

Figures 7.2A and B. With a trocar of given sharpness a firmly distended abdominal wall. A: will be less indented before it gives way than a less well distended one B: reducing the chance of injury to viscera with the trocar tip

directly without previous insufflation (Figure 7.3). This may be done after merely incising the skin and elevating the abdominal wall.[1] This technique is not a guarantee of avoiding bowel injury.[2] There is one randomized trial in the literature comparing direct insertion of the primary trocar with insertion after Veress needle insufflation.[3] No major complications occurred, but minor complications of omental trauma and emphysema were more common in the insufflation group with prior Veress needle insertion.

- Special care is needed if it is suspected that adhesions are present beneath the umbilicus (Figure 7.4), which might lead to injury even with the 'open' technique of Hasson. Insufflation with the Veress needle and insertion of a 5 mm trocar and endoscope at an alternative site through which a hysteroscope lens is inserted to allow direct inspection of the underside of the abdominal wall. The main trocar can then be inserted under direct vision after division of adhesions if necessary.[2]

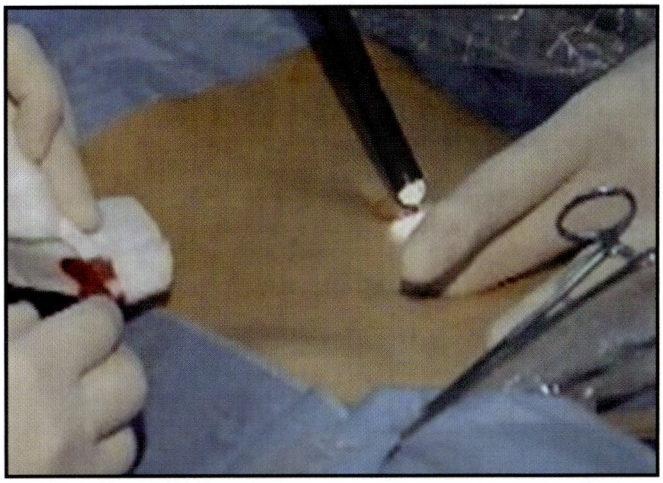

Figure 7.3. Primary trocar insertion without insufflations of abdominal cavity

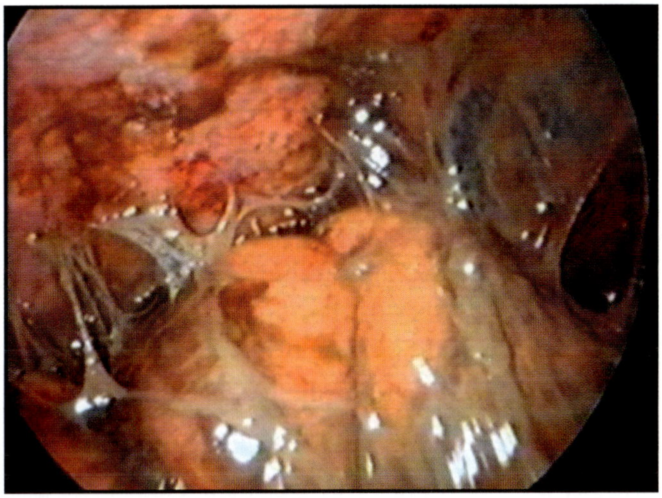

Figure 7.4. Adhesions beneath the umbilicus

- Today dispute also arises about the merits of disposable primary trocars with and without safety shields (Figure 7.5). The question is, are these trocars with safety shields safer than reusable trocars? It has been shown that the force needed to insert a new sharp disposable trocar is half that needed to insert a reusable trocar.[4] Complications are also more

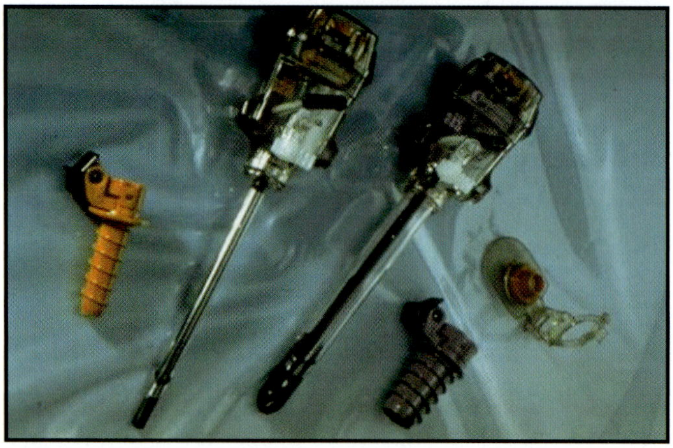

Figure 7.5. Trocars with safety shields

common if dull reusable trocars are used requiring greater force and multiple attempts at insertion.[5] But Soderstromin 1993 has published that trocars with a so-called safety shield are no guarantee of avoiding bowel trauma, and may even lead to a false sense of security.

- Another technique to avoid bowel injury is to perform percutaneous ultrasonography to identify adhesions of bowel to the abdominal wall based on the demonstration that the position of adherent viscera will not alter during deep inspiration.[6]
- Having gained entry to the abdomen, it should be possible to insert all subsequent ports under direct vision (Figures 7.6A to C).
- Adhesions tethering a portion of bowel to the underside of the abdominal wall can be readily identified, and an appropriate site free of adhesions can be selected for ancillary ports. Ensuring an adequate pressure of pneumoperitoneum should help avoid the bowel residing beneath the common sites for secondary ports. In modern practice visceral trauma sustained during secondary port placement is avoidable and consequently difficult to defend.
- It is prudent to remove the umbilical trocar with the tip of the laparoscope slightly protruding to observe one's exit and hopefully detect any unnoticed through and through bowel injury (Figure 7.7) and to prevent bowel herniation into the umbilical site.

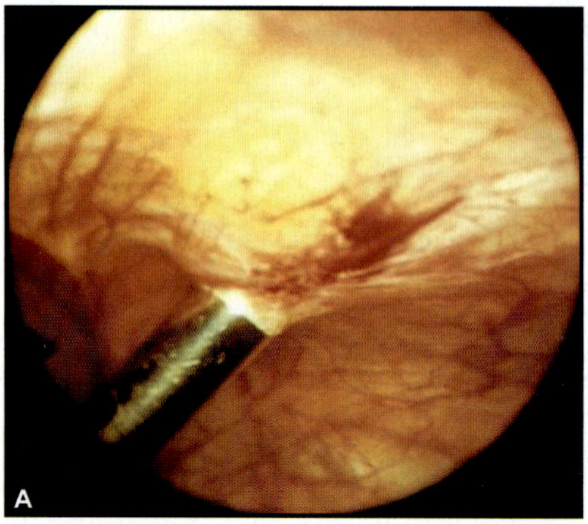

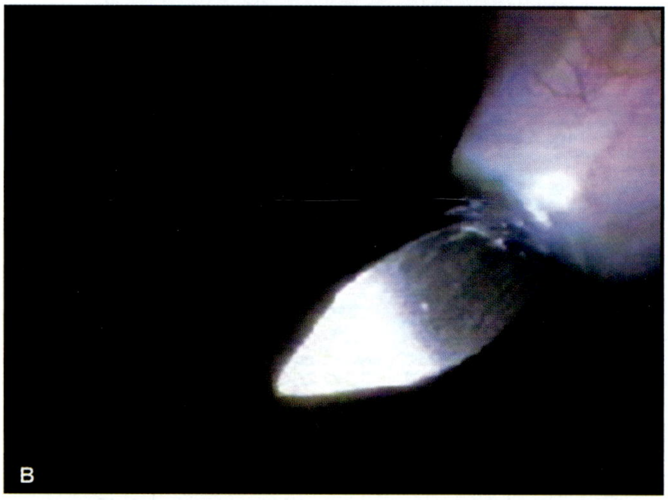

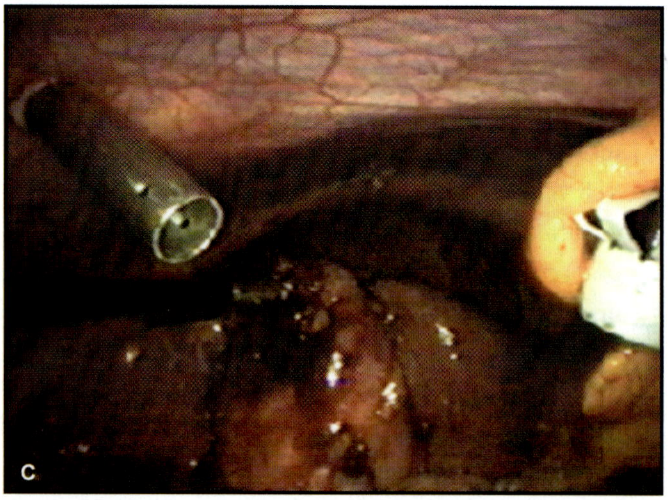

Figures 7.6A to C. A and B: Insertion of tocar and cannula under vision, C: Insertion of instruments under vision

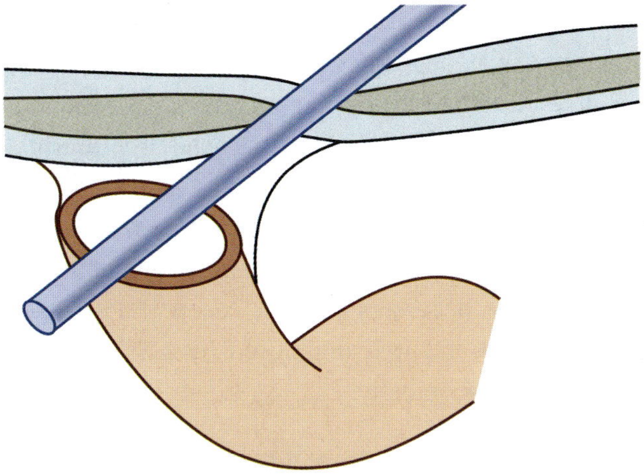

Figure 7.7. A through and through injury to a loop of bowel may be detected only by removing the laparoscope under direct vision to catch a glimpse of the bowel lumen

- The major compounding factor in many cases of bowel trauma at laparoscopy is the failure to appreciate the injury during the procedure. Bowel trauma with the Veress needle or primary trocar often goes unnoticed at the time and during the rest of the procedure. Only depressing site of the bowel lumen will immediately identify such a problem. Hints that injury may have occurred include fecal contamination on the tip of an instrument or in the abdomen, an intestinal odor at any time, and gradual distension of the bowel due to gas entering through the perforation. In only 60 percent of cases is the diagnosis made at the time of surgery, with the remaining 40 percent presenting over the next few days or even weeks, in varying states of ill health. It is unfortunate that the first signs that all is not well and that bowel trauma may have occurred may not arise for days or even weeks after the original surgery. The trend towards ever-earlier discharge of all surgical patients, most notably those having had major procedures through small incisions, increases the potential for misdiagnosis and delayed repair. Patients should get progressively better after laparoscopic surgery and if a patient describes worsening or even just persistent abdominal pain, bowel trauma must be considered early and actively excluded. It is far better to explore a patient suspected of having a bowel injury and have an occasional negative finding, than to delay the diagnosis through procrastination.

Although it is reasonable to manage a case of bowel trauma with the Veress needle conservatively provided the defect is small and there is no contamination, larger punctures or lacerations caused by a trocar or instrument require primary closure or resection. Some experienced operators are prepared to repair damage to the large bowel laparoscopically,[7] but most would advocate laparotomy.

SPECIFIC PROCEDURES AND BOWEL INJURY

Three operative procedures warrant special mention with respect to bowel trauma, namely:

- Adhesiolysis.
- Treatment for severe endometriosis.
- Posterior colpotomy.

The laparoscopic management of severe intestinal adhesions should only be practiced within the confines of units with advanced experience and expertise. Even with great experience complications will be relatively frequent in such cases.

Advanced endometriosis with complete obliteration of the cul-de-sac is characterized by the morbid adherence of the small and large bowel, and the absence of identifiable tissue planes. It is not difficult to cause partial or full thickness damage to the bowel wall without being aware of one's proximity to the bowel lumen. If an injury to the sigmoid colon or upper rectum is suspected, the integrity of the bowel wall should be tested. This can be achieved quite simply by placing a Foley catheter with a 30 ml balloon in the lower rectum and infusing an antiseptic solution such as povidone-iodine above the balloon, while observing the bowel closely from above. Small tears and partial thickness damage are probably amenable to laparoscopic suture repair, but a bowel surgeon at laparotomy may better deal with larger holes and cases of fecal contamination.

Tissue retrieval is often a tiresome part of a major laparoscopic operation. The desire to avoid extending one of the abdominal incisions has made posterior colpotomy a frequently used alternative. This is often performed using cutting monopolar diathermy with a wet swab in the posterior vaginal fornix. The danger comes when the pouch of Douglas is not deep in the antero-posterior diameter, with the anterior rectum in a more anterior position than suspected. Failure to direct the incision towards the back of the cervix increases the chance of damaging the rectum.

Prevention of Injury to Vessels in Abdominal Wall

Bleeding from vessels at the incision site, rarely gives rise to concern and usually stops with firm pressure. Superficial bruising at the site of trocar insertion is common but resolves in few days. Bleeding from injury to deep inferior epigastric vessel may occur during insertion of secondary trocars. Injury may be avoided by Transillumination of the abdominal wall before insertion of the trocars. In an obese patient it may be impossible to visualize the vessel. In such instance the vessels may be avoided by inserting the trocars in the lower quadrant lateral to the rectus sheath and above the line joining the anterior superior iliac spines, taking care to angle them medially to avoid the external iliac vessels. Injury to inferior epigastric is recognized by blood dripping or spurting into the abdomen from the site of secondary trocar. At times a large abdominal wall hematoma may develop. At times simply rotating the trocar sleeve by 360° or levering it against the abdominal wall will tamponade the bleeding and if this is successful pressure maintained for 5 minutes. The other strategy is to insert a Foley's catheter through the trocar, and then inflate the balloon and apply traction after removing the trocar by pulling up into the insertion site to tamponade the bleeding. If this fails large retention suture is taken through the entire abdominal wall under direct vision.

Prevention of Injury to Omental or Mesenteric Vessels

Insertion of primary trocar and cannula may injure omental or mesenteric vessels. Injury from insertion of secondary instruments can occur only if they are not kept under constant visual control. The bleeding vessels can be grasped and ligated or coagulated with bipolar forceps. If injury is caused by Veress needle to a mesenteric vessel, it may go unnoticed as the telescope is usually directed into the pelvis or the bleeding is hidden behind loops of bowel. These patients usually present 24 to 48 hours later with abdominal pain, pallor and tachycardia. Laparotomy is necessary in these cases. If a hematoma has developed and it is diagnosed by USG, it can be drained laparoscopically.

Prevention of Injury to Great Vessels

Laceration of a major abdominal blood vessel is one of the most devastating and immediately life-threatening complications of diagnostic and operative laparoscopy. Perforations of the aorta, vena cava, common, left and right iliac arteries and veins, have been reported. The true incidence of great vessel injury is unknown since the vast majority of these cases go unreported. Patients at highest risk for vascular injury on initial trocar insertion have been young, thin, nulliparous women with well-developed abdominal musculature. In these women not only does the aorta lie less than one inch (2.5 cm) below the skin at the umbilicus, but the fascia and abdominal wall are tense and inelastic creating a tough barrier to insertion of instruments.[8,9] Obesity may play a role as well in that identification of anatomic landmarks may be compromised and the surgeon, in an effort to avoid preperitoneal placement of the insufflating needle or trocar, may overzealously thrust the instrument in a perpendicular fashion and impale the retroperitoneal vessels against the sacral promontory. Elderly and chronically ill patients with poor tissue turgor or patients with multiple previous abdominal operations represent other groups with risk factors for vessel injury. Both blunt trocars and disposable sharp trocars have been implicated as predisposing to major vessel trauma.[10,11] Operator inexperience also contributes to higher incidence of great vessel injuries.[8] Technical surgical errors may be associated with catastrophic injury in the retroperitoneum including:

- Failure to adequately stabilize the abdominal wall.
- Forceful thrusting motion for insertion.
- Perpendicular or lateral insertion of the needle or trocar.
- Failure to note anatomic landmarks.
- Abnormal or inappropriate patient positioning.

Placing patients in the Trendelenburg's position before insertion of the insufflating needle or trocar increases the risk of retroperitoneal injury by rotating the sacral promontory into a position closer to the umbilicus.[12] The angle of insertion must be adjusted to avoid the great vessels. It is wise to test the Veress and trocar to assure its proper function. During insertion of a Veress needle, be sure that the valve is open, it allows immediate recognition of possible intravascular placement and prevent gas insufflation into the circulation. Manual elevation of the abdominal wall may facilitate needle or trocar placement by stabilizing the tissues and increasing the distance to the retroperitoneum.[13] With the abdominal wall manually stabilized or elevated the Veress needle or trocar should be firmly, but gently guided at 45° towards the hollow of the sacrum or towards the fundus of the elevated uterus if the anatomy has been difficult to palpate. With any trocar insertion, it is best to control the depth of penetration of the trocar tip with stabilizing guidance from the surgeon's nondominant hand. Marketing of disposable trocars with 'safety shields' has created a false sense of security among surgeons. The 'safety shield' is designed to lock in place covering the sharp trocar once the initial resistance has been decreased. Damage to major vessels may also occur during the operative procedure after trocars have been safely placed. Dissection of the retroperitoneum for lymph node sampling, excision of endometriosis and extensive adhesiolysis place the pelvic sidewall vessels and the great vessels at risk. Sharp dissection, electrosurgery and lasers have all created unintended openings in major vessels. Extreme caution must be exercised when operating near the pelvic sidewall or in the vicinity of the great vessels.

Significant damage to retroperitoneal vessels may not be immediately apparent to the surgical team due to:

- Increased intra-abdominal pressure (pneumoperitoneum).
- Decreased venous pressure due to the Trendelenburg's position.
- Retroperitoneal dissection and tamponade.

Major vessel injury should be suspected whenever blood returns from the open insufflating needle. In addition, inspection of the abdomen directly underneath the area of trocar insertion immediately upon placement of the laparoscope may demonstrate a small amount of bleeding. At times a hematoma of upto 4 liters may develop without intraperitoneal spillage as posterior abdominal wall peritoneum is loosely attached to the anterior surface of aorta and inferior vena cava. Sudden deterioration in vital signs (decrease in end-tidal carbon dioxide, decreased blood pressure and increased heart rate) in a previously stable patient after needle or trocar insertion should be considered to be due to a vascular accident until proven otherwise. Immediate resuscitation and laparotomy must be carried out and a vascular surgeon called. Vessels should be sutured with silk or vicryl after placing soft clamps above and below the injury.

Prevention of Bladder Injury with Veress and Trocar

Laparoscopic injuries to bladder result from Veress needle or lower abdominal trocar insertions. The risk of bladder perforations increases with previous abdominal surgery, previous bladder surgery congenital anomalies or a full bladder. Routine bladder catheterization before surgery or continuous bladder decompression in selected patients with residual urine or previous surgery may prevent bladder injuries. One has also to master the art of correct needle and trocar placement.

Prevention of Incisional Hernia

This is a rare complication caused by trocar site fascial defect.[14] Defects that are 10 mm or larger or use of cannula anchoring devices that increase the diameter of incision by as much as 3 mm carry a higher risk. Stretching of the incision when removing large surgical specimens may also increase the incidence. Other implicated factors include pre-existing umbilical hernias, poor abdominal relaxation on removing the ports, and excessive coughing during reversal of anesthesia. The bowel or omentum usually passes through the unopposed or inadequately repaired incision. At times omentum or bowel may be trapped in the incision and present 3-5 days postoperatively, as Richter's hernia, may result in perforation, peritonitis and death.

Methods to Prevent Incisional Hernia

- Whenever possible use small diameter cannulas for secondary ports.
- The Z-track insertion method offsets skin and fascial incision, which potentially reduces the incidence of incisional hernia.
- Trocar incision should be done at an angle so that the fascial wound is not at the center of the incision. This reduces the risk of weakening of the abdominal wall.
- Removal of all ancillary cannula under direct vision to ensure that bowel is not drawn into the incision.
- Insertion of obturator into the primary cannula before removal prevents suction of bowel or omentum into incision.
- Closure of fascia either with a simple or figure of eight suture reduces the incidence.

Injuries from Energy Sources—Electrosurgery or Laser

Many complications of laparoscopic surgery occur secondary to the use of electrical energy. One must be familiar with the properties of any energy source used. The effect depends on the power, and area and duration of contact. Therefore it is important to impart minimal amount of thermal injury with ideal waveform and power output. It has been demonstrated that tissue damage can be caused up to:

a. 5 cm beyond the point of contact using monopolar electrosurgery.[15]
b. 5 mm for bipolar electrosurgery.[16] Bipolar cautery has a less risk of distant burns, but risk of burning adjacent tissue by direct spread of heat remains.
c. 5 mm for endocoagulation.[17]

Thermal trauma can be classified into three categories.

- Unintended thermal injury through use of active electrode. Can be prevented by the surgeon having the direct control of electrode activation, and by removing all electrosurgical instruments from the peritoneal cavity when not in use. It is also important to have all operating instruments in good working condition with intact insulation.
- Diversion of current to another path, causing injury at a distant area from the main operating field. This can be prevented by properly earthed monitoring system and by properly applied or fault free return plate.
- Injury at the site of dispersive electrode.

Operator error accounts for more cases of bowel injury associated with the use of energy sources than equipment failure. In electrical injuries there is an absence of the neovascularization seen in cases of trauma. Also, because of the coagulation necrosis and cooptation of the surrounding vascular bed, in electrosurgical injury there is a paucity of white cell infiltration; the opposite is found in traumatic injuries to the bowel.

The extent of damage extends beyond the confines of the visible serosal injury and the extent of the damage is related to the energy form used. Successful surgery on the bowel is closely related to the vascularity of the affected segment. With monopolar electrosurgery, the current will preferentially flow down vascular channels, leading to devascularization to a wider extent than the visible serosal injury. This means that local or excisional repair should involve wide margins of safety. It has been proposed that a similar thermal injury might be caused by leaving the laparoscope inside the abdomen during prolonged periods of loss of pneumoperitoneum: tissue lying against the tip of the laparoscope could become heated even with the use of modern 'cold' light sources. To date, there are no confirmed cases of bowel damage due to this cause.

With regard to electrosurgery, there's a new device that's referred to as active electrode monitoring which adds dimension of safety to electrocautery by giving more insulation and overcoming some of the problems of capacitance of generation of electrical current.

With this we can almost exclude electrosurgical complications except those due to surgeon error, and we're not able to take the human error out of things but we can try to diminish the technical errors as much as possible.

LASER

In contrast to electrosurgery, the use of lasers during laparoscopy has a deserved reputation for a low incidence of visceral trauma.[18] CO_2 and Nd: YAG laser is commonly used to treat endometriosis or to lyse adhesions. It has been demonstrated that tissue damage that can be caused is up to 2.7 mm for the CO_2 laser.[19] A non-contact laser injury causing a blanched area to appear on the bowel wall will be characterized by vascular damage to all of the blanched area.

Using a backstop and not firing the laser inadvertently can prevent laser burns.

SAFETY AT USE OF OPERATIVE INSTRUMENTS – PREVENTION OF INJURIES TO BOWEL, URETER AND BLADDER

The commonest organ to be injured by scissors is bowel. This is liable to occur during adhesiolysis as a result of PID or endometriosis, when loops of bowel may be adherent to the uterus, tubes, ovaries, and cul-de-sac or each other. In such cases dissection is preferably done either by blunt /mechanical or hydrodissection, avoiding sharp dissection or use of laser or electrosurgery to avoid risk of thermal or laser injuries.

The bowel may also be traumatized by traction with forceps, which is usually evident immediately but may be missed with complications of fecal fistula or peritonitis.

All patients and more so if the patient is suspected to have adhesions involving the bowel require a thorough preoperative bowel preparation.

Apart from secondary trocar injuries, bladder may be injured during dissection off the vagina during laparoscopic hysterectomy and during vaginal closure of the cuff following laparoscopic bladder dissection. One could identify bladder lacerations by identifying the appearance of gas or blood in the Foley's catheter drainage bag.

Ureteric injuries are rare during diagnostic or minor laparoscopic surgery, but more common with advanced operations. Knowledge of the ureter's path through the pelvis and the vulnerable points are key to preventing injuries. The intrapelvic segment of the ureter is close to the broad ligament, ovaries and uterosacral ligaments, and injuries often occur in these areas. The surgeon should note the ureter's course through the peritoneum. Ureteral injury can occur:

- During sharp dissection of an ovary adherent to the pelvic sidewall.
- In uterosacral transection.
- During ligation, transection or coagulation of the uterine arteries.
- When removing endometriotic implants or fibrosis from the ureter.
- While trying to control bleeding vessels.

Unrecognized anomalies in the location of the ureter may predispose the patient to injury. To avoid such injuries, the tissue being destroyed or removed and the location of the ureter must be identified before irreversible action is taken. Meticulous and continuous attention to the location of the ureter will reduce complications.[20] Endometriosis and severe pelvic adhesions can thicken the peritoneum, obscuring the location of the ureter, especially near the uterosacral ligaments. If the ureter cannot be clearly identified through the peritoneum, it must be located by retroperitoneal dissection. Using hydrodissection, a horizontal incision is made in the

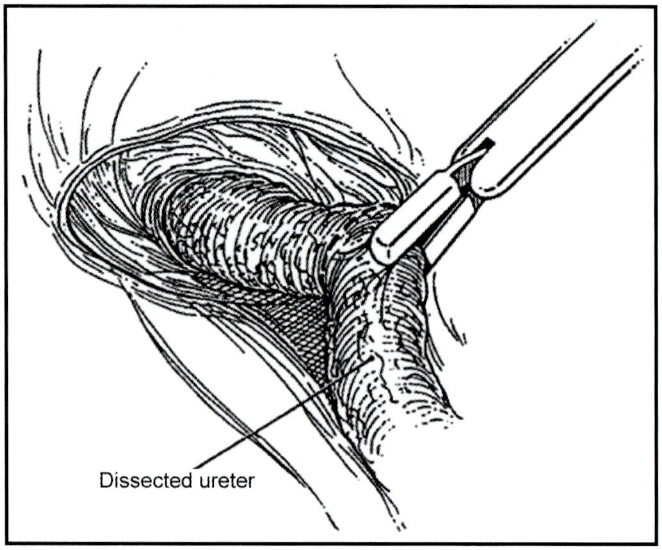

Figure 7.8. Ureterolysis is performed and the ureter involved with endometriosis and fibrosis is dissected and pulled medially

peritoneum midway between the ovary and uterosacral ligament. The lower edge of the peritoneum is grasped and pulled medially. Blunt dissection with the suction/ irrigator probe helps locate the ureter lateral to the peritoneum (Figure 7.8). If the peritoneum is involved with endometriosis and there is retroperitoneal fibrosis, the ureter can be attached to the peritoneum. The horizontal incision in the peritoneum is extended as necessary.[21] The ureter displaced laterally, provides a plane for safe ablation of endometriotic implants, lysis of adhesions or resection of the involved peritoneum.

Additionally, the fluid absorbs the laser energy, decreasing the risk of thermal damage to underlying tissue. This procedure is only applicable when the peritoneum is not densely adherent to the underlying ureter. During uterosacral transection, a backstop can be placed between the lateral aspect of the uterosacral ligament and ureter. Before using the bipolar forceps during adnexectomy, the infundibulopelvic ligament must be put under traction to identify the ureter and avoid thermal damage.

The routine use of preoperative intravenous pyelography is controversial and no prospective study confirms that this prevents ureteral injury. However, for selected patients, it may level ureteral obstruction or displacement and allow appropriate surgical planning. The routine use of ureteral catheters is not warranted, but we find a ureteral catheter useful in rare cases of severe endometriosis or adhesions with retroperitoneal fibrosis and displacement of the ureter.

Prevention of Bladder Injury

Bladder injury is rare and usually occurs in patients who have had laparotomies or whose bladder is not emptied before surgery. Under these conditions, sharp instruments such as trocars and uterine manipulators can perforate or lacerate the bladder. Electricity and lasers can cause thermal injury and blunt instruments can cause a laceration. Certain laparoscopic procedures increase the risk of bladder injury:

- The Veress needle can perforate a distended bladder.
- A misplaced Rubin's cannula can perforate the vagina and bladder with upward pressure.
- Accessory trocar insertion can injure a full bladder, or one with distorted anatomy by previous pelvic surgery, endometriosis or adhesions, or if insertion is less than 4 cm above the symphysis pubis.
- Coagulation or laser ablation of endometriotic implants or adhesiolysis in the anterior cul-de-sac can predispose the patient to bladder injury. Hydrodissection or a backstop used with the carbon dioxide laser decreases this possibility.
- During a laparoscopic hysterectomy (LH) or laparoscopic assisted vaginal hysterectomy[22] (LAVH) the bladder may be lacerated or torn, specifically if blunt dissection is used to free the bladder from the pubocervical fascia, particularly in women who have had a previous cesarean delivery, severe endometriosis[23] or lower segment myomas.
- Bladder injury can also occur while entering and dissecting the space of Retzius before laparoscopic bladder neck suspension.

To prevent injury, a Foley's catheter is placed to drain the bladder. The position of the bladder should be assessed during the initial examination with the laparoscope. If the boundaries of the bladder are not clear, particularly when pelvic anatomy is distorted, the bladder should be filled with 350 ml of fluid to delineate its position. Care should be used when performing LH or LAVH and the assistant should push the uterus cephalad during bladder dissection.

POSTOPERATIVE WOUND INFECTIONS OR PELVIC INFLAMMATORY DISEASE

Wound infections following laparoscopic procedures are rare. Wound abscess, cellulites and necrotizing fasciitis may occur, particularly when the patient is obese or subcutaneous tissue is exposed to infected material. Judicious use of antibiotics will prevent this complication. Thorough rinsing of instruments in normal saline after removing them either from formalin or gluteraldehyde solution avoids chemical suppurative lesions.

There is a small risk of producing or exacerbating PID by any procedure involving insufflation or surgery on tubes. The incidence is lower with laparoscopy as compared of conventional surgery.

Tumor Seedlings

Port and drain site metastasis have been reported following laparoscopic surgery. Use of warmed humidified air and less peritoneal damage, should have fewer incidence of port metastases and spread of the tumor. Care should be taken in removing malignant lesions through incisions during laparoscopy. Protective sheaths and adequate opening should allow removal of specimen without squeezing, which will minimize metastasis.

SUMMARY

The need for safety in laparoscopic surgery has gained more importance due to increase in operative as opposed to diagnostic procedures where a larger number of trocars are inserted for each surgical case. One must be aware of the potential contributing factors that exist at all parts of the surgical process. Constant vigilance and scrupulous adherence to recognized practices and techniques should serve to limit the danger to our patients. However, our colleagues, our patients, and we must be aware of the pitfalls as well as the benefits of this exciting surgical revolution.

SAFETY ASPECTS OF HYSTEROSCOPY

Operative hysteroscopy is a new and valuable technique in the treatment of non-malignant conditions of the uterine cavity. As with any other surgical technique, operative hysteroscopy requires an intensive training period. It is therefore advisable that a surgeon starting hysteroscopic surgery should have performed at least 250 diagnostic procedures before embarking on operative work. Use of sharp instruments, monopolar electric current or laser makes operative hysteroscopy a risky procedure.

All advanced hysteroscopic surgeries must be combined with either a laparoscopy or an ultrasound examination.[24-26] It is very important to rule out any contraindications that may make the procedure unsafe. The absolute contraindications are inexperienced endoscopist, pelvic infection and cervical malignancy. There is no area of gynecologic surgery that can result in such sudden and catastrophic disaster as a result of a lack of adequate supervised training. The relative Contraindications are cardiorespiratory disease, metabolic acidosis, pregnancy, uterine bleeding, and occult cervical malignancy.

To avoid significant complications, the physician should take a careful history and perform a thorough pelvic examination and ultrasound to rule out any contraindications. The hysteroscopic equipment should be disassembled, rinsed and flushed, and disinfected before each examination. Efficiency should be instituted at every step of surgery to prevent complications right from dilation of cervix to therapeutic procedure.

SAFETY AT ANESTHESIA

Hysteroscopy can be done either under local or general anesthesia. Provided the dosage of local anesthetic drug is within accepted limits and care is taken to avoid an intravascular injection, complications are rare, although toxic reactions can occur. General anesthesia should be administered with controlled positive pressure respiration and an endotracheal tube for all diagnostic and operative hysteroscopies and for combined laparoscopy and hysteroscopy.

PREOPERATIVE PREPARATION

All patients who undergo operative hysteroscopy should have bowel preparation. The least expensive is a combination of an oral laxative the morning and the evening of the day preceding the hysteroscopy and an enema approximately two hours before the procedure.

DILATION OF THE CERVIX

The use of rigid instruments may damage the cervical canal if appropriate care is not taken. The cervix can be lacerated by the tenaculum due to excessive traction during dilation.[27] Dilation itself can provoke bleeding. A certain amount of force is often necessary to dilate a cervical canal up to Hegar 9. The use of Hegar dilators increasing by half a size at a time or Pratt dilator is less traumatic. Pharmacological cervical dilatation like laminaria stents, and prostaglandins are useful in overcoming these problems.

HAZARDS OF DISTENSION MEDIA

CO_2 and Other Gases

For operative hysteroscopy where the time used for the procedure is longer than for a classical diagnostic hysteroscopy it is mandatory to have a reliable and calibrated hysteroflator. The flow should not exceed 80 ml min.[28] The insufflation pressure should not exceed 200 mg Hg. The use of cervical cups is contraindicated as it prevents the outflow of gas through the cervical canal.

The physical properties of CO_2 are such that mixing with the blood and the mucus of the endocervix and the endometrium creates bubbles. Bubbles impair vision, but invariably disappear when the physical reaction of mixing ends. However, this can take a long time and CO_2 is less appropriate for hysteroscopic surgery since liquid distension media are safer and provide good visibility for the surgeon. Air and other gases must never be used for uterine distension. Fatal air embolism has been recorded with both tubal persufflation and with hysteroscopy.[29]

Liquid Distension Media

Liquid distension media are absorbed and intravasated into the uterine vessels, especially if the latter are transected during operative hysteroscopy. Transtubal intra-abdominal spillage occurs to a lesser extent, though peritoneal absorption occurs over a long period of time and aspiration of the spilled fluid by concomitant laparoscopy may be helpful in preventing overload.

High-viscosity Fluids

Intravascular reabsorption of high-viscosity fluids like dextran has been linked to anaphylactic shock and non-cardiogenic pulmonary edema[30,31] and should be avoided. Dextran 70 has been associated with coagulation disorders. Disseminated intravascular coagulation has been reported after Hyskon hysteroscopy. The antithrombotic effect of dextran is thought to be secondary to decreased platelet adhesiveness to the endothelium. Dextran may also alter fibrin clot structure making it more susceptible to lyses. It also reduces the activity of fibrinogen, clotting factors V, VIII and IX, and the factor VIII-von Willebrand complex.

Low-viscosity Fluids

A variety of symptoms associated with the absorption of large volumes of distension media - bradycardia and hypertension followed by hypotension, nausea, vomiting, headache, visual disturbances, agitation, confusion and lethargy. These symptoms are the result of hypervolemia, dilutional hyponatremia and decreased osmolarity. If untreated the result may be seizures, coma, cardiovascular collapse and death. The inflow and outflow of liquid media must be carefully measured to avoid complications.[32] Therefore care should be taken even when glycine is used as a distention media.

MECHANICAL COMPLICATIONS

Perforation

Perforations do occur when using dilators to dilate the cervix or when inserting the hysteroscope. Usually the hemorrhage stops on its own but if hemostasis fails to occur laparoscopic endocoagulation, diathermy or sutures can stop it, but occasionally it is necessary to perform a laparotomy or even a hysterectomy. Visual control makes perforation unlikely. Simultaneous laparoscopy reduces the consequences of accidental perforation in selected patients. Moreover when observation is limited because of intrauterine disease, the endoscope should be advanced slowly and gently and always under direct vision.

Instrumental and Electrosurgical Injuries

Mechanical injury is circumscribed and mostly easy to detect with the laparoscope. If a perforation occurs during instrumentation (Figures 7.9A to D), the operation must

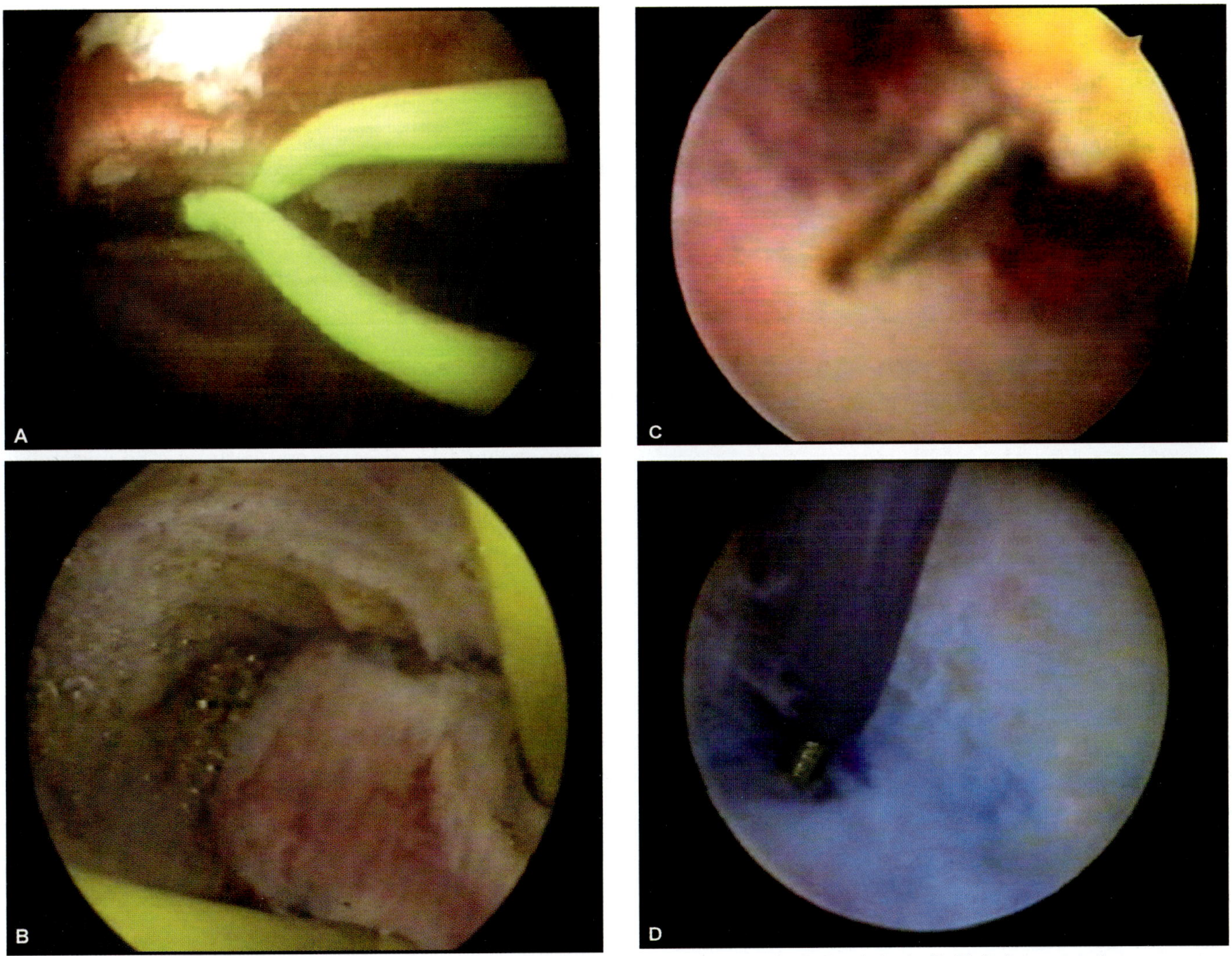

Figures 7.9A to D. A: Septal resection, B: Resection of submucous myoma, C: Adhesiolysis D: Tubal cannulation

be terminated immediately. On no account must a laser or electric current be activated if perforation is suspected. Most serious complications occur when instruments have been used without proper vision due to poor distension or to bleeding. The surgeon has to ascertain that there has been no major vessel injury and withdraws the hysteroscope only after removing the ancillary instruments.[33] A possible complication of perforation is fluid overload due to massive absorption of the distension medium at the time of the perforation. The rate of fluid absorption is increased 20-fold. Therefore a strict watch has to be kept on the cardiovascular and respiratory system, once perforation is diagnosed. Injuries to the bowel-mostly colon or rectum due to electric current are often not so obvious and require some expertise to be detected. If the current is activated during the perforation the results are more spectacular and require immediate intervention. If at the time of perforation the current is not been activated, injury will be a thermal injury and sometimes it will take several days before the bowel perforates and the patient will present with a septic peritonitis. For this reason if perforation is suspected the patient should be kept under close observation in hospital for several days.

The procedure is best performed with a passive resectoscope.[34] The automatic advancement of the loop can cause a perforation if the resectoscope is held too close to the uterine wall. The passive resectoscope automatically retracts the loop towards the end of the hysteroscope and requires an active movement from the fingers of the surgeon to move it outwards, thus reducing the danger of perforation. When using a resectoscope the active phase should always be towards the lens so that the surgeon is able to control the section at all times. As long as the loop, the ball or the knife is not completely visible the current should not be activated.

We are aware that electricity has an effect beyond the visual field of the surgeon. Coagulation and devitalization occur up to 6 mm into the tissues. This has serious implications in the region of the uterine cornua where the safety margin before reaching the serosa is only approximately 8 mm.[35]

Inside the cavity the zona compacta of the myometrium, situated directly under the endometrium, is approximately 6-8 mm thick, and beneath this lies the vascular bed. Perforation of this layer causes intensive bleeding. Secondary bleeding one week or more after surgery has been reported due to the deep devitalization of the tissues after overzealous coagulation.[36] In presence of adenomyosis resection has to be done carefully as crypts of endometrial tissue infiltrate the myometrium and facilitate conduction of both electricity and laser energy far deeper than would be expected in myometrium. The leads to delayed healing of the endometrial wound.

Laser procedures take much longer than electrosurgery; hence they increase the risk of fluid overload and should therefore only be used with continuous flow hysteroscopes or flexible hysteroscopes, which require less fluid. Flexible hysteroscopes, however, are more difficult for the beginner to use.[37] The power setting needed for intrauterine laser surgery is high, so damage can be extensive, moreover if fiber has perforated the uterus and the laser has been activated the bowel and major vessels may be damaged and therefore the laser should be used with caution in hysteroscopic surgery.

Care should be taken during insertion of probes into tubal ostia for tubal recanalization. If done improperly it can create false passage and perforate the uterotubal junction. It is also important that tubal recanalization for proximal tubal obstruction, must be carefully controlled visually, either by concomitant laparoscopy or fluoroscopy.[38,39] A hydrosalpinx can rupture during CO_2 insufflation and gaseous medium can pass into leaves of broad ligament.

POSTOPERATIVE COMPLICATIONS

Postoperative complications in the form of hemorrhage, infection, hematometra and pain, although rare may arise during the first few hours or days after hysteroscopy.

Hemorrhage if mild or moderate can be treated conservatively, while sever may require insertion of Foley's catheter for uterine tamponade. Rarely uterine or iliac artery ligation or hysterectomy may be required. Patients undergoing endometrial or myometrial resection should be stringently monitored.

Infection can be prevented in all patients by prophylactic antibiotics. Those at a risk of infection viz, sexually transmitted diseases, vaginal or cervical infection, and those with past history of PID should be started on antibiotics 48 hours prior.

Formation of hematometra can be prevented by insertion of IUCD following hysteroscopic surgery to prevent adhesions and avoiding resection of endometrium down till the cervix, which may result in cervical stenosis.

SUMMARY

Careful case selection, correct choice of media for distention and efficient safe surgery will reduce the incidence of complications of hysteroscopic surgery.

REFERENCES

1. Phipps JH. Avoidance of complications of laparoscopic hysterectomy. In Sutton CJG (Ed.) Baillière's Clinical Obstetrics and Gynaecology: Advanced Laparoscopic Surgery, London: Baillière Tindall 1995;9(4).
2. Soderstrom RM. Bowel injury litigation after laparoscopy. Journal of the American Association of Gynecologic Laparoscopists 1993;1:74-7.
3. Nezhat FR, Silfen SL, Evans D, et al. Comparison of direct insertion of disposable and standard reusable laparoscopic trocars and previous pneumoperitoneum with Veress needle. Obstetrics and Gynecology 1991;78:148-51.
4. Corson SL, Batzer FR, Gocial B, et al. Measurement of the force necessary for laparoscopic trocar entry. Journal of Reproductive Medicine 1989;34:282-4.
5. Baadsgaard SE, Bille S, Egeblad K. Major vascular injury during gynaecological laparoscopy. Report of a case and review of published cases. Acta Obstetricia et Gynecologica Scandinavica 1989;68:283-5.
6. Marin G, Bergamo S, Miola E, et al. Pre-laparoscopic echography used to detect abdominal adhesions. Endoscopy 1987;19:147-9.
7. Reich H, McGlynn F, Budin R. Laparoscopic repair of full thickness bowel injury. Journal of Laparoendoscopic Surgery 1991;1(2):119-22.
8. Hulka JF. Major vessel injury during laparoscopy. American Journal of Obstetrics and Gynecology 1980;138:138-590.
9. Kurzel FB, Edinger DD. Injury to the great vessels. A hazard of transabdominal endoscopy. Southern Medical Journal 1983;76:656-7.
10. McDonald PT, Rich NM, Collins CJ, et al. Vascular trauma secondary to diagnostic and therapeutic procedures:Laparoscopy. American Journal of Surgery 1979;136:651-5.
11. Shin CS. Vascular injury secondary to laparoscopy. New York State Journal of Medicine 82:935-6.
12. Lynn SC, Katz AR, Ross PJ. Aortic perforation sustained at laparoscopy. Journal of Reproductive Medicine 1982; 27(2):17-9.
13. Corson SL. Major vessel injury during laparoscopy. American Journal of Obstetrics and Gynecology 1980;138: 589.
14. Kadar N, Reich H, Liu CY, Manco GF, Gimpleson R. Incisional hernia following major laparoscopic gynecological procedures. American Journal of Obstetrics and Gynecology 1993;168:1493.
15. Wheeless CR. Thermal gastrointestinal injuries. In Phillips JM (Ed): Laparoscopy. Baltimore: Williams and Wilkins 1977;231-5.
16. Ryder RM, Hulka JF. Bladder and bowel injury after electrodesiccation with Kleppinger bipolar forceps: A clinicopathological study. Journal of Reproductive Medicine 1993;38:595-8.
17. Semm K, Freidrich ER (Eds). Operative Manual for Endoscopic Abdominal Surgery. Chicago: Year Book 1987.
18. Ewen SP, Sutton CJG. Complications of laser laparoscopy. Eleven years experience. Minimally Invasive Therapy 1995;4:27-9.
19. Martin DC. Tissue effects of lasers. Seminars in Reproductive Endocrinology 1991;9(2):127-37.
20. Chaffkin L, Luciano AA. Ureteral injuries. In Corfman RS, Diamond MP, DeCherney AH (Eds): Complications of Laparoscopy and Hysteroscopy. Boston, MA: Blackwell Scientific Publications, Inc. 1993;134.
21. Nezhat C, Nezhat F, Luciano AA, Siegler AM, Metzger DA, Nezhat CH (Eds): Operative Gynecologic Laparoscopy: Principles and Techniques. New York: McGraw-Hill 1995a.
22. Nezhat C, Nezhat F, Nezhat CH, Admon D, Nezhat A. Proposed classification of hysterectomies involving laparoscopy. Journal of the American Association of Gynecologic Laparoscopists 1995b;2:427-9.
23. Nezhat CH, Seidman DS, Nezhat F, Rottenberg H, Nezhat C. Laparoscopic management of intentional and unintentional cystotomy. Journal of Urology 1996a;156:1400-2.
24. Sugimoto O, Ushiroyama T, Fukuda Y. Diagnostic and therapeutic hysteroscopy for traumatic intrauterine adhesions. In Siegler AM, Lindemann HJ (Eds): Hysteroscopy, Principles and Practice. Philadelphia: JB Lippincott 1984;58-62.

25. Taylor PJ, Leader A, George RE. Combined laparoscopy and hysteroscopy in the investigation of infertility. In Siegler AM, Lindemann J (Eds): Hysteroscopy, Principles and Practice. Philadelphia: JB Lippincott 1984;207-10.
26. van Herendael BJ. Hysteroscopy in infertility. Pakistan Journal of Obstetrics and Gynaecology 1988;1:136-47.
27. Siegler AM. Risks and complications of hysteroscopy. In Van der Pas H, van Herendael B, Van Lith D, Keith L (Eds): Hysteroscopy. Lancaster: MTP Press 1983;75-80.
28. Porto R. Hysteroscopie- In Encyclopidia, Paris, Medici-Chirurgie 1974.
29. Baggish MS, Daniell JF. Death caused by air embolism associated with Nd:YAG laser surgery and artificial sapphire tips. American Journal of Obstetrics and Gynecology 1989;161:877-8.
30. Kaplan AI, Sabin S. Dextran 70- another cause of drug induced non-cardiogenic pulmonary edema, Chest 1975; 68:376.
31. Zbella EA, Moise J, Carson SA. Noncardiogenic pulmonary edema secondary to intrauterine instillation of 32 percent dextran 70, Fertility Sterility 1985;43:479.
32. Leake JF, Murphy AA, Zacur HA. Noncardiogenic pulmonary edema—a compliction of operative hysteroscopy, Fertility Sterility 1987;48:497.
33. Haning RV, et al. Preservation of fertility by transcervical resection of a benign mesodermal uterine tumor with a resectoscope and glycine distension medium. Fertility Sterility 1989;39:209.
34. DeCherney AH, Diamond MP, Lavy G, Polan ML. Endometrial ablation for intractable uterine bleeding: Hysteroscopic resection. Obstetrics and Gynecology 1987;70:668-70.
35. Neuwirth RS, Amin HK. Excision of submucous fibroids with hysteroscopic control. American Journal of Obstetrics and Gynecology 1976;126:95-7.
36. DeCherney A, Polan MH. Hysteroscopic management of intrauterine lesions and intractable uterine bleeding. Obstetrics and Gynecology 1983;61:392-7.
37. Baggish MS, Baltoyannis P. New techniques for laser ablation of the endometrium in high risk patients. American Journal of Obstetrics and Gynecology 1988;159:287-92.
38. DeCherney AH. Anything you can do I can do better or differently! Fertility Sterility 1987;48:374.
39. Rosh J, Thurmond AS, Ucjida BT, et al. Selective transcervical fallopian tube catheterization: Technique update, Radiology 1988;168:1.

8 Endoscopic Instrumentation

Manish Banker, Pravin Patel, Manish Shah

INTRODUCTION

Laparoscopy in this modern era is not only a diagnostic tool but also a means to perform complex surgical procedures. Various instruments have been designed to allow wide range of operations to be performed. Although it is not necessary to have the complete range of instruments to perform diagnostic or operative laparoscopy; it is necessary to have the correct instruments. Optical systems as well as hand instruments are so important in laparoscopy that visualization and tactile exploration of the operative field is always indirectly achieved through these. Technical details of all the instruments allow the surgeon to overcome a series of dysfunctions or malfunctions, which are very common in laparoscopic surgery.

Instruments are divided basically in to basic instruments, hand instruments and advanced instruments.

BASIC INSTRUMENTS

Insufflator

The first and foremost requirement of laparoscopy is the provision of safe pneumoperitoneum. This is achieved with the help of an insufflator. An insufflator helps in creating a pneumoperitoneum by injecting gas at a desired flow rate to maintain a pre-designated pressure. In surgical laparoscopy, compensation for considerable volume losses must be made in a relatively short period of time, e.g. due to frequent suction of irrigating solutions using high performance irrigation/suction units. Fully automatic high flow electronic insufflators have totally replaced mechanical pneumoflators (Figure 8.1). Technical characteristics include its capacity to insufflate up to 15-30 liters per minute and to maintain a constant intra-abdominal pressure without exceeding the safety limit of 12-16 mm Hg. Continuous control of the intra-abdominal pressure helps prevent complications related to an incorrectly positioned Veress needle. The insufflator has a display which gives continuous information to the surgeon on the following:

a. The patient's intra-abdominal pressure. This can be preselected to a maximum limit, generally 12 mm Hg.
b. Flow rate of CO_2. The maximum flow rate can be preset. This is as high as 20 liters/min in the new generation high flow insufflators.
c. Total amount of gas insufflated
d. The gas reserve.

Newer generation insufflators are also equipped with an integrated preheating element, which keeps the insufflated gas at body temperature, in order to prevent the patient from hypothermia (Figure 8.2). It also prevents continuous fogging of the optics and maintains a clear vision.

Telescopes

The development of the rod lens in 1953 by Professor Hopkins of Reading has improved the performance of

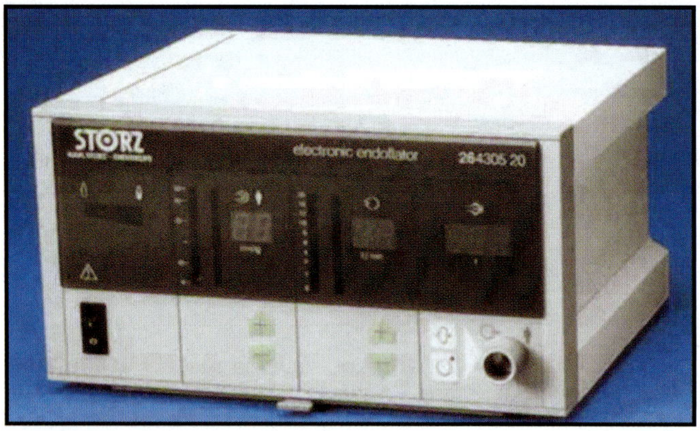

Figure 8.1. Electronic insufflator

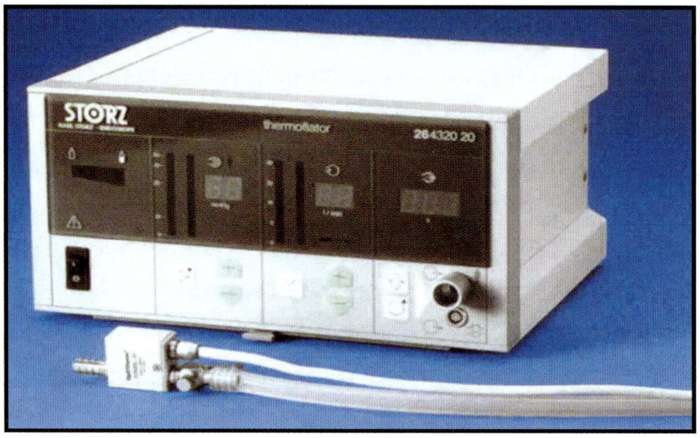

Figure 8.2. Electronic thermoflator

laparoscope giving brighter image with better definition and wider viewing angle (Figure 8.3). The lens system of scope provides double magnification, which can be further increased by use of video monitoring with high definition digital video cameras and monitors. There are two important aspects of a telescope: Its diameter and its viewing angle.

a. 0° straight forward telescope: The direction of view corresponds to the natural approach and facilitates orientation.
b. 30° forward oblique telescope: This can be rotated to enlarge the field of vision and is advantageous during dissection in the pouch of Douglas.

For simple diagnostic and minor operative procedures, 5 mm laparoscope is adequate. It also serves the basic purpose of minimal invasiveness of laparoscopy.

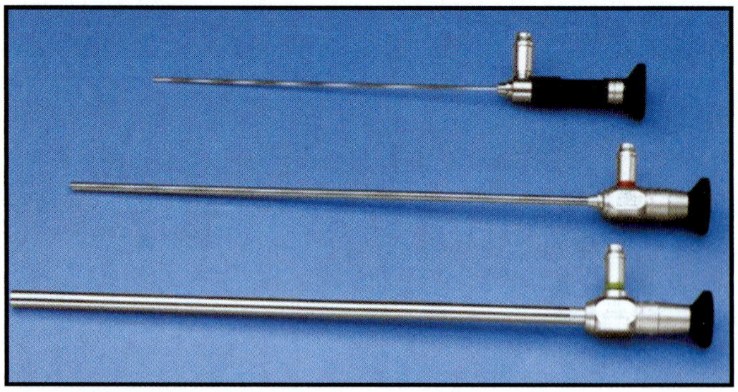

Figure 8.3. Telescopes

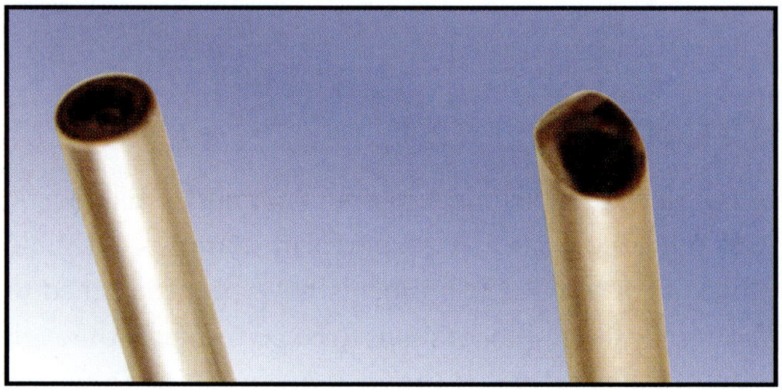

Figure 8.4. 4°C and 30° scopes

10 mm scope is preferable for major video-operative laparoscopic surgical procedures. Although 0° laparoscopes are most preferred, 30° laparoscopes enable the surgeon to see aspects of organs which are hidden from direct view (Figure 8.4). Operative laparoscope has parallel channel for introduction of instruments to perform operative work. However, narrow lens system in this type of scopes decreases the intensity of light. The new Bettocchi design microhysteroscope with an operating channel reduces the need of excessive dilatation of the cervix and provides the same operative facilities.

Light Sources

As operative laparoscopy is performed with endocamera vision, the quality of the light source is very important for providing good vision. Light sources are either xenon or halogen. Each type of light source generates light of slightly different color and intensity. The more powerful the source, the greater the temperatures increase. 175 watts xenon light source is generally sufficient for

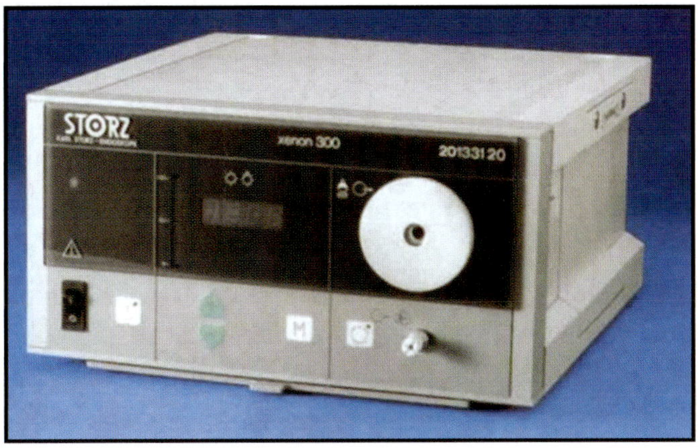

Figure 8.5. Xenon light source

routine interventions. For special interventions and while using scopes of smaller diameters, 300 watts are required (Figure 8.5). Halogen light source of more than 200 watts is sufficient to do operative laparoscopy but it is necessary to do proper white balancing because it generates yellow light.

Light Cables

The light cable transmits light from the light source to the abdominal cavity. The light cables may be fiberoptic or liquid gel with a diameter between 3.5 mm and 6 mm, and a length ranging from 180 to 350 cm. The light carrying capacity of the cable depends on the number of fiberoptic bundles.

Camera Equipment

There are several types of video camera systems. The technical criteria for good quality camera are: Resolution expressed in number of lines or pixels, sensitivity expressed in lux [1 lux is equivalent to illumination of one candle light], number and quality of video outputs. Most cameras are either single chip or three chip and both images are acceptable in quality for routine surgery. But three-chip camera is very helpful in surgeries where finer work is necessary with tissue identification at magnified view (Figure 8.6). An image-processing module with even a single chip camera gives equally good resolution as in digital camera.

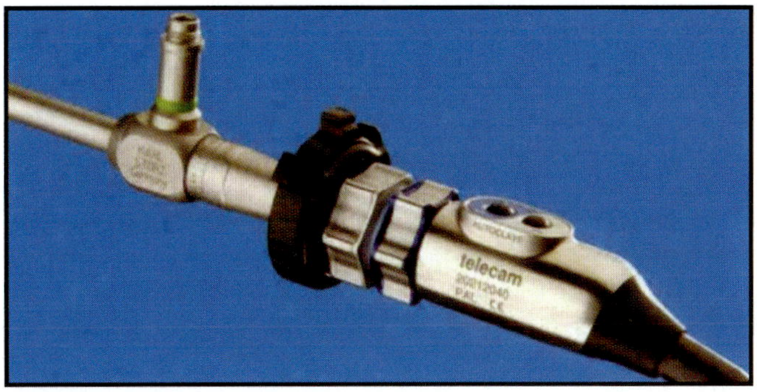

Figure 8.6. 3-chip camera

HAND INSTRUMENTS

Veress Needle

Veress needle is used to inject gas in the abdominal cavity to create a pneumoperitoneum (Figure 8.7). It has a spring mechanism which protects the viscera from the sharp needle edge. The Veress needle must be kept in perfect condition to ensure that the mandrel can be slid easily in to the protection sleeve. When the needle is inserted through the abdominal wall, passage through the fascia and peritoneum should be recognized as a tactile sensation.

Trocar

Trocars serve as a pathway into the abdominal cavity through which laparoscopic surgery is performed. The trocar carrying the telescope is usually introduced via the umbilicus (Figure 8.9). It is introduced blind after creating the pneumoperitoneum with the Veress needle.

Pyramidal tip trocar is easier to insert but is more likely to perforate blood vessel in the abdominal wall. The conical trocar tip requires a stronger thrust to insert. The flap valve trocar open and close automatically with passage of instrument. In trumpet valve trocar, a spring

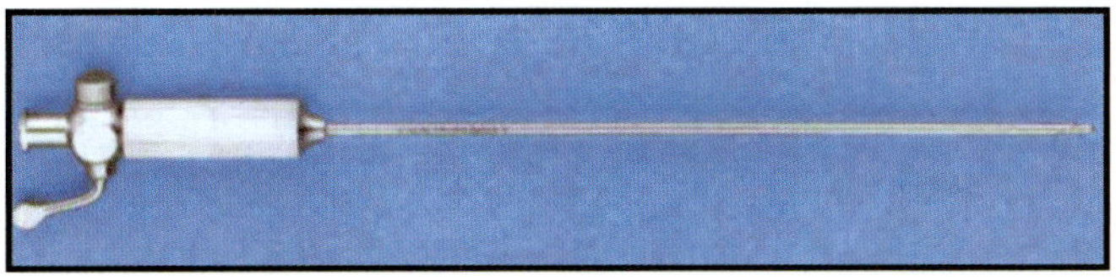

Figure 8.7. Veress needle

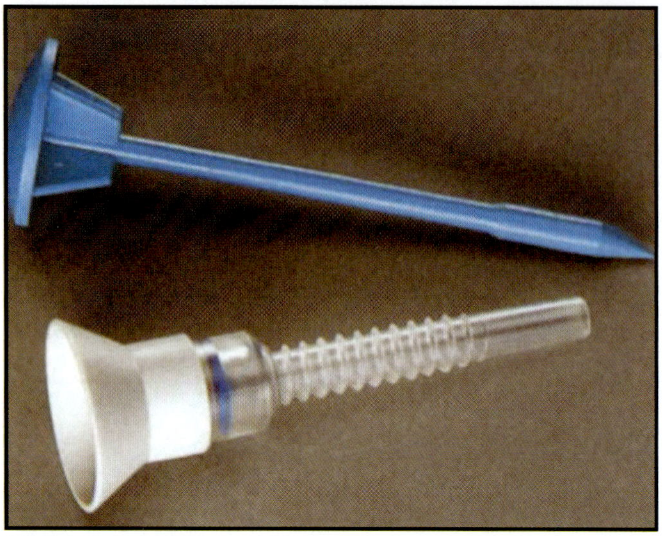

Figure 8.8. Ancillary trocars

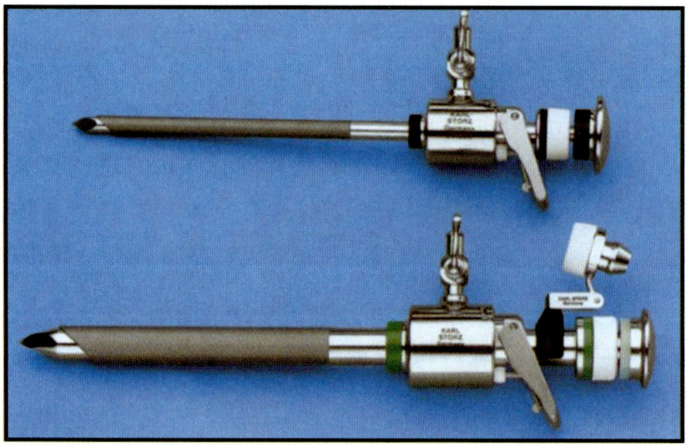

Figure 8.9. Primary trocars: 5 mm and 10 mm

system closes the valve and it must be held open for introduction of instruments. Introduction of auxiliary (Figure 8.8) trocar is always carried out under visual control. It is also very important to have a retention system at the trocar so as to avoid unexpected removal of trocar while changing instruments or during surgical maneuvers. Trocars come in different diameters for introduction of 3, 5 or 10 mm instruments. Special reducers are available to reduce the diameter from 10 to 5 mm or 5 to 3 mm. Trocars can be of metal or plastic. If electrical current is to be passed from the instrument inserted through the trocar, proper insulation needs to be carried out.

Graspers/Forceps

Atraumatic and grasping forceps are available in different sizes shapes and are very important for stabilizing during surgeries. Ideal grasper should be medium sized with a rounded tip and serrated jaws so that it can grasp tissue for exposure, act as a blunt probe with jaws closed, allows dissection with jaws open (Figure 8.10). Maryland dissector resembles the curved hemostat of the open surgery. It is also useful for blunt dissection. Atraumatic grasping forceps [multi serrated] are designed for atraumatic and precise tissue grasping (Figure 8.11). Grasping forceps [2 × 4 teeth] are used to grasp and liberate solid organs. Sturdy grasping forceps are used to fix ovarian capsule or remove tissues in an endobag.

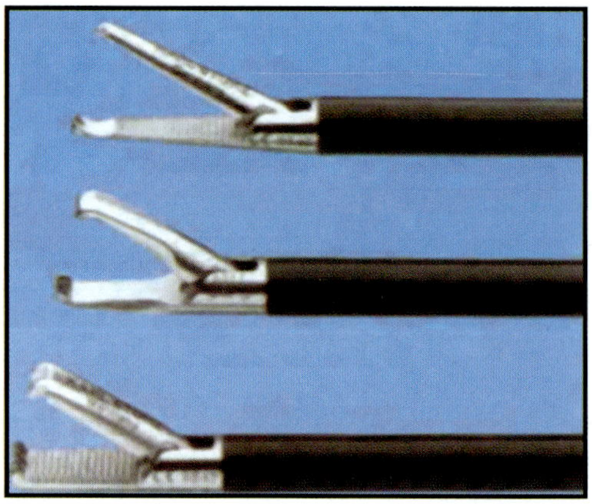

Figure 8.10. Traumatic graspers

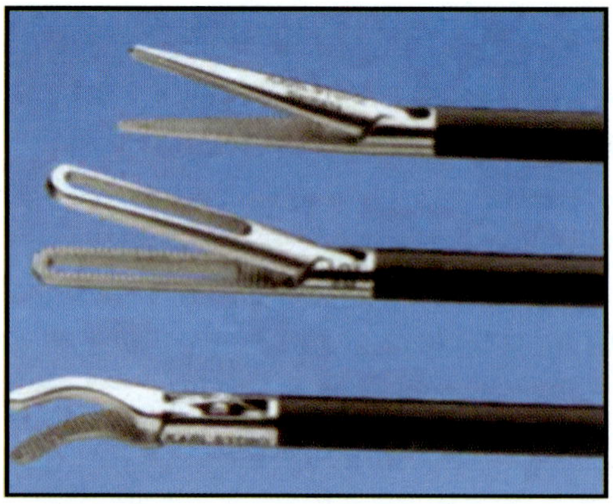

Figure 8.11. Atraumatic graspers

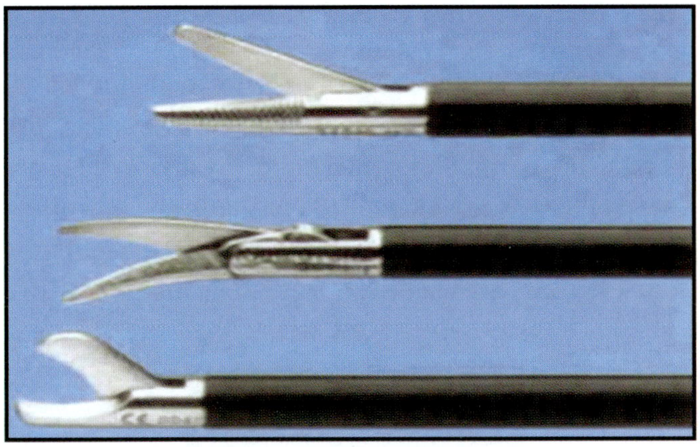

Figure 8.12. Scissors

Scissors

They can be curved or straight (Figure 8.12). Hook scissors are suitable for cutting ligature fibers and for tissue transaction. Delicate dissection can be carried out with straight scissors. Some scissors have adaptor for attaching the cautery with scissor. However, this type of use may hamper the sharpness of scissors.

Suction and Irrigation Apparatus

Controlled suction and irrigation is vital for maintaining the clear field of vision during laparoscopy (Figure 8.13). A simple suction cannula is usually of 5 mm in diameter with two-way channel system with suction and irrigation function. Hydrodissection with high-pressure water is also used for division of tissue layers and spaces.

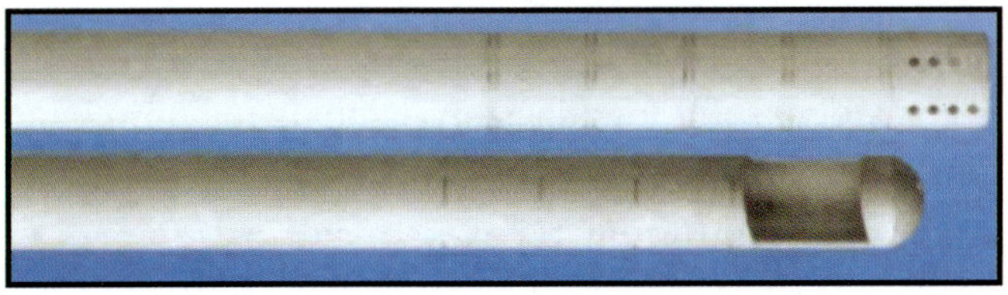

Figure 8.13. Suction and irrigation apparatus

Myoma Screws

They are required while doing laparoscopic myomectomy. They have a screw to fix the myoma and are available in 5 mm and 10 mm size (Figure 8.14). They allow stabilizing fibroid, maneuvering the myoma and applying traction with improved visibility and access.

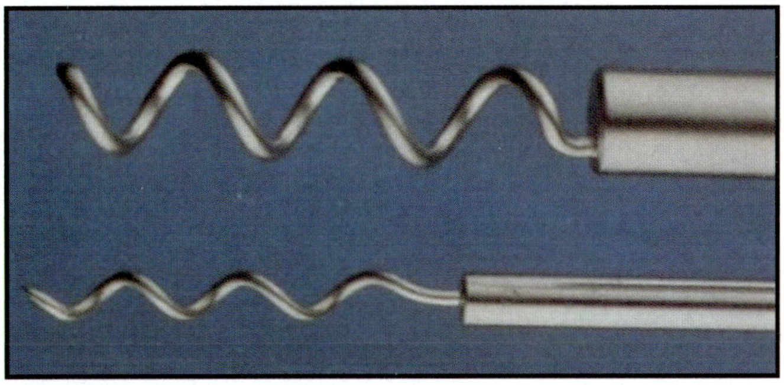

Figure 8.14. Myoma screws

Monopolar Hook and Needle

A very fine needle with spring control is routinely used for PCO drilling, cyst puncture and linear salpingostomy for unruptured ectopic pregnancy. Monopolar hook or spatula is routinely used for precise incision during myomectomy or cyst wall enucleation (Figure 8.15).

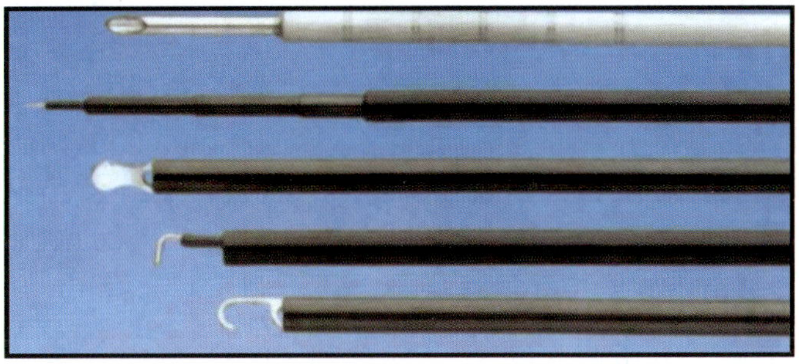

Figure 8.15. Different monopolar electrodes

Bipolar Forceps

Bipolar forceps are used for coagulating the bleeding vessels, endometriosis or for coagulating the pedicles during hysterectomy. For gynecological surgery, forceps within 3 mm wide electrodes are preferred. Current research is moving towards increased use of bipolar forceps and also giving them the functions of grasping, cutting and dissection. The aim is to minimize the number of instrument changes (Figure 8.16).

SPECIALIZED DEVICES

Electrocautery

In monopolar system, the current flows from the unit to the active electrode (tip of the hook or scissors) and from this electrode the current is conducted through the tissue

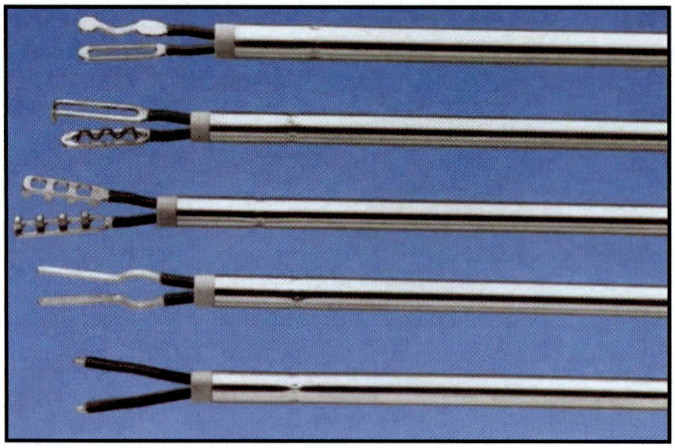

Figure 8.16. Bipolar forceps

to the return electrode and back to the unit. As path of the electrons traveled is not known, use of this system is dangerous. It can be used for pure cutting, coagulation and cutting using a blended (mixed) current. The coagulative current is characterized by intermittent pulses of current and causes cellular dehydration and protein coagulation. The pure cutting current is continuous flow of electrons causing rapid rise in intracellular temperature leading to an explosion of the cell. In bipolar system, the current flows from one jaw of the bipolar forceps through the tissues to the other jaw (Figure 8.17). In this system, path is always known, so there is no risk of electrical burns. However, there is risk of spreading of the heat generated to the organs other than desired. So energy should always be applied with short exposure times and at an adequate distance away from vulnerable structures.

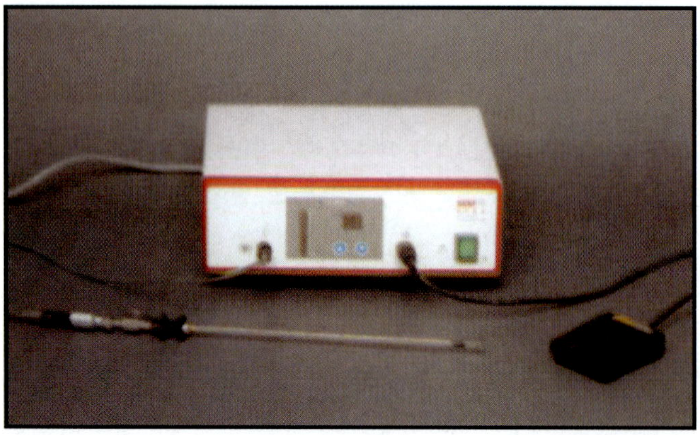

Figure 8.17. Bipolar electrocautery

Laser

CO_2 and Nd: YAG laser systems are most commonly used laser systems. They are more precise and cause less thermal injury than electrocautery. CO_2 laser is more effective for tissue vaporization and cutting but not effective for coagulation. Nd: YAG laser has good coagulation properties but poor vaporization properties (Figure 8.18).

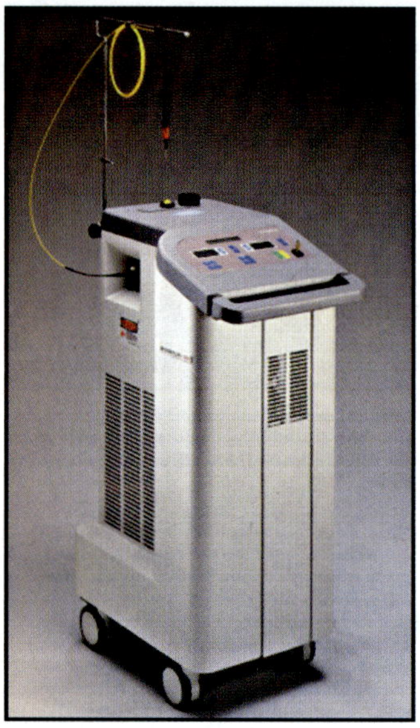

Figure 8.18. CO_2 laser system

Ultrasound Systems (Harmonic Scalpel)

In this system, cutting and coagulation is achieved by ultrasound waves. Advantage is no risk of electrical injuries and minimal thermal spread to adjacent organs. It is mainly useful for adhesiolysis involving bowel and adnexa. Ultrasound waves are transferred from the generator to different types of hand instruments to produce the desired tissue effect (Figure 8.19).

SPECIALIZED INSTRUMENTS

Suturing Instruments

Two suturing methods are routinely used, extracorporeal and intracorporeal. In extracorporeal suturing, once the tissue is sutured, the needle is withdrawn out of trocar

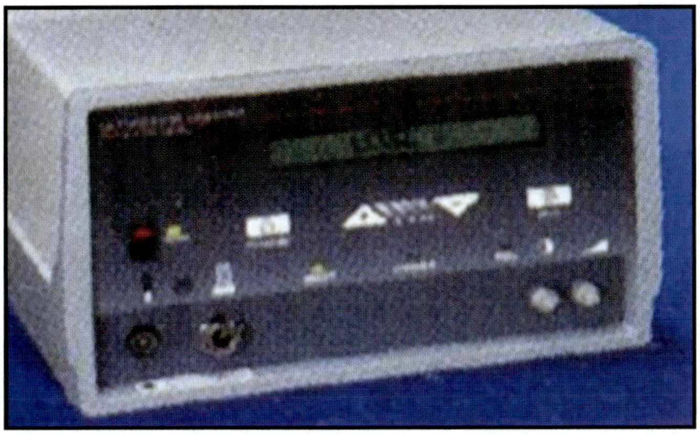

Figure 8.19. Harmonic scalpel

and knot is tied extracorporeally and then knot is pushed using knot pusher (Figure 8.21). For intracorporeal suturing, two specialized needle holders: one with flat serrated ends and the other with parrot beak or flamingo beak tip are essential (Figure 8.20). The ideal needle holder is the one with lightweight and with good grasp.

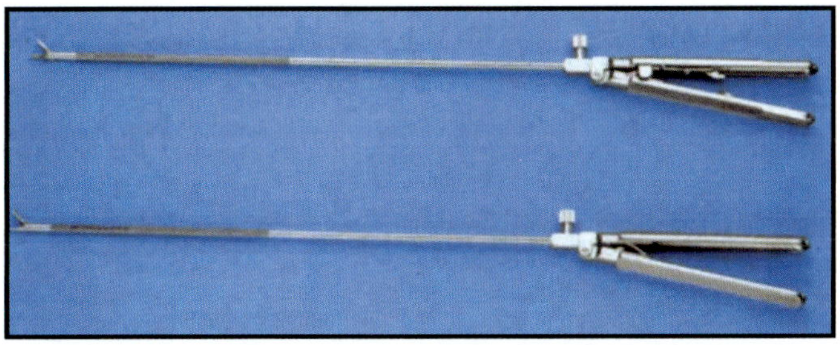

Figure 8.20. Needle holders for intracorporeal suturing

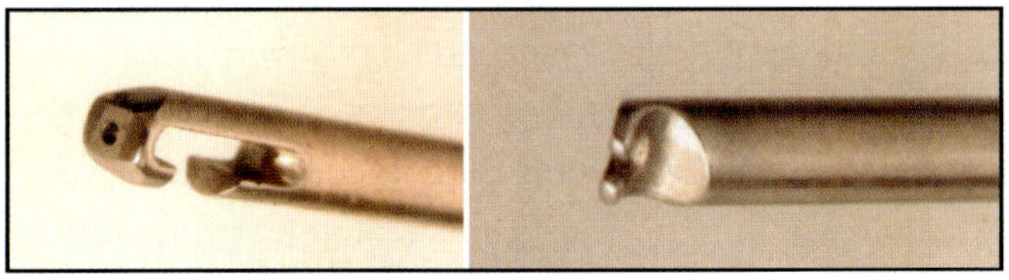

Figure 8.21. Knot pushers for extracorporeal suturing

Uterine Manipulators

Various method of uterine manipulation can be used to mobilize or stabilize the uterus and adnexa during laparoscopic surgery. Simple Rubin's Cannula along with tenaculum is useful method for minor surgeries. More sophisticated and effective manipulators such as KOH –

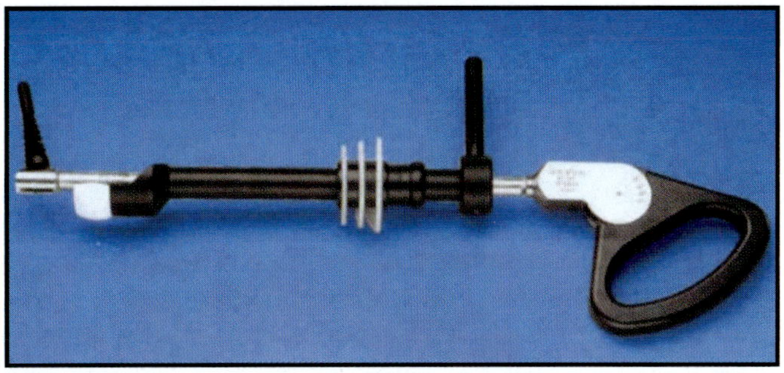

Figure 8.22. Clermont-Ferrand uterine manipulator

manipulator or Clermont-Ferrand manipulator are required when surgeries like hysterectomy or rectovaginal endometriosis is performed (Figure 8.22).

TISSUE RETRIEVAL METHODS

Morcellator

Advent of this devise has revolutionalized the concept of tissue retrieval during laparoscopy that was considered to be surgeons' most dreaded nightmare. It has outdated earlier crude methods of tissue retrieval such as colpotomy, mechanical morcellation and minilaparotomy. It grasps and cuts the specimen into small parts, which are then removed through the hollow part of the instrument. They are available in 10, 12, 15 and 20 mm size (Figure 8.23).

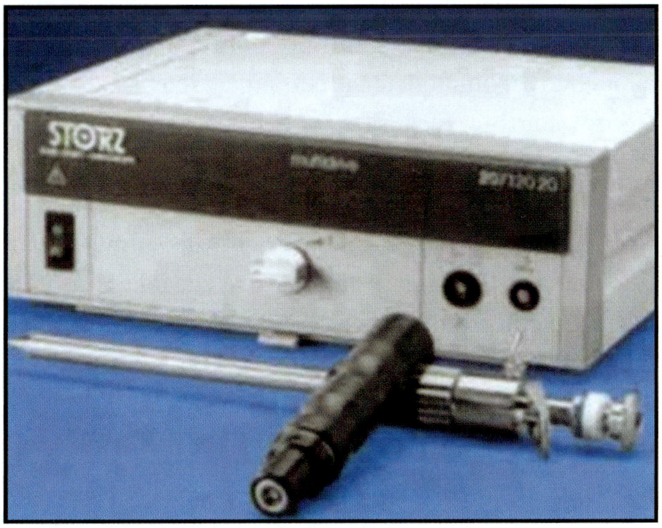

Figure 8.23. Electronic tissue morcellator

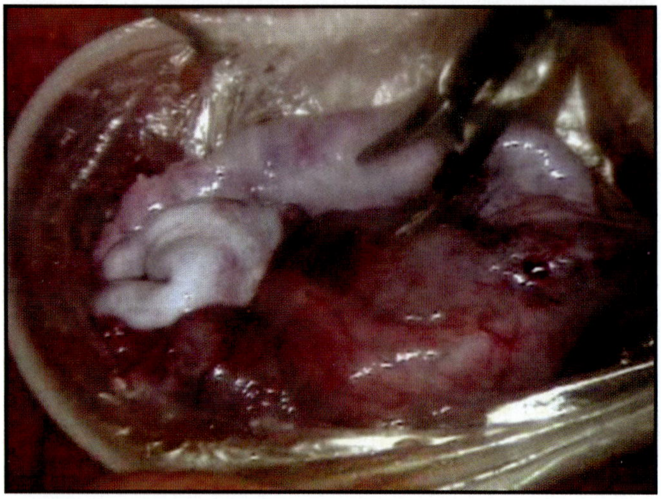

Figure 8.24. Mass removal using endobag

Endobag

These are very important for avoiding the contamination of the abdominal wall and peritoneal cavity during extraction of specimens such as endometriosis, Ectopic pregnancy, suspected malignant mass, dermoid cysts (Figure 8.24).

OPERATING ROOM SET-UP

Endoscopic surgery requires a precise technological environment. A very well organized operating room is not only essential for successful laparoscopy, but also reduces costs. The operating room should be large enough to accommodate the equipment that is necessary. Before starting surgery it is necessary to check the instrumentation and particularly the insufflation device, as well as the coagulation and the aspiration system. It is indispensable that all members of the surgical team (including the surgeon) be trained and capable of solving all technical problems which could occur before and during the intervention.

MAINTENANCE AND STERILIZATION OF INSTRUMENTS

Reusable surgical instruments must be safely cleaned and sterilized after surgery. Instruments must be dismantled before cleaning. After decontamination, every small piece and space must be cleaned and dried with water and compressed air. For lenses and telescope, alcohol or special soap should be used. Most modern instruments are designed for sterilization in the autoclave at 134°C. Other systems of sterilization are currently available.

1. Chemical sterilization is generally performed by immersing the instruments and telescopes in a glutaraldehyde solution. This solution can render HBV, HCV and HIV viruses inactive after 20 minutes immersion. However, to ensure complete sterilization, 10 hours immersion is necessary.
2. Sterilization via autoclave is the most widely used and inexpensive system. Unfortunately lenses, telescopes and instruments with plastic parts cannot be sterilized in autoclaves. In the case of telescopes and instruments expressly made and sold as autoclavable, sterilization cycles of 121° C for 20 minutes or 134° C for 7 minutes should be used.
3. Gas sterilization with ethylene oxide should be the ideal system, because it is carried out at low temperature and is not detrimental to endoscopic instrumentation. Unfortunately this technique is expensive and time consuming (72 hours before the instruments can be used).

NEWER DEVELOPMENTS

So far the focus of research was increasing the patient safety and comfort. Today the trend is towards increasing the comfort of the operating surgeon. As laparoscopy is coordinated effort involving the surgeon and the assistant, it requires a quality of assistance along with quality of surgery. Various artificial assistance devices have been developed starting from laparoscopic holding system to the fully automatic robotic enhancement of instrument manipulating system (Table 8.1). Robotic system answers the need of making some fine movements even more precise, essentially microsuturing (Figure 8.25). Although technology developed in this field is far more sophisticated and costly, it requires regular maintenance and specialized training of operating room staff.

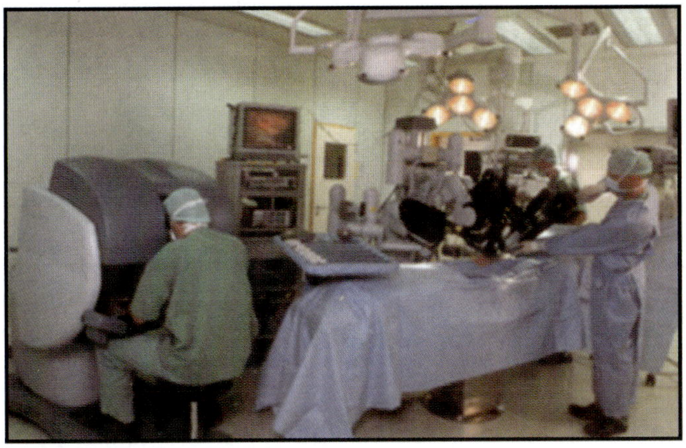

Figure 8.25. Da Vinci Robot system

Table 8.1. Classification of laparoscopic artificial assistance devices

A. Laparoscope holders: Holds the laparoscope only		
1. Static: The surgeon moves the laparoscope holder manually		
	Examples	Static holders
		Kronner
		Passist
		Siska
2. Dynamic: The surgeon moves the laparoscope holder by voice, finger, or head control		
	Example	Aesop (computer Motion): voice
		Image Track (Olympus): finger
		Lapman (Medsys): finger
		Endosista (Armstrong): head
		FIPS
B. Laparoscope holders and instrument manipulators		
		Zeus (Computer Motion)
		Da Vinci (Intuitive)

Source: J Donnez and M Nisolle; An Atlas of Operative Laparoscopy

FULLY INTEGRATED OPERATING ROOM (FIGURE 8.26)

Several companies have focused their research work into integrating the management of the operative laparoscopic surgery theater in to a fully surgeon controlled environment. Insufflation, light source, coagulation, camera control, image capture, operative protocol edition, theater

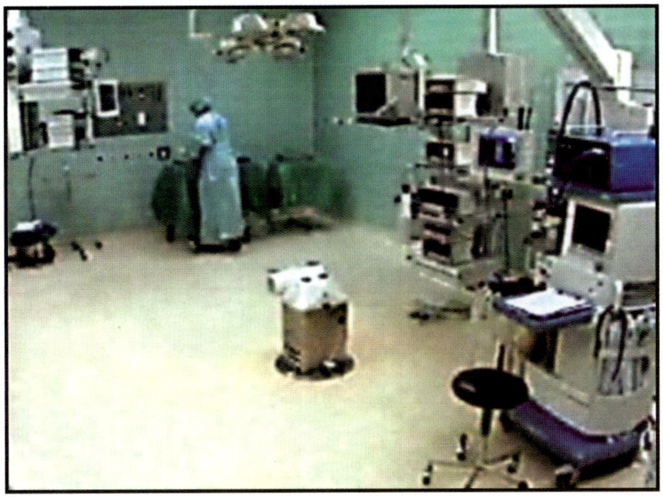

Figure 8.26. Fully integrated operating room

lighting, and internet and telephonic consultation are centralized at the surgeon's command through PC technology controlled by voice or by a sterile draped tactile touch screen.

CONCLUSION

As newer and better instruments are being invented and manufactured, the preceding list is less than exhaustive. However, it is necessary that for any basic gynecological laparoscopy, the basic instruments should be available. Any diagnostic procedure may develop into an operative laparoscopy if the surgeon has the skill and the instruments to perform that surgery. The instruments should be acquired gradually as the skill of surgeon develops.

SUGGESTED READING

1. Donnez J, Nisolle M. An Atlas of Operative Laparoscopy and Hysteroscopy.
2. Jain N. State of the Art Atlas of Endoscopic Surgery in Infertility and Gynecology.
3. Luca Mancaglia, Arnaud Wattiez. Manual of Gynecological Laparoscopic Surgery.
4. Trivedi P. Beyond the boundaries of endoscopic surgery.

9 Anesthetic Management of Endoscopic Surgeries—Laparoscopy and Hysteroscopy

Ravi Kumar

INTRODUCTION

Laparoscopic procedures have been improved to reduce trauma to the patients, mortality and morbidity,hospital stay and thereby to reduces health care costs.

The development of better equipments and understanding of anatomy pathology have allowed the development of endoscopy for diagnostic and operative procedures. Since about 1970, various pathologic gynecologies conditions have been diagnosed and treated by use of laparoscopy. This endoscopic approach has now been extended to gastrointestinal surgical procedures such as appendectomy, cholecystectomy, adhesiolysis, inguinal hernia repair and many more other surgical procedures.

PREANESTHETIC EVALUATION

History

Through medical,surgical and previous exposure to anesthesia and anesthetic complications has to be taken.

Physical Examination

General Examination

Pulse, blood pressure, pedal edema, cyanosis, and pallor.

Systemic Examination

- Respiratory system
- Cardiovascular system
- Per-abdomen

Airway Assessment

Laboratory Investigation

Routine—Complete hemogram, Random blood sugar, Blood urea, Serum creatinine, ECG, Chest X-ray.

Specific investigation should be asked for depending on medical problems.

Patient aged above 65 years 2D echo should be done to assess left ventricular function.

ANESTHETIC TECHNIQUES

- Local anesthesia (LA)
- Regional anesthesia (RA)
- General anesthesia (GA)

Local Anesthesia (LA)

Local anesthesia offers several advantages reduced anesthesia time, quick recovery, decreased postoperative nausea and vomiting , early awareness of complications, and less hemodynamic changes. Sequelae of GA such as sore throat, muscle, pain, and airway trauma, can be avoided. However, this anesthesia approach requires precise and gentle surgical technique and may result in increased patient anxiety, pain and discomfort during the manipulation of pelvic and abdominal organs. For these reasons LA is regularly supplemented with IV sedation. Success with LA requires a relaxed and co-operative patient, a supportive operating room staff, and a skilled surgeon.

Intra-abdominal pressure(IAP) should be as low as possible to reduce pain and ventilatory disturbances. Any laparoscopic procedure that requires multiple puncture sites, considerable organ manipulation, steep tilt and large pneumoperitoneum makes spontaneous respiration difficult for the patient, results in discomforts, and must not be managed with LA.

Regional Anesthesia (RA)

RA such as subarachnoid block is mainly used for hysteroscopic procedure. Epidural technique combined with the head-down position can be used for gynecologic laparoscopy. Globally, epidural and LA share the same benefits and disadvantages.

General Anesthesia (GA)

GA with endotracheal intubation and controlled ventilation should be used for long laparoscopic procedures. This technique provides good muscle relaxation, the ability to control ventilation, protection from aspiration of gastric contents, complete analgesia and a still operative field. IAP should be monitored, kept as low as possible to reduce hemodynamic and respiratory changes and not allowed to exceed 20 mm Hg.

The laryngeal mask airway (LMA) results in less sore throat and might be proposed as an alternative to

Diagnostic hysteroscopy
- Local anesthesia
- Regional anesthesia
- General anesthesia

Operative hysteroscopy
- Regional anesthesia
- General anesthesia

Diagnostic laparoscopy
- Local anesthesia with IV sedation
- Regional anesthesia with IV sedation
- General anesthesia

Operative laparoscopy
- General anesthesia with controlled ventilation

(Figures 9.1 and 9.2)

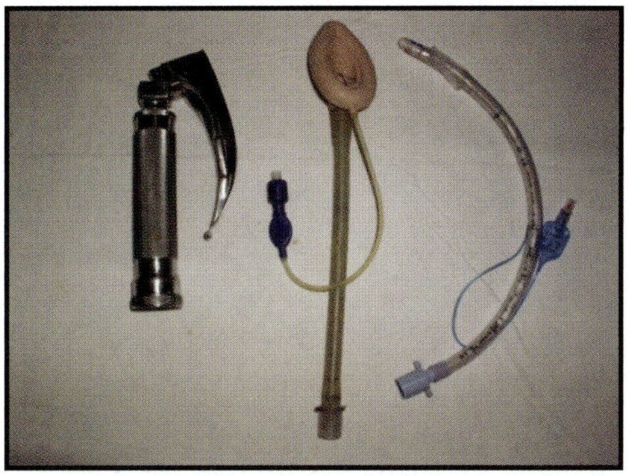

Figure 9.1. Equipment used for GA

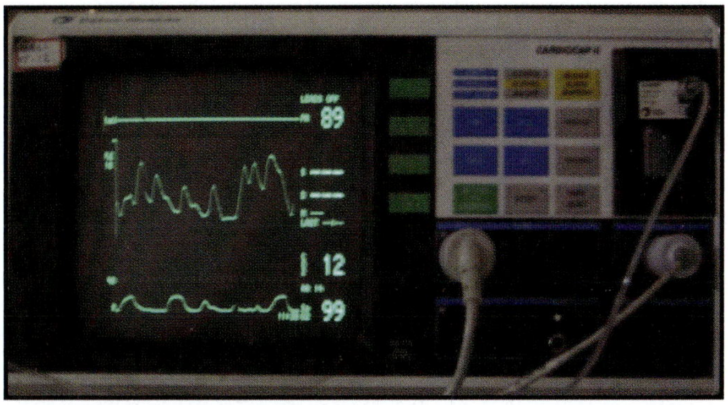

Figure 9.2. Multiparameter monitor

endotracheal intubation, but this device does not protect the airway from aspiration of gastric content.

PROBLEMS DURING LAPAROSCOPY

Ventilatory Problems

Three main ventilatory problems may occur during laparoscopy increased in $PaCO_2$ pneumothorax and gas embolism.

Increased in $PaCO_2$

Causes

1. Absorption of CO_2 from the peritoneal cavity.
2. V/Q mismatch: increased physiological dead space
   Abdominal distension
   Position of the patient
   Controlled mechanical ventilation
   Reduced cardiac output

3. Increased metabolism
4. Depression of ventilation by anesthetic (spontaneous breathing)
5. Accidental events
   CO_2 embolism
   Pneumothorax
   CO_2 emphysema (subcutaneous or body cavities)
   Selective bronchial intubation.

Pneumothorax Pneumomediastinum and Pneumopericardium

Movement of gas during the creation of pneumoperitoneum can produce subcutaneous emphysema, pneumomediastinum, unilateral and bilateral pneumothorax and pneumopericardium. Gas may dissect retroperitoneally through congenital foramina and produce a pneumomediastinum. There are potential channels of communication, embryonic remnants, between the pleural, peritoneal cavities and pericardial sacs and these can open when intraperitoneal pressure increases. Defects in the diaphragm or weak points in the aortic and esophageal hiatus may allow gas diffusion into the thorax. Pneumothorax may also develop secondary to surgical procedures at the level of gastroesophageal junction. Pre-existing pulmonary bullae can rupture because of increased alveolar inflation secondary to increased minute ventilation during pneumoperitoneum, leading to pneumothorax.

These complications are potentially serious and may lead to respiratory and hemodynamic changes. Pneumothorax should be suspected in the presence of cyanosis, decreased SPO_2, subcutaneous emphysema and increased airway pressure. Diagnosis must be confirmed by auscultation of the chest and radiology when pneumothorax develops during laparoscopy following guidelines are recommended:

1. Stop N_2O administration
2. Adjust ventilator setting to correct hypoxemia
3. Apply peak end-expiratory pressure (PEEP)
4. Reduce IAP as much as possible
5. Maintain close communication with the surgeon
6. Avoid thoracocentesis unless necessary since pneumothorax will spontaneously disappear after desufflation.

Gas Embolism

Although gas embolism is rare, but most feared and fatal complication of laparoscopy. Intravascular injection of gas may follow direct needle or trochar placement into a vessel or as a consequence of gas insufflation into an abdominal organ. Early recognition and treatment of gas embolism reduces the size of the embolism and thus the severity of its effects and sequelae . CO_2 is used most frequently for laparoscopy because it is more soluble in blood than air, CO_2 or even N_2O. A dose of equivalent to 1 liter of CO_2 in humans can be given intravenously before cardiac output is altered. Therefore, peritoneal insufflation with CO_2 should be started slowly at a rate not higher than 1 liter/minute to allow early recognition of gas embolism.

The diagnosis of gas embolism depends on the detection of gas emboli in the right side of the heart or recognition of physiological changes secondary to emboli, when the size of the embolus increases, tachycardia, cardiac arrhythmias, hypotension, increased central venous pressure, mill wheel murmur, cyanosis, and ECG changes right heart strain pattern can develop. Pulmonary edema can also be an early sign of gas embolism.

Treatment of CO_2 embolism consist of immediate cessation of the insufflation and release of pneumoperitoneum. The patient is placed in a steep head-down and left lateral decubitus (Durant's) position. Discontinue N_2O will allow 100 percent O_2 ventilation to correct hypoxemia. Hyperventilation increases CO_2 excretion. If these measures are not effective, a central venous or pulmonary artery catheter later may be introduced for aspiration of the gas.

Risk of Aspiration of Gastric Contents

Usually seen in patients undergoing laparoscopy. Risk factors include: Increased intra-abdominal pressure

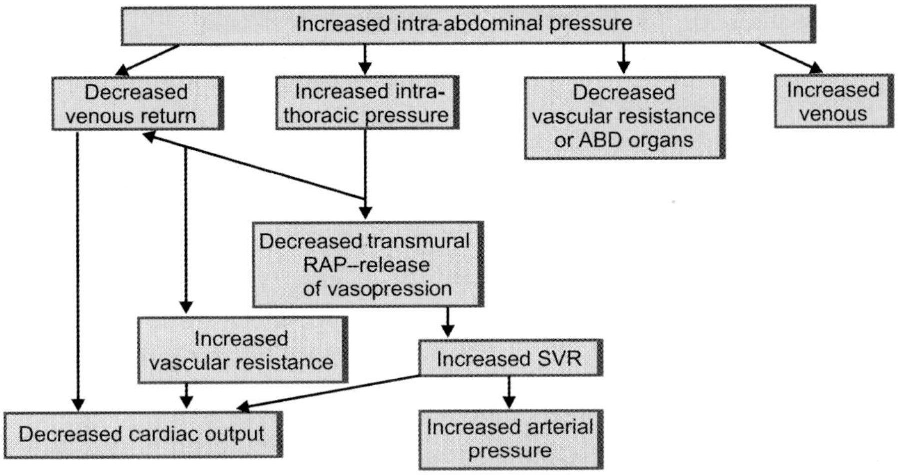

Figure 9.3. Hemodynamic changes during pneumoperitoneum

(IAP). The head-down position should help to prevent regurgitated fluid from entering the air way.

Hemodynamic Problems

Hemodynamic problems results from the combined effect of pneumoperitoneum and patients position. Peritoneal insufflation of IAP higher than 10 mm Hg induce significant alternation in hemodynamics, decreased cardiac output, elevation of arterial pressure and increase of systemic and pulmonary vascular resistances. The decreased in cardiac output, is proportional to the increase in IAP and steepness of the tilt. The mechanism of the decreased cardiac output is multifactorial (Figure 9.3), increase of IAP results in pooling of blood in the legs and reduces the venous return to the right atrium. The subsequent decline in venous return parallels the decrease in cardiac output. Cardiac filling pressures however, increases during peritoneal insufflation. Since intrathoracic pressure also increases consequent to the pneumoperitoneum, transmural right arterial pressure, actually decreases, which is indicator of venous return. The increase in systemic vascular resistance also contribute to the decreased in cardiac output. The release of humoral factors like catecholamines, Prostaglandins, the rennin-angiotensin system and vasopressin are potential mediators for increased SVR.

Intra-abdominal organs are particularly sensitive to the increased IAP. When IAP is increased to 20 mm Hg, renal vascular resistance increases by more than 500 percent and RBF (Renal blood flow) and glomerular filtration decreases less than 25 percent of normal. Increased IAP also results in a significant decrease in mesenteric artery blood flow and intestinal mucosal blood flow increases in IAP significantly decreases organ blood flow (OBF) in all intra-abdominal organs except the adrenal gland. Cardiovascular monitoring routinely used during anesthesia blood pressure, Heart rate, capnography and pulse oximetry gives no accurate information on the changes in SVR and cardiac output.

Cardiac Arrhythmias

Hypercapnia due to peritoneal insufflation of CO_2 known to precipitate arrhythmias during halothane anesthesia and spontaneous ventilation, therefore use of controlled hyperventilation was recommended. Enflurane and isoflurane are less arrhythmogenic than halothane in the presence of increased circulating catecholamines and have been used safely in patients, breathing spontaneously.

Sudden stretching of the peritoneum may result in reflex increase in vagal tone, bradycardia, cardiac arrhythmias and even asystole may develop. Electrocoagulation of fallopian tube can stimulate a vagal reaction. These events are easily and quickly reversible by interruption of insufflation, administration of atropine, and deepening of anesthesia after recovery of heart rate.

PROBLEMS RELATED TO PATIENT POSITION

Patient positioning depends on the site of surgery; head-down tilt is used for pelvic and submesocolic surgery. The head-up position is prefered for supramesocolic surgery. In addition, the patient is often placed in the lithotomy position. These positions may be responsible for or contribute to the development of pathophysiologic changes or injury during laparoscopy.

Cardiovascular Effects

In normotensive patients, the head-down position results in an decreased in central venous pressure and cardiac output. However, central blood volume and blood pressure changes are greater in patients with coronary artery disease, leading to a increased myocardial O_2 demand. The Trendelenburg's position also affect the cerebral circulation resulting in elevated intracranial pressure. The head-down position although decreases transmural pressures in the pelvic organs, reducing blood loss by increasing the risk of gas embolism.

In case of head-up position, a decrease in cardiac output and mean arterial pressure is observed secondary to the reduction in venous return. This decrease in cardiac output compounds the hemodynamic changes induced by pneumoperitoneum. "Steeper the tilt larger the decrease in cardiac output".

Venous stasis in the legs occurs in the head-up position and may be aggravated by the lithotomy position with the lower legs in flexion. Pneumoperitoneum further increases blood pooling in the legs. Venous stasis may lead to venous thrombosis and pulmonary embolism particularly during prolonged laparoscopic procedures. Any additional contributing to circulating dysfunction should be avoided, the legs must be freely supported and not tightly strapped, and pressure on the popliteal space must be prevented.

Respiratory Effects

Steep head-down position results in decreased functional reduced capacity (FRC) total lung volume (TLV) and pulmonary compliance (PC), also facilitates the development of atelectasis, a PEEP of 5 cm H_2O may minimize this complication. These changes are more marked in obese, elderly, or debilitated patients, who may not tolerate these changes.

During the head-down position the ETT can move into the right main stem bronchus resulting in one lung ventilation, therefore the cuff of the ETT must be positioned just below the vocal cords and the correct position of the ETT must be verified after any change in patient position.

The head-up position is unsually considered to be more favorable to respiration.

NERVE INJURY

Nerve compression is a potential complication in the head-down position. The lower extremity neuropathies (peroneal neuropathy, meralgia paresthetica, femoral neuropathy) have been reported after laparoscopy. The common peroneal nerve is vulnerable during lithotomy position, should be protected during prolonged procedures. Over extension of the arm must be avoided, which may lead to brachial plexus injury. Prolonged operative laparoscopies can result in lower extensively compartment syndrome.

POSTOPERATIVE BENEFITS AND CONSEQUENCES OF LAPAROSCOPY

The intraoperative problems faced may be counter balanced by multiple postoperative benefits. In contrast to laparotomy, improved and earlier recovery and feeling of wellbeing. Plasma concentration of C- reactive protein and interleukin-6, which reflects the extent of tissue damage are less after laparoscopy than after laparotomy. Laparoscopy avoids prolonged exposure and manipulation of the intestines, consequently postoperative fasting, duration of intravenous infusion and hospital stay are significantly reduced after laparoscopy.

Surgical trauma contributes to pain and pulmonary dysfunction. The nature of pain varies depending on the surgical techniques after laparotomy, patients complains more of parietal pain (abdominal wall), whereas after laparoscopy patients report visceral pain and shoulder tip pain resulting from diaphragmatic irritation.

Upper abdominal surgeries results in postoperative pulmonary changes, which is less after laparoscopy. Incidence of PONV is more after laparoscopy, which can be controlled by use of antiemetics.

COMPLICATIONS

Occasional catastrophic complication indicates that procedure is not without risk. Cardiac arrest occurs during the induction of pneumoperitoneum because of gas embolism. The improvement of anesthetic techniques, a better understanding of the pathophysiologic changes induced by laparoscopy, and also the improved training and experience of surgeons, declines in the mortality rate. The rate of major complications is usually between 1 and 2 percent, large vessel injury (aorta, IVC and iliac vessels) can lead to emergency situation. Retroperitoneal hematoma can develop insidiously and result in large blood loss without major intraperitoneal effusion, leading to delayed diagnosis. Parietal hemotoma can develop consequent to vessel injury during trocar placement.

The second major traumatic complication consists of visceral injury usually gastrointestinal perforation, which may require conversion to laparotomy. This complication frequently occur during the creation of pneumoperitoneium and the introduction of trocars. Other complications such as pneumothorax, pneumoperitoneum and subcutaneous emphysema have been explained earlier.

Recovery and Postoperative Monitoring

Hemodynamic monitoring should be continued in the postoperative ward. If postoperative shivering occurs oxygen should be administered. Hypothermia which may occur because of use of cold irrigation fluid, lead to delayed recovery, hence irrigation fluid should be warmed.

Finally prevention and treatment of nausea, and vomiting and pain are very important.

SUMMARY

Laparoscopy results in multiple postoperative benefits, including less trauma, less pain, less pulmonary dysfunction, quicker recovery, and slower hospital stay. These advantages are regularly emphasized and explain the increasing success of laparoscopy, now proposed for many surgical procedures.

10 Anesthesia for Endoscopic Surgery in Infertility

Chong Jin Long

Over the past two decades, there is an increase in the number of surgical procedures for infertility. This is due to the higher success rate and an increasing use of surgical endoscopies to perform the procedures. In addition, many procedures are done as an outpatient procedure making it more acceptable to patients because of lesser pain, and the accompanying lesser down time from work. The benefits of using a endoscopic approach to surgery is primarily the reduction in tissue trauma. This results in lesser postoperative pain and improvement in post-operative ventilatory mechanics and reduced time for recovery. This also leads to decrease significant savings for the health care system and an earlier return to work results in a global benefit to the work economy.

This is due, in no small way, to improved technology in instrumentation and video-visualization. That these procedures are being done on the outpatient basis is also due to the improvement of anesthetic techniques and medications. In this chapter we will discuss these anesthetic considerations.

ANESTHESIA FOR ENDOSCOPIC SURGERY

Laparoscopic Surgery

The laparoscopic procedure is covered in our chapters of this book. It is basically the inspection of the abdominal cavity through an endoscope. It is also called minimally invasive surgery or endoscopic surgery. In the traditionally described technique, a pneumoperitoneun is first created using carbon dioxide insufflation into the abdomen. A Trendelenburg, reversed Trendelenburg and Lithotomy position is used to facilitate surgical access and view. The surgical manipulation require good hand eye co-ordination with the use of visual image on a monitor instead of directly at the surgical site makes surgical times longer than conventional surgery. The learning curve for surgeons is also longer.

The types of infertility laparoscopic surgery ranged from myomectomy and tubal reanastomosis in females to varicocelectomy in males.

The anesthetist has to be aware that there are risks associated with laparoscopic surgery. The risks of laparoscopic surgery are linked to the insertion of the trocar and/or Verres needle or the complications resulting from pneumoperitoneum. The incidence of complications have been reported to vary from 0.05 to 0.38 percent. Complications include subcutaneous emphysema, mediastinal emphysema, pneumothorax, bleeding, gastrointestinal perforation, solid visceral injury, avulsion of adhesions, cardiac arrhythmia, and incisional hernia at trocar insertion sites.

Major vascular injury during the initiation of the pneumoperitoneum is well recognized, with a reported mortality rate as high as 15 percent.[1] Its incidence is between 0.02 to 0.26 percent. Minor vascular injuries occur slightly more frequently wit incidence of

0.7-2.6 percent but with significantly less morbidity associated with them. Bowel injury is the third most common cause of death after major vascular injury and anesthesia. Conversion to open surgery occurs in 2.5 to 10 percent and is often due to uncontrolled bleeding or extensive tissue injury an inadequate accessibility.

Physiologic Changes Associated with Laparoscopy

The patient's position and the introduction of a pneumoperitoneum may result in marked physiologic disturbances. The Lithotomy position together with the pneumoperitoneum may cause ventilatory and respiratory alterations with changes in circulation that may compromise the patient wellbeing.

The insufflation of carbon dioxide and the induction of pneumoperitoneum are the events responsible for most of the changes seen in laparoscopic surgery. Although there are alternatives to the use of carbon dioxide insufflation and pneumoperitoneum, they have no gained widespread use. These include the use of an inert gas such as helium or argon or the use of gasless laparoscopy utilising abdominal lifting devices.

Arterial CO_2 partial pressure increases progressively over the first 30 minutes of insufflation.[2] With the use of general anesthesia and controlled ventilation this is often managed with hyperventilation. However, if the patient is breathing spontaneously hypercarbia develops rapidly. If performed under local anesthesia, the patient responds to hypercarbia by increasing the respiratory rate.[3]

Capnography should be used to monitor the carbon dioxide levels, although it must be borne in mind that there are reports that showed a widening difference between end-tidal carbon dioxide and arterial carbon dioxide tension with laparoscopy.[4] Thus end-tidal capnography may not reveal the actual carbon dioxide levels in the arterial blood. This is more pronounced in the sicker patients.

Although the increase in $PaCO_2$ during laparoscopy is multi-factorial, it is largely due to absorption of CO_2 during insufflation. Due to the increase in carbon dioxide, a range of humoral agents such as cathecholamines, renin-angiotensin and vasopressin are released. This is associated with the increase in blood pressure and reduced systemic vascular resistance. There is also a fall in renal blood flow and a reported 50 percent in glomerular filtration rate. The use of clonidine and dexmedetomidine can attenuate these changes.

The increase in CO_2 tension also results in increased intracranial pressure due to the cerebral vasodilator effects of carbon dioxide. Pneumoperitoneum also results in increased intrathoracic pressure and decrease thoracopulmonary compliance by 30-50 percent. With diaphragmatic elevation and splinting, the functional residual capacity of the lungs will decrease and cause airway closure and ventilation-perfusion mismatch. The young healthy patient should tolerate these changes well but patients with pre-existing respiratory disease may not be able to compensate. The head-down position affects respiratory mechanics and also a tendency towards atelactasis.

In addition to the respiratory changes, the increased abdominal pressure leads to the reduction of cardiac output. This is largely due to the decrease in venous return of blood to the heart. In a minor way the increase systemic vascular resistance also reduces cardiac output. Venous pooling due to the increased venous resistance in the inferior vena cava also contributes to the reduction of cardiac output.

Selection of Patients and Location of Surgery

Most patients are young and relatively healthy and are able to tolerate the physiological changes associated with the lithotomy position and pneumoperitoneum. Patients with restricted lung diseases and cardiac diseases should be properly assessed before the operation. Referral to a internal medicine physician for optimization of the medical condition. Where appropriate the cardiologist and respiratory physician should be consulted.

The location of surgery should be carefully considered, as a major vascular accident will require the urgent services of a vascular surgeon. In stand-alone ambulatory centers, this may not be immediately accessible.

PREOPERATIVE EVALUATION

Anesthetists perform preoperatively visits to develop rapport, appraise themselves of and optimize the patient's clinical condition, formulate an anesthetic plan, and inform the patient of proposed procedures and risks of anesthesia. All patients should have a proper evaluation of the suitability for anesthesia since these surgeries are always elective in nature. The American Society of Anesthesiologist Physical Classification score provides a screening guide to the risk of surgery. ASA I is a patient without any medical problems. ASA II being the present of mild systemic disease. ASA III being the presence of severe systemic disease with a life-threatening condition. ASA IV being a moribund patient.

Patients in the ASA I and II Physical Classification are associated with low risk for postoperative morbidity and mortality.[5-7] The risk of hospital death in ASA I and II patients are 0 and 0.04 percent respectively. The risk for death in a ASA III patient is 0.59 percent.[8] In a larger study in France during the years of 1978-1982 in 198,103 patients reported the incidence of events related to anesthesia was 1 per 2,387 cases. Anesthesia was totally responsible in 61 percent of these cases. (28% during induction of anesthesia,and 30% during maintenance, and 42% occurred during the postanesthetic period). The main complications totally attributable to anesthesia were anaphylactic shock, inhalation of gastric contents and postoperative respiratory depression.[9] Patients with an uncontrolled systemic disease that is a threat to life should not have the procedure done as an outpatient. Diabetic and hypertensive patients should have their conditions controlled prior to surgery. Medications should be continued to have effective control until the morning of operation. Patients with thyroid disorders should have their thyroid function assessed, rendered clinically euthyroid before anesthesia is induced.

The airway must be assessed prior to surgery since most patients would undergo general anesthesia with controlled ventilation. Overweight patients pose a higher risk for intubation and ventilatory problems during anesthesia and surgery. The respiratory system should be thoroughly investigated in this group of patients. Problems associated with this group of patients include Obstructive Sleep Apnea syndrome posing problems in the recovery period.

ANESTHESIA TECHNIQUES

General anesthesia is the most common mode of anesthesia for laparoscopic surgery.

The advantage is the flexibility general anesthesia offers in terms of extension of the duration of surgery and the possibility of handling major complications should it arise. The major disadvantage is the effects on recovery times and its complications of nausea and vomiting thus delaying of early discharge.

If general anesthesia is used, the patient's ventilation is controlled and a muscle relaxant is used. This will allow the abdomen to be relaxed adequately for appropriately large pneumoperitoeum, A controversy is the use of laryngeal mask airway (LMA) for ventilation. The concern is the relatively theoretical insecure airway from the LMA in preventing aspiration of gastric content. The other argument against it was that a displaced LMA under the drapes during surgery may cause the stomach to inflate and hence post the risk of damage by the trocar. However, recent studies from the Britain have proven the safety and efficacy of using the LMA during laparoscopic surgery.

Monitoring

All patients should be monitored using a continuous ECG, non-invasive blood pressure monitor, pulse oximetry and end-tidal capnography during the anesthetic.

Choice of Anesthetic Drugs

The classic anesthesia technique is a balanced anesthesia technique where a combination of hypnotics and muscle relaxant is used to maintain anesthesia. In this technique, the hypnotics include the use of an induction agent like intravenous pentothal or propofol. This is followed by maintenance agents like the inhalational anesthetics, e.g. isoflurane, sevoflurane or desflurane.

Induction agent Propofol is the agent of choice for the induction of anesthesia because there is no prolonged post-anesthesia cerebral depression. It can be used as a total intravenous anesthesia technique (TIVA) where no inhalational agents are used. TIVA is touted as a suitable alternative to conventional anesthetic technique. Its advantage is still in controversy. Times to neuromuscular recovery is improved because of the conventional inhalational anesthetic prolongs neuromuscular recovery. However, studies showed mixed results of shorter postoperative recovery times. It produces less post-operative nausea and vomiting reducing delay in post-anesthesia discharge. However, there are arguments against TIVA. It was postulated that propofol-based anesthesia might be associated with vestibular disturbances. There is also the lack of assessment of depth of anesthesia with this technique. Using hemodynamic parameters seems a crude method of determining hemodynamic depth.

Volatile agents Isoflurane, sevoflurane and desflurane are all suitable volatile agents available for ambulatory laparoscopic surgery. Desflurane have been reported to have earlier emergent from anesthesia compared to isoflurane and sevoflurane but the readiness for home discharge times were similar. Using depth of anesthesia monitors, like Bispectral Index monitor or auditory-evoked potential monitor, to assess depth and titrating the amount of anesthesia given have been shown by research workers that any of the agents are suitable for ambulatory laparoscopic surgery. The caveat here is that a suitable anti-emetic must be given prior to the anesthesia induction. It is known that ambulatory laparoscopic surgery is associated with a high incidence of postoperative nausea and vomiting.

Nitrous oxide Nitrous oxide is a popular gas in the anesthetic mixture because it is inexpensive and easy to administer. However, there are controversies to its use. These controversies have involved some reports of adverse occupational effects on health care providers, its effect on postoperative nausea and vomiting, its effect on expanding air-filled spaces such as lung cyst, air-emboli and bowel. Debate on the occupational hazard of nitrous oxide had been going on for decades. The discussion is beyond the scope of this book. There is some evidence that nitrous oxide contributes to postoperative nausea and vomiting. But the study that reported this had a small sample size and a definite conclusion cannot be reached. In a large study utilizing a TIVA technique with or without the use of a nitrous oxide did not show any difference in the postoperative nausea and vomiting. It did show that the amount of propofol can be reduced if nitrous oxide is used, the conclusion being that propofol reduces PONV and that the use of nitrous oxide will reduce usage of propofol and that translate to cost saving.

Muscle relaxants Good surgical condition demands that the muscle relaxation must be adequate. In addition, laparoscopic surgery should be done under controlled ventilation and hence the need for muscle relaxation. The choice of relaxant is controversial. Succinylcholine use is controversial. There is a significant postoperative myalgia with the use of succinylcholine. Most use a non-depolarizing muscle relaxant for ambulatory surgical patients. A rapid onset agent is suitable-like rocuronium. However, its incubating dose of 0.6 mg/kg although achieving excellent intubating conditions within 90 seconds may last too long for the short surgery. A shorter agent-like mivacurium using a dose of 0.25 mg/kg is a suitable alternative. The onset of block is delayed, achieving excellent intubating condition only after 180 seconds.

EPIDURAL/SPINAL ANESTHESIA

The use of regional anesthesia for laparoscopy is not widely practiced. Some studies have reported the use of this technique.[10] Many use a spinal anesthesia technique utilizing hypobaric solution of lignocaine (10-20 mg) with either sufentanil (10 μg) or fentanyl (25 μg).[11] Side effects include pruritus and shoulder tip pain in 50 percent of patients. There is also a 20 percent incidence of nausea. However, the use of selective spinal anesthesia have economic savings. Lennox et al reported cost savings of using spinal anesthesia versus desflurane anesthesia.[12]

Epidual anesthesia have also been described for laparoscopy.[13] The induction time for epidural is often longer than the surgical procedure. However, there is a lower incidence of postoperative nausea and vomiting compared to general anesthesia in one study. In a study at Virginia Mason Clinic, epidural anesthesia was used in 50 percent of the laparoscopic procedures. Many of the patients have anxiety when the abdomen is insufflated and some respiratory compromise occurs. The patients also cannot tolerate the head-down position and the shoulder-tip pain was troublesome.

INTRAOPERATIVE COMPLICATIONS

Despite being minimally invasive, complications can be life-threatening. Complications requiring surgical intervention occur in 1 in 660 cases with mortality of 1 in 2000 cases.[14,15]

Adequate training, reduced surgical duration, proven safer techniques, improved technology, a high index of suspicion, and prompt appropriate intervention will reduce these complications. In serious life-threatening complications, deflation of the peritoneum may result in good outcome. Technically, lower intra-abdominal pressure, and shorter surgical duration contribute to lower risks for complication.

Cardiorespiratory Complications

Pneumothorax occurs in 0.03 percent of cases and usually requires no treatment but in severe cases will lead to decreae in ventilation and hypoxia. This will compromise the cardiac function. Life-threatening surgical emphysema and hypercarbia can be sign of pneumopericardium, although this complication has been reported without the evidence of surgical emphysema.

Arrhythmias are the most common cardiac intraoperative events, with a 47 percent incidence. Ventricular ectopics is the most common arrhythmia. It is observed more with the use of CO_2 insufflation and associated with acidosis and catecholamine release. Often the presence of arrhythmia is evidence of a more serious underlying complication, such as pneumothorax, embolism or hypoxemia.

Gas embolism occurs in 0.002-0.016 percent of cases and can be fatal. It usually occurs within 10 minutes of initiating insufflation and is due to inadvertent venous cannulation. Presenting features may be dysrrhythmias and raised central venous pressure and hypoxia. Cardiac arrest may also occur. Management consists of stopping insufflation and attempt aspiration of the emboli and cardiac support.

PAIN MANAGEMENT AFTER THE SURGERY

Many extremely painful procedures can now be performed in an ambulatory setting with aggressive postoperative pain control techniques. The intensity of early acute postoperative pain may be an important predictor of the development of chronic pain. A multimodal strategy for postoperative analgesia should begin prior to the surgical procedure because patient preparation and education may improve postoperative outcome.[16] Patients should also benefit from counseling them how much pain and where to expect pain after surgery. Pain that occurs after this procedure is much less and of shorter duration than after a similar procedure done with open laparotomy. Pain after laparoscopy may occur in the upper abdomen, lower abdomen, back, or shoulders regardless of the surgical site and may persist for many days postoperatively. The greatest incidence of pain is in the upper abdomen. The highest pain scores are in the first 24 hours after surgery and usually subside after that. Rapid distention of the peritoneum may be associated with tearing of blood vessels, traumatic traction of nerves, and release of inflammatory mediators. The persistence of shoulder pain suggests excitation of the phrenic nerve. Patient should receive instruction on the importance of coughing, deep breathing and ambulation after surgery to reduce the possible complications.

Preemptive analgesia is an antinociceptive treatment that prevents establishment of altered processing of afferent input that amplifies postoperative pain. Crile formulated the concept of preemptive analgesia on the basis of clinical observations. He postulated that the use of regional blocks, in addition to general anesthesia, could prevent intraoperative nociception and the formation of painful scars, caused by changes in the central nervous system during surgery. The concept of preemptive analgesia refers to the administration of an analgesic prior to tissue trauma to produce a greater effect compared to that when administered after the injury.[17] Anti-inflammatory analgesic medication, local anesthetic wound infiltration or nerve block or small doses of opioid analgesics are administered prior to surgical incision to take advantage of this preemptive effect.[18]

The concerns of potential perioperative bleeding from the effects of NSAIDs on platelet function have led to the reduction of use of this group of drugs in the postoperative setting. COX-2 drugs have a safer profile on platelet function. The NSAIDs have reduced the need or the amount of opioid analgesics in the postoperative period. Some conflicting evidence of the effects of the safer COX-2 NSAIDs on cardiac failure have led to the withdrawal of some of these drugs from the market.

The local anesthetics used for infiltrating surgical wounds include lignocaine, bupivacaine or ropivacaine. All the trocar punctures should have local anesthetic infiltration before or after the surgery starts. Because of the small wounds involved, toxic levels would not be exceeded in these cases.

I would recommend the routine use of local anesthetic infiltration, acetaminophen together with a traditional NSAID, or Celecoxib, without contraindications to their use in the management of postoperative pain in this group of patients.

CONCLUSIONS

The advance of endoscopic surgery is relentless. The next decade will bring newer technologies into this advancing field of surgery. The challenge for anesthesiologists is to keep up with the changes. The improvement of surgical techniques will lead to more and more operation being performed as an ambulatory surgery technique. The anesthesiologist role is to provide a safe anesthesia with rapid recovery and good postoperative analgesia for these operations. Public demand will push us into making this possible. Previously large uterine myoma were performed under laparotomy, now many are done under day surgery laparoscopic procedures. Pain relief is vital for the success of this technique. Good anesthesia care is the answer.

REFERENCES

1. Nordestgaard AG, Bodily KC, Osborne RW Jr, Buttorff JD. Major vascular injuries during laparoscopic procedures. Am J Surg 1995;169(5):543-5. Review
2. Mullet CE, Viale JP, Sagnard PE, et al. Pulmonary CO_2 elimination during surgical procedures using intra or extraperitoneal CO_2 insufflation. Anesth Analg 1993; 76:622.
3. Hodgson C, McClelland RMA, Newton JR. Some of the effects of the peritoneal insufflation of carbon dioxide at laparoscopy. Anesthesia 1970;25:382.
4. Fitzgerald SD, Andrus CH, Bauddendistel LJ, et al. Hypercarbia during Carbon dioxide pneumoperitoneum. Am J Surg 1992;163:186.
5. Cohen MM, Duncan PG, Tate RB. Does anesthesia contribute to operative mortality? JAMA 1988;260:2859
6. Lunn JN, Farrow SC, Fowkes FGR, et al. Epidemiology in anaesthesia I. anaesthesia practice over 20 years. Br J Anaesthesia 1982;54:803-9.
7. Vacanti CJ, Vanhouven RJ, Hill RC. A statistical analysis of the relationship of physical status to postoperative mortality in 68,388 cases. Anesth Analg 1970;49:564.
8. Forrest JB, Rehder K, Goldsmith CH, et al. Multicenter study of general anaesthesia. 1. Design and patient demography. Anesthesiology 1990;72:252.

9. Tiret L, Desmnts JM, Hatton F, et al. Complications associated with anaesthesia: A prospective study in France. Can Anesth Soc J 1986;33:336.
10. Vaghadia H, Viskari D, Mitchell GWE. Selective spinal anesthesia for outpatient laparoscopy. 1 Characteristics of 3 hypobaric solutions. Can J Anaesth 2001;48:256-60.
11. Lennox PH, Vaghadia H, Henderson C, Martin L, Mitchell GW. Small-dose selective spinal anesthesia for short-duration outpatient laparoscopy: recovery characteristics compared with desflurane anesthesia. Anesth Analg 2002;94(2):346-50.
12. Lennox PH, Chilvers C, Vaghadia H. Selective spinal anesthesia versus desflurane anesthesia in short duration outpatient gynecological laparoscopy: a pharmaco-economic comparison. Anesth Analg 2002;94(3):565-8.
13. Collins LM, Vaghadia H. Regional anesthesia for laparoscopy. Anesthesiol Clin North America 2001;19(1): 43-55.
14. Fishburne J. Anesthesia for laparoscopy: considerations, complications and techniques. J Reprod Med 1978;21:37-40.
15. Bongard F, Dubecz S, Klein S. Complications of therapeutic laparoscopy. Current Problems Surg 1994;31:857-924.
16. Acute Pain Management Guideline Panel. Acute Pain Management: Operative or Medical Procedures and Trauma; Clinical Practice Guideline. Rockville, Md: Agency for Health Care Policy and Research, Public Health Service, US Department of Health and Human Services; 1992.
17. Dahl JB, Kehlet H. The value of preemptive analgesia in the treatment of postoperative pain. Br J Anaesthesia 1993; 70:434-9.
18. Dahl JB, Kehlet H. Non-steroidal, anti-inflammatory drugs; rationale for use in severe postoperative pain. Br J Anaesth 1991;66:703-12.

Section Two

UTERUS

11 Hysteroscopic Myomectomy

Christopher Chen

INTRODUCTION

Fibroids or leiomyomas of the uterus are the most common solid pelvic tumors in the female and can occur among 20-40 percent of women in the reproductive age group (Wallach[1]). They can grow in various locations of the uterus and are described as subserous, intramural, or submucous (Figure 11.1). The submucous variety forms about 5 percent of the total and can cause infertility, abnormal uterine bleeding, or become infected. The submucous fibroid can develop as a sessile growth or become polypoid, or even grow out of the cervix as a fibroid polypus.

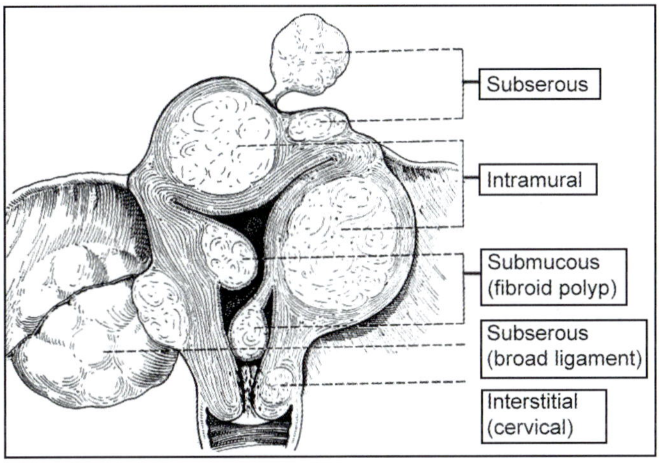

Figure 11.1. Uterine fibroids

DIAGNOSIS OF SUBMUCOUS FIBROIDS

Submucous fibroids are often discovered through gynecological pelvic examination. They may be seen as polypoid growths in the cervical canal or may even protrude out of the cervix into the vagina. Transvaginal ultrasonography provides a good way for their detection.

Hysterography (HSG) is another method for their detection, and are seen as filling defects, with accompanying distortion of the uterine cavity. Crescentric formation also occurs as contrast material surrounds the myoma during hysterographic dye injection. Vascular intravasation may also sometimes be observed. The procedure of sonohysterography may also be used in place of hysterography.

Occasionally MRI can be employed, especially to differentiate between the fibroid and adenomyosis (Murase[2]).

Generally, submucous fibroids are of a size that can be removed through the cervical canal after prior dilatation. Larger growths may not be possible by this route and the alternative will then be by hysterotomy and removal through the laparoscope (see chapter on **Laparoscopic Myomectomy**).

HYSTEROSCOPIC MYOMECTOMY

Before surgery is embarked upon, the location and size of the fibroids require to be determined, as part of surgical planning. This is usually done by transvaginal ultrasonography. The hysteroscopic operation is then performed, usually combined with laparoscopy such as for the removal of intramural or subserous fibroids, or pelvic endometriosis. The combined procedures of hysteroscopy and laparoscopy have the advantage of identifying any complications, such as uterine perforation, during the hysteroscopic operation, which can be seen through the laparoscope and repair then performed immediately.

Hysteroscopic myomectomy is regularly done as a day surgery procedure and the patient goes home the same day. The patient is positioned in the lithotomy position under general anesthesia. After cleansing of the vulva and vagina with antiseptic solution, the cervix is grasped with a vulsellum and a uterine sound passed to determine the length of the uterine cavity. In our Center, a flexible hysteroscope is used, after dilating the cervical canal to Hegar 6, and then distending the uterine cavity with normal saline for examination of the submucous fibroids. A 3-chip video camera attached to the scope and a TV monitor allow magnification of the findings and recording of the surgery. A thorough examination of the site, size and numbers of the submucous fibroids is done. Any subserous or intramural fibroids present are examined by simultaneous laparoscopy and laparoscopic myomectomy. An important advantage of this combined procedure is safety, since any occurrence of perforation during hysteroscopic myomectomy is immediately identified and surgical repair performed.

Having identified the submucous fibroids, their removal is then done with the resectoscope (Figure 11.2). The cervix is first dilated to Hegar 10 and the resectoscope then passed into the uterine cavity which is then distended with glycine. A 3-chip video camera is attached to the eyepiece and visualization obtained on the TV monitor.

Each submucous fibroid is systematically shaved in pieces down to the plane of the endometrial wall by drawing the wire loop of the resectoscope towards the operator. The pieces of floating fibroid are then removed

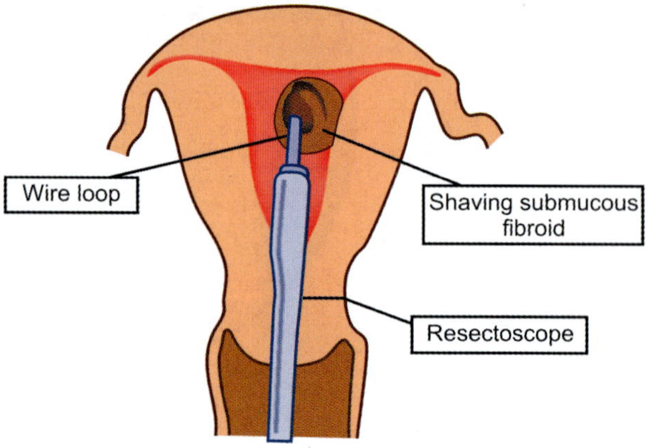

Figure 11.2. Hysteroscopic myomectomy

with forceps, or simply flushed out of the uterine cavity through the cervical canal. Using a grasping forceps, the rest of the fibroid can be enucleated by grasping and pulling on that portion of the growth that protrudes above the uterine wall. This can be done either blind or under direct vision (Please refer to the video recording which accompanies this book for a demonstration of hysteroscopic myomectomy using the resectoscope).

One difficulty with hysteroscopic myomectomy is clouding of the field of surgery by blood as a result of the procedure. This can be minimized by coagulating the tissue surrounding the fibroid prior to cutting into it. Pitressin injected into the cervix can also reduce the bleeding and cloudiness of the glycine distension medium. Opening the outlet tap of the resectoscope partially allows gentle flushing of the uterine cavity which clears the field of surgery of cloudiness by blood.

It is necessary to be aware of the relative thickness of the uterine wall at various levels so that one does not cut too deeply, and result in perforation. The Table 11.1 shows various thicknesses of the uterine wall.

Table 11.1. Uterine wall thickness

Site	*Thickness (mm)*
Fundus	19.5
Anterior wall	22.5
Posterior wall	21
Isthmus	10

Table 11.2. Summary of studies reporting on the reproductive outcome after hysteroscopic myomectomy

Reference	*No. of cases*	*Pregnancy rate (%)*	*Delivery rate (%)*
Donnez et al[3]	24	67	67
Valle[4]	16	62	50
Corson and Brooks[5]	13	77	61
Hucke[6]	14	28.7	–
Goldenberg et al[7]	15	47	40
Preutthipan and Theppisai[8]	12	16.7	–
Giatras et al[9]	41	60.9	48.7
Varasteh et al[10]	36	52.8	36.1
Vercellini et al[11]	40	37.5	32.5
Hernandez et al[12]	59	27.1	10.0

The amount of medium used requires to be monitored because of the risk of intravasation with resulting fluid overload and intoxication. Hence an account must be kept of the quantity of fluid infused and the amount flowing out of the uterus through the outlet tap.

Bleeding during or after hysteroscopic myomectomy may be encountered at a rate of 2-3 percent. This can be controlled by the tamponade effect of the distending medium or by electrocoagulation. Postoperative bleeding may be controlled by introducing a Foley's catheter and distending the balloon up to 30 ml and leaving it for 24 hours before its removal.

Regularly the patient is discharged home the same day, or the next day, and may take 2 to 7 days to recover at home, depending on the extent of the surgery.

The operating time can vary, depending on the difficulty of the operation. On the average the time is about 1 hour.

RESULTS AFTER HYSTEROSCOPIC MYOMECTOMY

The overall risk of recurrence of fibroids after hysteroscopy myomectomy varies between 20 to 30 percent.

Many cases requiring hysteroscopic myomectomy also have infertility problems. Overall, the pregnancy rates are about 60 percent. The Table 11.2 summaries 10 studies done between 1990 to 2001. The study sizes varied between 12 to 59 patients and the pregnancy rates ranged from 16 to 67 percent. The birth delivery rates occurred from a low of 10 percent to a high of 67 percent.

REFERENCES

1. Wallach EE, Vlahos NF. Uterine myomas: An overview of development, clinical features, and management. Obstet Gynecol 2004;104(2):393-406.
2. Murase E, Siegelman ES, Outwater EK, et al. Uterine leiomyomas: Histopathologic features, MR imaging findings, differential diagnosis, and treatment. Radiographics 1999;19(5):1179-97.
3. Donnez J, Mathieu PE, Bassil S, et al. Fibroids: Management and treatment. The State of the Art. Hum Reprod 1996;11:1837-40.
4. Valle RF. Hysteroscopic removal of submucous leiomyomas. J Gynecol Surg 1990;6:89-96.
5. Corson SL, Brooks PG. Resectoscopic myomectomy. Fertil Steril 1991;55:1041-4.
6. Hucke J, Campo RL, De Bruyne F, Freikha AA. Hysteroscopic resection of submucous myoma. Geburtshilfe Frauenheilkd, 1992;52:214-8.
7. Goldenberg M, Sivan E, Sharabi Z, et al. Outcome of hysteroscopic resection of submucous myoma for infertility. Fertil Steril 1995;64:714-6.
8. Preutthipan S, Theppisai U. Hysteroscopic resection of submucous myomas: Results of 50 procedures at Ramathibodi Hospital. J Med Assoc Thai 1998;81:190-4.
9. Giatras K, Berkeley AS, Noyes N, et al. Fertility after hysteroscopic resection of submucous myoma. J Am Assoc Gynecol Laparosc 1999;6:155-8.
10. Varasteh NN, Neuwirth RS, Levin B, Keltz MD. Pregnancy rates after hysteroscopic polypectomy and myomectomy in infertile women. Obstet Gynecol 1999;94:168-71.
11. Vercellini P, Zaina B, Yaylayan L, et al. Hysteroscopic myomectomy: Long-term effects on menstrual pattern and fertility. Obstet Gynecol 1999;94:341-7.
12. Hernandez F, Sefrioui O, Virelizier C, Gervaise A, Gomel V, Frydman R. Hysteroscopic resection of submucosal myomas in patients with infertility. Hum Reprod 2001;16(7):1489-92.

12 Laparoscopic Myomectomy

Christopher Chen

INTRODUCTION

Uterine fibroids, also known as leiomyomas or myomas, are benign growths composed primarily of smooth muscle. Their frequency varies but is found to be present among at least 25 percent of women.[1]

They are usually asymptomatic but some present with menorrhagia, metrorrhagia, pain, and pressure effects on the bladder or rectum. They are frequently present in women with infertility or repeat abortions. Between 27 to 40 percent of women with multiple fibroids are found to be infertile.[1] The incidence of spontaneous abortion secondary to fibroids is possibly 2 times the incidence in the normal population.[1]

Fibroids may be present as solitary growths or as multiple ones. They do not remain static in size but tend to be progressive in their growth, ultimately becoming very large, e.g. 22 weeks pregnancy size.

Fibroids may grow from various locations in the uterus and are classified as subserous, intramural, or submucous.

Traditionally laparotomy with open myomectomy is still widely practised.[2] Most of these gynecologists cite the concerns of fear of intraoperative technical difficulties, and hemorrhage with laparoscopic myomectomy. There is apprehension over the ultimate status of the uterine scar after laparoscopic repair. They also express uncertainty about the occurrence of postoperative adhesion formation, especially with gut and omentum. They doubt the reproductive performance after laparoscopic surgery, and the possibility of recurrence of the fibroid(s).

Clearly these concerns apply, whether the myomectomy is done by laparotomy or laparoscopy. The results of the surgery must be influenced by the skill of the surgeon.

Compared to laparotomy, laparoscopic myomectomy when skillfully done, results in less blood loss, very little need for hospitalization, fewer complications, a speedier recovery, and a superior cosmetic scar.[3-9] The majority of patients are treated as day surgery cases and go home the same day.

PATIENT SELECTION AND PREPARATION

Contrary to concerns over the maximum size of fibroids that can be dealt with by laparoscopy, the limiting factor is the depth of vision and the available space for the performance of the myomectomy. A practical maximum size may be about 16 weeks pregnancy size. Fibroids in excess of this size will require to be shrunk down to this size at least. This can be achieved using gonadotropin releasing hormone (GnRH), agonist long-acting such as Zoladex, which will reduce the fibroid size after 3 to 4 monthly injections.[3] The maximum percentage reduction in size is about 50, after this period of medical therapy. There is no further significant reduction even if treatment is carried beyond this period.

The clinical diagnosis of uterine fibroid is always confirmed by pelvic ultrasound. Their number, size, and location are thus determined. If necessary magnetic resonance imaging (MRI) may also be performed.

Patients with large fibroids tend to be anemic. Their hemoglobin should be measured, and if anemic, treated with hematinics and the hemoglobin levels brought up to safe levels before embarking on surgery as inevitably there will be bleeding and blood loss during the surgery.

CLINICAL STUDY

A study was performed at my Center involving women who presented with fibroids exceeding 4 cm in diameter on transvaginal ultrasound scanning. May of these patients presented with very large intramural fibroids which were quite challenging and daunting to remove laparoscopically, their sizes varying from 12 to 20 weeks pregnancy size. Indeed many surgeons would have opted to do a laparotomy instead. Their clinical presentation included infertility, a history of miscarriage, a complaint of a swelling in the abdomen which was increasing in size, heavy menstruation, whilst some of them were simply detected during routine gynecological check-up. My experience is that many of these women with very large fibroids have associated anemia which required to be corrected before surgery. Large sized fibroids were reduced by depot GnRH analogue, e.g. Zoladex. A total of 250 patients were treated with an age range between 18 and 55.

LAPAROSCOPIC MYOMECTOMY TECHNIQUE

The myomectomy operation performed in the study involves the patient as a day surgery case unless she requires admission, frequently for not more than one night in hospital.

The patient has a general anesthetic and is positioned in the lithotomy and Trendelenburg's position.

The bladder is catheterized after antiseptic cleansing of the abdominal skin, vulva, and vagina.

The cervix is grasped with a vulsellum and the uterine cavity sounded, followed by cervical dilatation to Hegar 6, allowing entry of a flexible hysteroscope. The uterine cavity is examined using a 3-chip camera and TV monitoring system.

The tubular orifices are identified on each side of the cavity and submucous fibroids looked for and to be dealt with by hysteroscopic myomectomy (see chapter on **Hysteroscopic Myomectomy**). The fallopian tubes are dye hydrotubated through the hysteroscope if infertility is an issue.

The operation then proceeds to the next stage, that of laparoscopy. A sharp Veress needle is inserted, taking care to puncture away from the uterus which is already enlarged. Carbon dioxide is insufflated to completely distend the abdomen. There must be loss of liver and splenic dullness. A 5 mm trocar is inserted through the umbilicus, after appropriate toilet and removal of dirt. No incision is made. The laparoscope is inserted through the trocar and a 3-chip video camera then attached to the laparoscope for detailed viewing and appraisal on the TV monitor.

The size of the uterus with its fibroid(s) is assessed in order to determine the site to make the lateral puncture holes (5 mm sizes) for use of the operative instruments. Where possible, the round ligaments, fallopian tubes, ovaries, and pouch of Douglas are examined for their health and status. Sometimes, the sizes of the fibroids may prevent a full examination to be performed at this stage.

To minimise bleeding, vasopressin may be injected into the uterine muscle but it has a limited duration of effect on uterine vasospasm.

Having determined the accessibility of the fibroids for myomectomy, the operation proceeds. Small fibroids are not problematical but large ones reduce the depth of vision so that visualization of the growths appears too near and too magnified. This causes a lack of spatial orientation on the part of the surgeon and a lack of space to perform the operation.

Strategies for the Myomectomy

Therefore, before one makes the first incision into the fibroid(s), careful decisive planning of the surgical steps are crucial toward a successful operation. The first principle is to remove the first few fibroids to improve and increase space for the continuation of the surgery. This can then lead to eventual complete removal of all the fibroids. In order that the fibroids do not become lost in the abdomen, it is wise to suture and string them along for their later removal through the trocar punctures. The second principle is skillful and speedy surgery, as there is a finite time of hemostasis before the effect of the vasopressin wears off. The third principle is to minimise bleeding and blood loss. This can be achieved by the administration of vasopressin, skillful suturing and repair, and good rapid knot-tying techniques. Where bleeding is profuse and extensive, the operation field becomes bloody and covered over with blood which hampers continuation of the surgery. Blood loss can pose a danger to the patient and can result in shock and potential mortality.

As the myomectomy proceeds, it may be judicious to suture the bed after the fibroid removal to stop bleeding. Where bleeding is profuse, packing the bed with surgicel and then suturing the bed will control the blood loss.

As each fibroid is removed, more and more space appears so that the surgery can proceed more easily with the new found room available, until all the fibroids are removed.

Procedure of Myomectomy

The uterine covering capsule over the fibroid may be incised, using a choice of approaches, and a needle point diathermy for cutting purposes. A transverse incision can be made and the fibroid removed. A cruciate incision may be more appropriate if the fibroid were larger to enable its enucleation. The most often-used is a circular incision followed by its extraction. An incision made somewhat transversely can convert into a "hood" for suture over the raw bed after removal of the fibroid should the raw surface be large and require covering it.

The fibroid is removed in a variety of ways. It can be extracted using a screw or claw. As the tumor is being shelled out of its bed, a bipolar electrode diathermises both tissue and blood vessels attached to its surface to minimise blood loss. The resulting bed is repaired in a purse-string fashion using Ethicon PDS II CT suture. The uterine wall, after completion of the myomectomy, is examined for the presence of any deep-seated ones and then incised into for their removal.

Large **submucous fibroids** that are too big for hysteroscopic myomectomy can be extracted by the laparoscopic approach after cutting through the uterine wall and pulling the growth out by using the myomectomy screw or claw. The endometrial cavity is carefully closed using a purse-string vicryl suture and the overlying myometrium sutured using PDS, also in purse-string fashion.

At the completion of the whole operation of myomectomy, the fibroids are taken out of the abdomen with an electric morcellator. Depending on the size of the fibroids, a 10 mm, 15 mm, or 20 mm instrument may be selected. The original 5 mm lateral trocar puncture wound is enlarged to accommodate the instrument. Great care is taken to avoid any injury to gut and other structures during the morcellation as the rotating blades can cause serious injury to these organs.

At conclusion of the whole surgery, the uterus is checked for any bleeding wounds and further sutures put in place to secure hemostasis. A thorough peritoneal toilet is done and where necessary, Interceed is used to cover any raw surfaces. Dexamethasone is instilled over the Interceed. The use of both of these materials helps minimise adhesion formation.

The patient is given intraoperative and followed by postoperative antibiotics for about 5 days.

The lateral abdominal puncture wounds are sutured, except the umbilical which is too deeply-seated and too small to require this. (A video recording of the technique of laparoscopic myomectomy accompanying this book can be viewed).

Four specific examples of my myomectomy technique among the 250 patients in the study are described. (Please view the enclosed DVD when reading the text).

Example 1 A patient presented with large fibroids measuring about 10 cm in diameter in one of them. A circular serosal incision was made towards the base of the fibroid in a circumferential manner. Using the claw, the fibroid was progressively enucleated and then cut off from its base attachment by electrocoagulation. The same technique was used for the rest of them. Deep purse-string sutures using No. 1 vicryl were introduced to repair the myometrial defect, as well as strengthening the myometrial wall. The defect was further mended by introducing a series of stitches to form a purse-string, resulting in a complete closure of the wound with hardly any raw surface exposed, thereby minimising adhesion formation, especially that with the colon and omentum. The fibroids were removed using an electric morcellator (Figure 12.1).

Example 2 Another huge fibroid growing from the posterior wall of the uterus. To minimise blood loss a circumferential sub-serosal suture was introduced towards the base of the fibroid and tied. A circumferential circular incision was made over the fibroid. The fibroid was progressively enucleated. The uterine defect was sutured using a series of sutures initially in longitudinal fashion, and then the raw surfaces being drawn together in such a way that very minimal exposure of raw surfaces resulted. The fibroid was morcellated and removed (Figure 12.2).

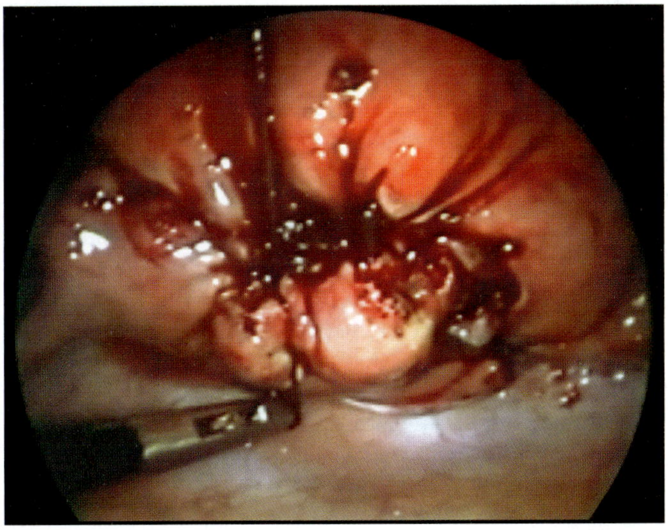

Figure 12.1. Deep purse-string sutures closing uterine wound

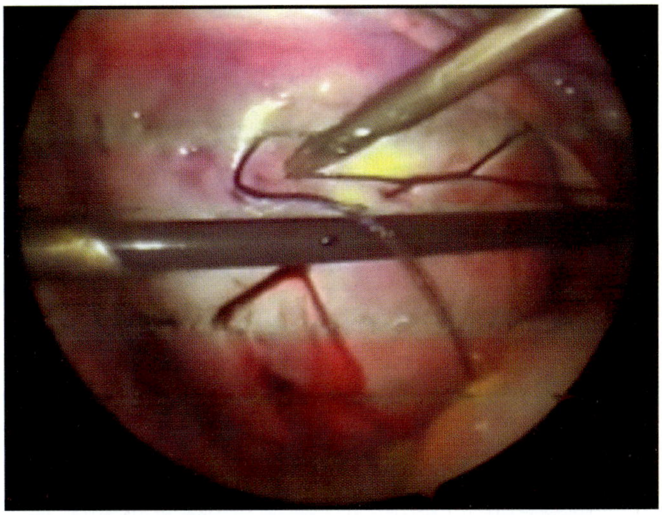

Figure 12.2. Tourniquet suture at base of large fibroid to reduce bleeding during myomectomy

Example 3 Another example of a large uterine fibroid measuring approximately 12 cm in diameter arising from the anterior wall of the uterus. Again, because of its size and vascularity the base of attachment of the fibroid was sutured using purse-string type sutures, tightening the sutures as the operation proceeded in order to achieve a tourniquet-like effect thereby minimising blood loss. The fibroid was removed and the defect progressively repaired and closed, again leaving very little raw surfaces which would attract adhesion formation. The blood loss was minimal (Figure 12.3).

Example 4 Large submucous fibroids that were too large to be removed by hysteroscopy were removed by the laparoscopic approach through an incision into the uterus and enucleating the fibroid using a claw. The endometrium and uterine incision were closed.

RESULTS OF THE STUDY

All 250 patients had their laparoscopic surgery successfully completed. There were none that required conversion to laparotomy.

The sizes of the fibroids ranged from 4 to greater than 20 cm, and the numbers removed per patient varied between 1 and 22. Some presented as an enlarging abdominal mass, others caused bladder pressure and

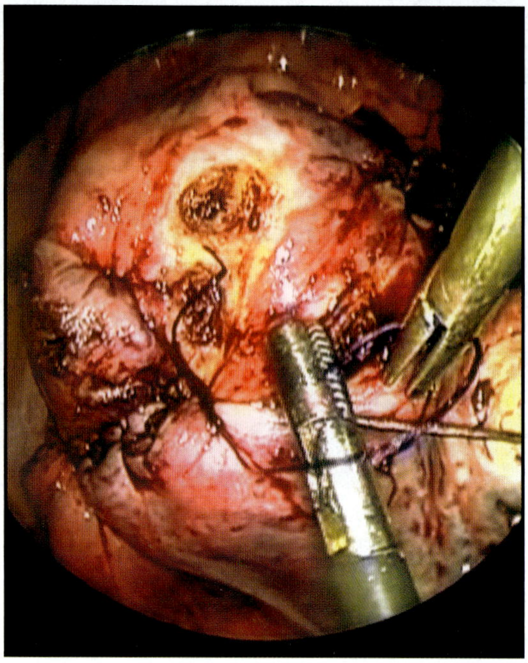

Figure 12.3. Purse-string sutures close defect in uterine wound

frequency of micturition, whilst still others produced rectal pressure and constipation. The larger fibroids and submucous ones caused menorrhagia and severe anemia.

On the average the operations were completed between 2 to 3 hours but the longest took 6 hours.

The average surgical blood loss was about 300 ml. But those with large fibroids lost as much as a liter of blood. However, there were no cases of hemorrhagic shock.

Recovery from the surgery was excellent and uneventful in all the patients. The convalescent time varied between 3 days to 1 week. They were having sexual intercourse 3 to 4 weeks later, and returned to work within a week to two. Because of the absence of a laparotomy wound and only small puncture holes their cosmetic result was excellent.

All the patients made an excellent recovery. I did not encounter any complications of the surgery itself or infection. No patients experienced uterine rupture or recurrence of fibroids during this period of study.

CONCLUSION

Laparoscopic myomectomy is an operation that is feasible for all sizes of fibroids, large and small. It replaces the need for laparotomy but requires the development of skill and experience by the surgeon. It is a safe operation, without complications, when skillfully done. Postoperative discomfort is minimal, patient acceptance is very high. There is also the advantage of cost savings, earlier ambulation, and a speedy return to the workforce. There is therefore much to recommend this method of myomectomy.

REFERENCES

1. Memarzadeh S, Broder MS, Wexler AS, Pernoll ML. Benign disorders of the uterine corpus. In DeCherney AH, Nathan L (Eds): Current Obstetric and Gynecologic Diagnosis and Treament, 9th edition. New York: Lange Medical Books; 2003;693-9.
2. Wallach EE. Myomectomy. In Thompson JD, Rock JA (Eds): Te Linde's Operative Gynecology, 7th edition. Philadelphia: JB Lippincott Co; 1992;647-62.
3. Chen C, Chua BL. Laparoscopic myomectomy and morcellation of huge fibroids. XXXIII World Congress of the International College of Surgeons. 2002, Taipei, Taiwan; Monduzzi Editore; 2002;273-6.
4. Nezhat C, Nezhat F, Silfen SL, et al. Laparoscopic myomectomy. Int J Fertil 1991;36(5):275-80.
5. Nezhat C, Nezhat F, Bess O, et al. Laparoscopically assisted myomectomy: A report of a new technique in 57 cases. Int J Fertil Menopausal Stud 1994;39(1):39-44.
6. Nezhat FR, Roemisch M, Nezhat CH, et al. Recurrence rate after laparoscopic myomectomy. J Am Assoc Gynecol Laparosc 1998;5(3):237-40.
7. Dubuisson JB, Chapron C. Laparoscopic myomectomy today. A good technique when correctly indicated. Hum Repro 1996;11(5):934-5.
8. Parker WH, Rodi IA. Patient selection for laparoscopic myomectomy. J Am Assoc Gynecol Laparosc 1994;2(1): 23-6.
9. Sinha R, Hegde A, Warty N, Patil N. Laparoscopic excision of very large myomas. J Am Assoc Gynecol Laparosc 2003; 10(4):461-8.

13 Laparoscopic Assisted Minilap Myomectomy

Nutan Jain

Myoma uteri are the most common benign uterine tumors encountered in gynecological patients. The incidence now appears to be higher due to better diagnostic facilities like high resolution transvaginal ultrasonography, CT and MRI. Novak et al[1] reported an incidence of 20-25 percent of sexually active and 30-35 percent of all women irrespective of their age. Other studies indicate an even higher incidence, stating that 20-30 percent[2,3] women above the age of 35 have at least one myoma. Another study noted leiomyoma in 50 percent of the females examined at the time of autopsy. A genetic and racial predisposition also exists, women of African origin have 3 to 9 times greater risk of developing uterine fibroids than Caucasian women who are more likely to have myomas compared to women of Asian origin. Overall myomas are responsible for about one-third of all gynecological admissions to hospital services.[4]

Most common indications for removal of fibroids are menorrhagia, pain and infertility. Patients in the younger age group with infertility often present symptomatic or at times big myomas without any symptoms. Their reason for seeking gynecological consultation is only infertility and myomas are diagnosed during the course of investigations. Other patients may present menorrhagia, which could be worse with pain and clots, short cycles amounting to loss of work and affecting day-to-day activities. Yet another presentation would be pain due to pressure symptoms or degenerating myomas. Pressure symptoms develop due to large myomas and size of the myomas increases rapidly.[5] Earlier the only treatment for myomas was hysterectomy, but now more recently, there has been a shift towards preserving the uterus and removing only the myoma. This has been possible with the advent of newer technologies which target the destruction of the myoma alone like myolysis.[6,7] Cryomyolysis and embolization[8,9] and laparoscopic uterine artery ligation.[10]

INDICATIONS

The most common indications of myomectomy appear to be:

1. Desire to conserve the uterus.
2. Severe menorrhagia.
3. Large myoma or multiple in number.
4. Pressure symptoms leading to abdominal pain.
5. Rapidly growing myomas.
6. Myomectomy for infertility in following situations.
   a. Altered tubo-ovarian relationship.
   b. Intracavitary fibroids.
   c. Significantly large, multiple intramural myomas.
   d. Cornual fibroids, pressing upon the utero-tubal junction.
   e. As an opportunity to assess other coexisting pelvic factors like, endometriosis and PID.

Compared to open myomectomy the occurrence of postoperative peritubal adhesions has been found to be

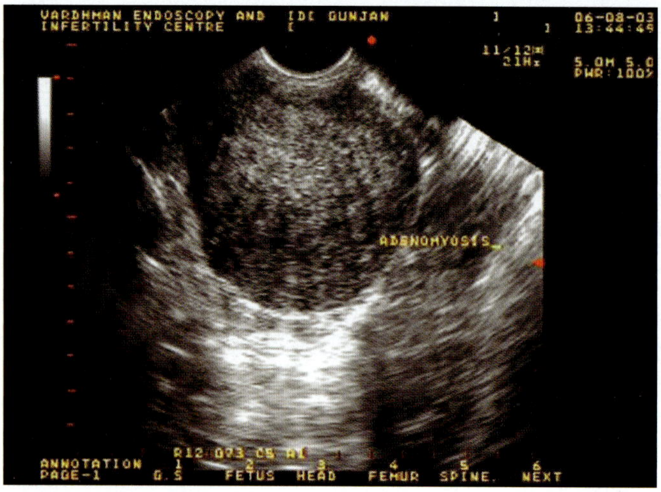

Figure 13.1A. Adenomyosis

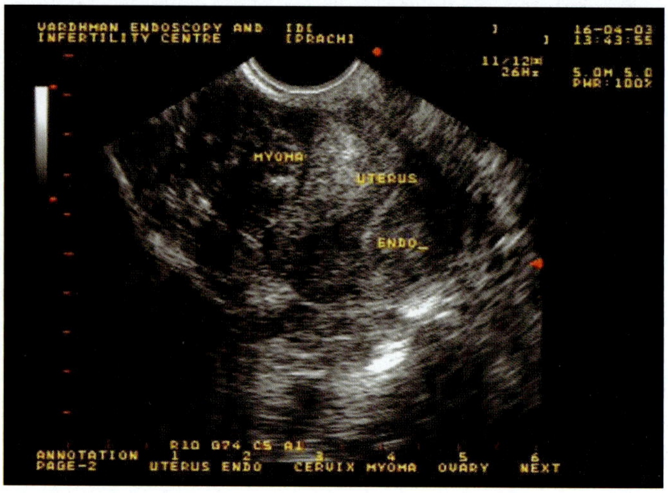

Figure 13.1B. Myoma

relatively low at 9.8 percent which shows that laparoscopic myomectomy or laparoscopic assisted myomectomy contributes to maintaining postoperative fertility. This along with the benefits of minimally invasive surgery are the main reasons for choosing them for the management of myomas.[11]

PREOPERATIVE EVALUATION

All patients must undergo a thorough sonography, which should be a combination of per abdomen, transvaginal and color Doppler sonography. It is mandatory to know the exact site, size, location and number of myomas. I attach so much significance to this that I always do it preoperatively myself to offset any chances of misdiagnosis between a myoma and an adenomyoma (Figures 13.1A and B).[12-15] I feel that preoperative workup before myomectomy is the single largest factor which determines the successful outcome of this technically demanding surgery. CT scan and MRI could be indicated in the face of multiple myomas to verify their location more precisely.

Size and number of myomas to be removed via laparoscopic route—laparoscopic myomectomy is definitely not for novices in the field of laparoscopy. It require greater skills and manual dexterity to complete a multilayer, sound anatomic closure of the myoma bed. For this reason alone, many authors have laid down guidelines regarding the size and number of myomas over which myomectomy should not be performed laparoscopically. All this appears due to the anatomical distortions provided by multiple fibroids and difficulty in suturing multiple myoma sites.[16] Though now several literature reports are appearing for laparoscopic myomectomy for large myomas.[17]

Keeping in mind the technical difficulties in enucleating and removing large myomas and most importantly, suturing the multiple, large myoma beds with precision such that they can bear the stretch and tension of subsequent pregnancy and labor, the concept of LAM (Laparoscopic Assisted Myomectomy) has come.[18-22] When posed with large and multiple fibroids and a surgeon having lesser technical skills this hybrid surgery becomes a very feasible option. A 12 cm myoma could be within the suturing skills of one surgeon but for another it may become too large to enucleate, remove and suture. So the indications for LAM appear to be relative, according to the surgeon's expertise. By and large the indications for LAM are:

i. Uterus size more than 20-22 cm (Figures 13.2A and B).
ii. Multiple, large myomas.
iii. Single, very large myoma.

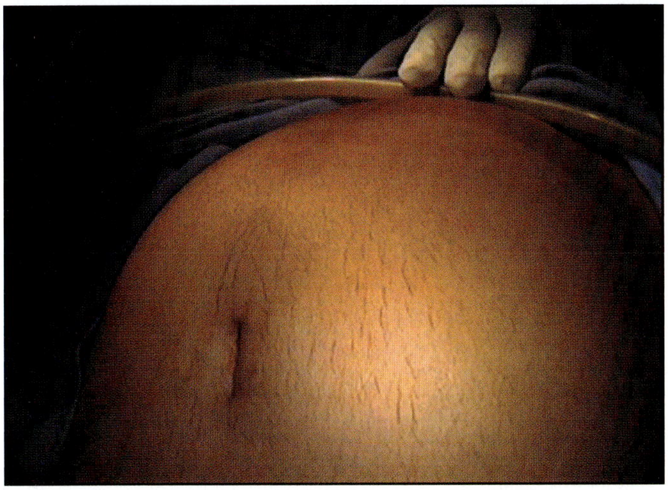

Figure 13.2A. Per abdomen picture of 26 wks size uterus

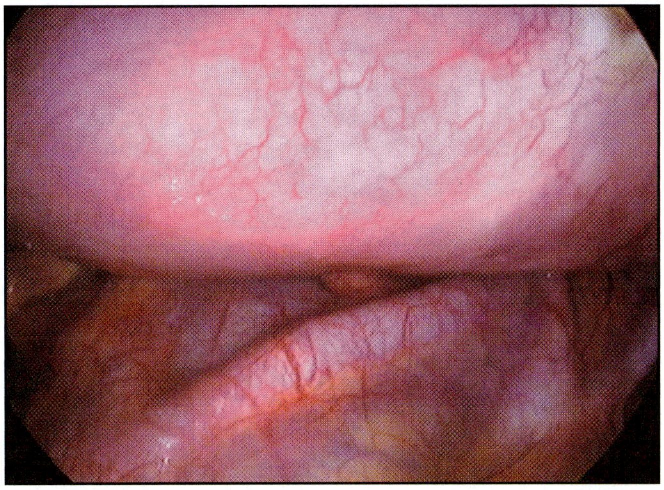

Figure 13.2B. Big myoma overlying the aortic bifurcation

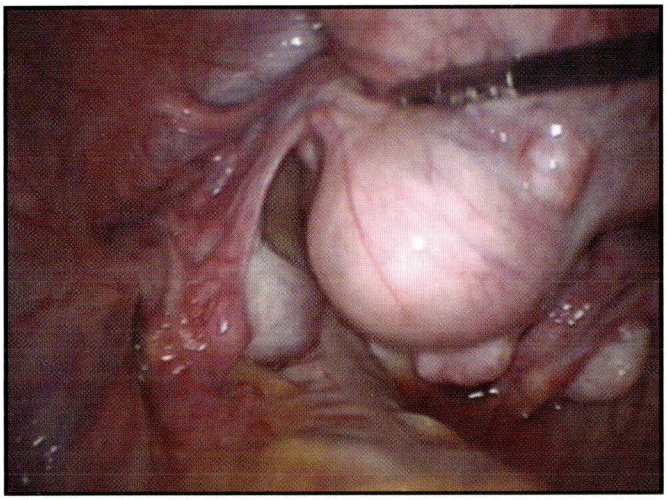

Figure 13.3A. Deep posterior wall myoma

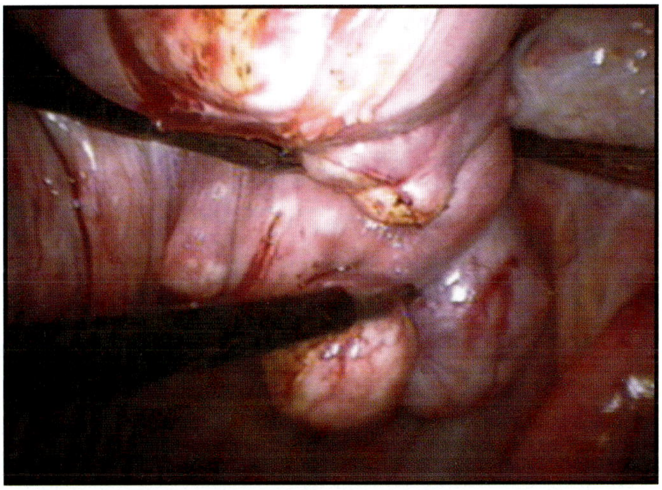

Figure 13.3B. Deep posterior wall myoma

iv. Myomas in more technically demanding positions like very deep posterior myomas (Figures 13.3A and B).

v. Any time when a surgeon is less versed in suturing and does not have access to a morcelator, and then he may choose to remove myoma by minilap incision.

Pretreatment with GnRH agonists before myomectomy remains controversial. In a systematic review of randomized, controlled trials of the use of GnRH analogs before hysterectomy and myomectomy, it was found that preoperative and postoperative blood counts were improved by GnRH agonist therapy, uterine and myoma volume decreased, and operative time and blood loss were reduced.[23] Reduction in leiomyoma size makes the procedure less time consuming because a smaller uterine incision can be made and less morcellation is required. The individual myomas, however, are softer, which often results in the Lahey clamps tearing through the tissue resulting in the loss of upward traction. This can result in increased bleeding. We have never used GnRH analogs in our practice, as I believe that removing a 10 cm or a 14 cm myoma does not make any difference if we work in a correct anatomical plane with a sound surgical technique.

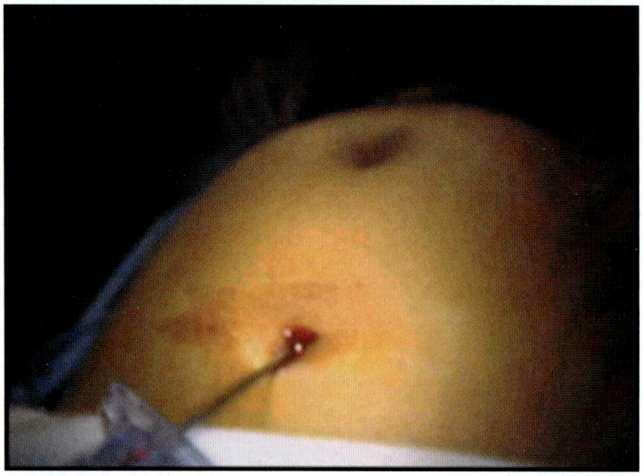

Figure 13.4. Veress needle insertion just beneath the xiphisternum

Procedure

Patient under GA, with nasogastric tube.

a. Modified lithotomy.

b. Primary umbilical port is shifted higher up anywhere between the umbilicus and xiphisternum according to the size of the myomas (Figure 13.4).

c. All accessory ports (3-4 in number) made higher up to accommodate the large and multiple myomas and make the enucleation easier.

d. After entry, a thorough inspection of entire pelvis is done and the preoperative scan findings are validated. Exact size and site of myoma is documented. In an Infertility patient all attempts are made to do gentle adhesiolysis and normalize the tube ovarian anatomy. Careful search is done to look for foci of endometriosis, which are fulgurated (Figure 13.5). A chromopertubation is done to check for tubal patency (Figure 13.6).

e. One ampoule of Pitressin diluted in about 100 ml of saline is injected subserosally in all the myomas.[24] It is important to enter the exact plane and inject a sufficient amount as Pitressin acts not only by decreasing bleeding from myoma bed but also by developing a handy plane of cleavage between the pseudo capsule and myoma. Since in minilap there are usually too many and large myomas, we dilute 1 amp of Pitressin in about 100 ml saline.

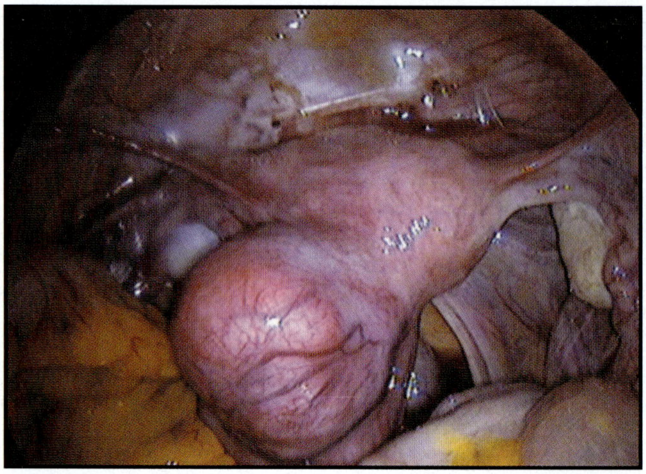

Figure 13.5. Endometriosis of UV pouch with sub serous myoma

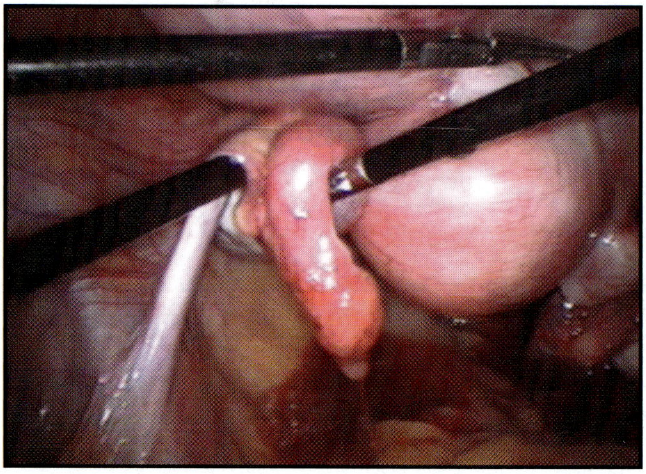

Figure 13.6. Chromopertubation before myomectomy

f. After injecting Pitressin I proceed to do a diagnostic hysteroscopy, which provides sufficient time for the Pitressin to be therapeutically effective. Hysteroscopy usually confirms the findings of prior transvaginal sonography.

SUBMUCOUS MYOMA

Fedele and colleagues[25] evaluated the accuracy of TVS in detection of small submucous myomas in patients who underwent both TVS and hysteroscopy. The sensitivity and specificity of TVS and hysteroscopy was same, TVS having sensitivity of 100 percent and specificity of 94

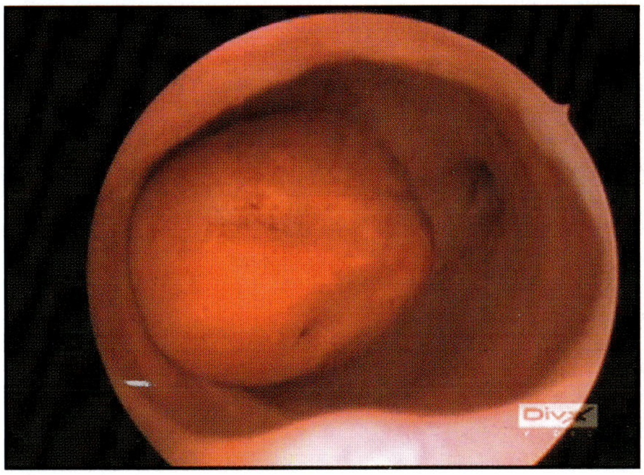

Figure 13.7. Fibroid polyps

percent and Hysteroscopy having sensitivity of 100 percent and specificity of 96 percent. The predictive value of an abnormal scan was 81 percent while that of abnormal hysteroscopy was 87 percent. TVS and hysteroscopy have found to have such good correlation and from here comes the reliance on it as a useful[26,27] diagnostic tool in the preoperative assessment of endometrial cavity.

If there is any small polyp (Figure 13.7), which was missed on the scan, it is removed. If there is a bigger myoma 3-4 cm then I prefer to leave it and remove it during the course of minilap myomectomy.

Laparoscopic Procedure

After injecting Pitressin and doing a hysteroscopy, we proceed to make a transverse incision on the biggest myoma. Transverse incision is usually preferred as it causes less blood loss since the incision goes in the line of radial arteries as they emerge from the uterine arteries (Figures 13.8A to F). A monopolar cautery hook or spatula is used to make and deepen the incision. Tissue harmonic scalpel can also be used. The myoma enucleation is started as soon as we reach the pearly white myoma. A myoma screw is applied over the most bulging part of myoma and enucleation progresses by means of sharp scissors dissection and preventive, prophylactic cautery by bipolar coagulation. This gives speed to the dissection. Thorough suction irrigation and lavage helps to keep the surgical field clear. Since now we will proceed for a minilap myomectomy it is not necessary to enucleate the entire myoma, it is rather much easier to let it remain attached to the uterus hooked by the myoma screw which makes it removal by minilap incision much easier and faster.

I personally prefer making incisions overall bulging myomas before proceeding for minilap myomectomy. Even a moderately deep, transverse incision made by monopolar cautery allows for a quick enucleation by a finger when minilap incision is given. As the incisions are made by monopolar cautery in the exact cleavage plane after injecting Pitressin, the incisions do not bleed. Hence, there is a no risk in giving incisions overall the myomas and then proceed for minilap incision.

Before proceeding to make a small 3-4 cm minilap incision, we ensure that, laparoscopically.

1. All myomas are conclusively located.
2. Their number is ascertained so that we can remove all.
3. All adhesiolysis, completed, chromopertubation done.
4. Biggest myoma is enucleated to some extent and myoma screw applied to it.
5. All other myomas have a transverse incision, which makes their location via minilap much easier and quicker, especially the deep posterior myomas.

Now with CO_2 pneumoperitoneum, a small 3 cm transverse incision is made just above the pubic hairline. The trick is to keep the skin incision smaller but to advance the rectus sheath incision 1-2 cm beyond the skin incision margins. This instantly gives a lot of space to work within. Some surgeons prefer to give a cruciate incision. Meaning thereby, that, the skin incision is transverse but the rectus sheath is opened vertically to a length of 6 cm by tunneling with a finger bluntly under the subcutaneous fat cranially towards umbilicus and caudally towards pubic bone. The myoma screw is already on the myoma so the peritoneum is incised vertically along it to quickly reach the largest myoma. Using a combination of vaginal manipulation, traction

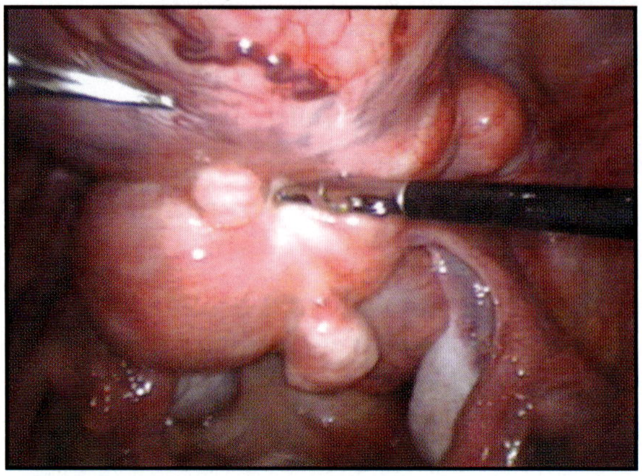

Figure 13.8A. Initial appearance of myoma

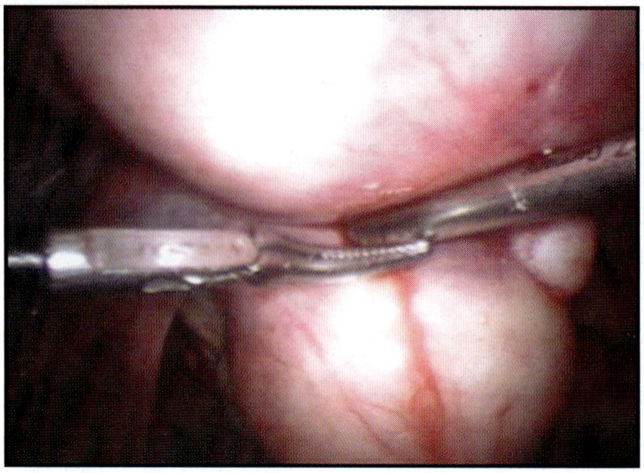

Figure 13.8B. Injecting Pitressin

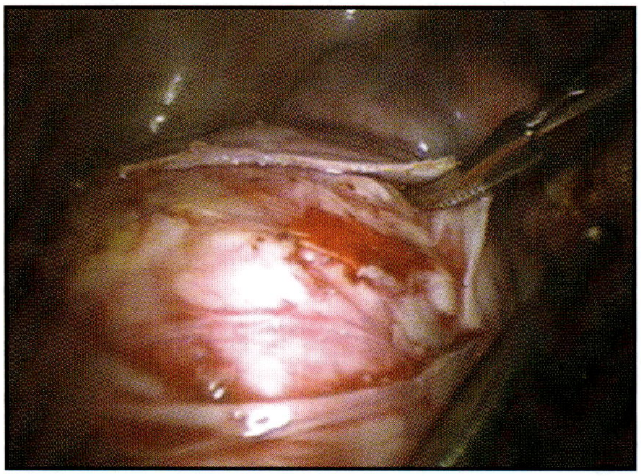

Figure 13.8C. Transverse incision

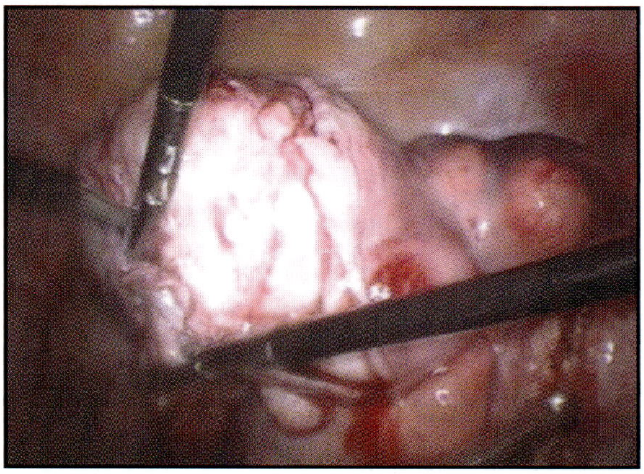

Figure 13.8D. Enucleation of myoma

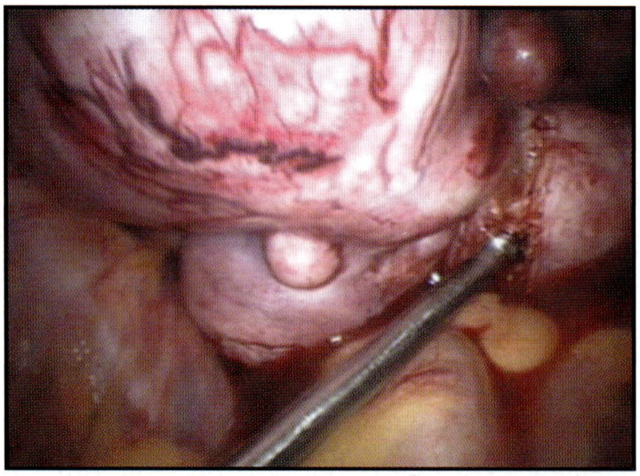

Figure 13.8E. Myoma screw applied over the posterior myoma

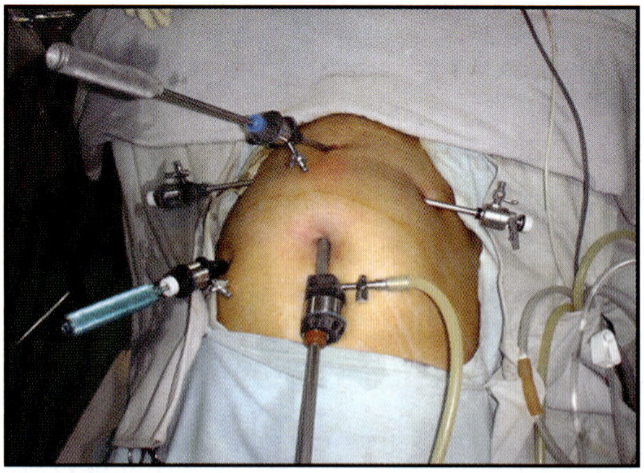

Figure 13.8F. Placing the two myoma screws, one over the largest myoma through the suprapubic port and other over the deepest posterior myoma through the left paraumbilical port

by myoma screw and surgeon's finger or knife handle, the myoma is enucleated . If it is too large we start reducing it piecemeal by cutting chunks of myoma using a conventional knife and keep removing them. Major debulking by cutting chunks of myoma tissue is done before removing a big myoma, so that the skin incision is not unduly widened. If we proceed patiently, it usually does not take too long, and adhering to the surgical plane causes hardly any bleeding. If at all the big myoma bed bleeds too much, then myometrial bed closure is done before proceeding to remove the other myomas. This is accomplished by using 1-0 vicryl on a curved needle. Very efficient closure can be done in two to three layers, starting from the base of myoma. Then the top most layer including subserosa and serosa is closed by 3-0 vicryl.

After making the peritoneal opening the CO_2 pneumoperitoneum is turned off. Now the procedure continues by the minilap route. One by one, all myomas are enucleated and removed by utilizing a tenaculum and surgeon's finger. After having first removed the biggest myoma, the smaller ones come out much more easily as the incision is widened by the removal of the first myoma. Irrigation and lavage continues by abdominal route. Suturing is done meticulously, trying to give a sound anatomic closure (Figures 13.9A to F), which will endure the stress of pregnancy and labor. All measures are taken to decrease adhesion formation like.

1. Minimal tissue trauma by gentle handling.
2. Avoidance of tissue drying.
3. Decreasing blood loss by controlled preventive bipolar coagulation and working in correct tissue planes.
4. Thorough suction irrigation and lavage to keep field clear.
5. Meticulous closure and use of fine sutures over the serosa.

I do not use any adhesion barriers and rely only on the above measures for postoperative reduction in adhesion formation.

After minilap, extraction of myomas and suturing is completed; (Figures 13.10A to C) we suture the small Pfannenstiel's incision and go back laparoscopically for a final inspection and clearing of the peritoneal cavity. All clots, fluids, debris and char is sucked out. All sutured myoma sites are visualized for any bleeding point, which is coagulated by using a bipolar forceps. The magnification offered by operative laparoscopy and the wide field of vision is more superior to minilap, so we routinely spend time on improving the cleanliness of the surgical field by laparoscopic means. At end we instill 2 liters of ringers lactate into the peritoneal cavity. The hospitalization ranges from 24-48 hours during which the patients are fully ambulatory and comfortable. The postoperative course does not appear to differ too much from that of laparoscopic myomectomy.

OTHER TECHNIQUES OF LAM

With technological advancements coming in, minilap myomectomy is carried out with the help of atraumatic elastic retractors with or without laparoscopic guidance. A small 4-6 cm incision is given and the elastic abdominal retractor is put in place.

The benefit of elastic retractor is that it gives a rounded opening in anterior abdominal wall. The retractor is soft and atraumatic to the tissue of the abdominal wall while it keeps subcutaneous fat, muscles and peritoneum out of the operative field. This needs a 4-5 cm incision.[28]

The study by Glasser et al comprises of 139 myomectomies, mean wt of myomas removed is 275 (rage 30-975 gm), 137 where discharged in less than 24 hours. The mean operating time was 110 minutes (rage 44-260 min) EBL (No-200 ml) with mid in of 300 L. Three hysterectomy performed one for hemorrhage and two for recurrent myomas. Pelosi et al[29,30] have described their technique for myomas of extreme sizes. Hand-assisted laparoscopic myomectomy (Figures 13.11A to D) fills the gap between conventional laparoscopic and laparoscopic assisted techniques and laparotomy for the massive fibroids. The ability to use an operative hand results in excellent laparoscopic exposure, effective myoma traction counter traction, digital feel and finer myoma enucleation, removal of myoma and suturing in full three layers. There are several hand-assisted

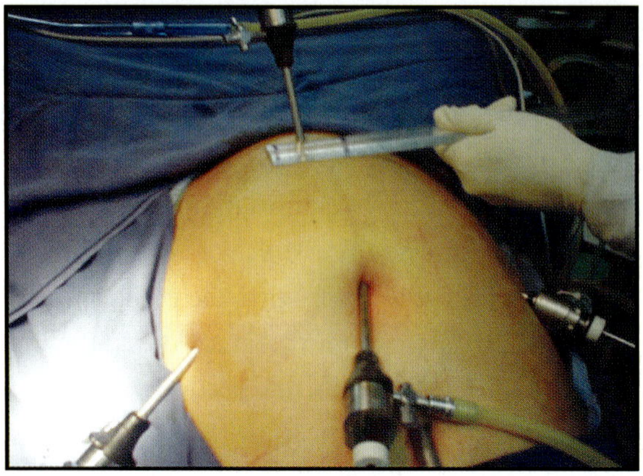

Figure 13.9A. Marking the minilap incision

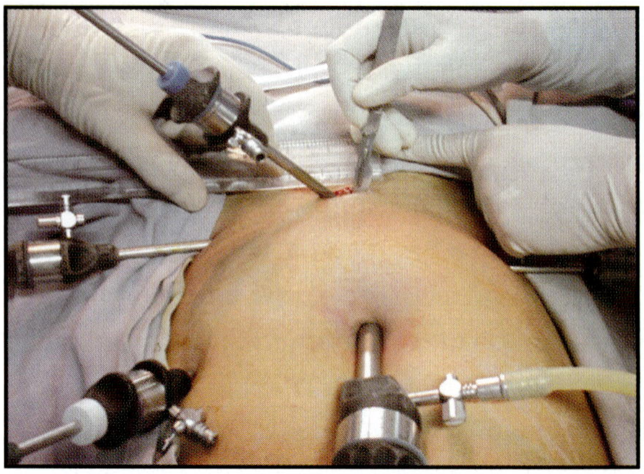

Figure 13.9B. Giving the minilap incision

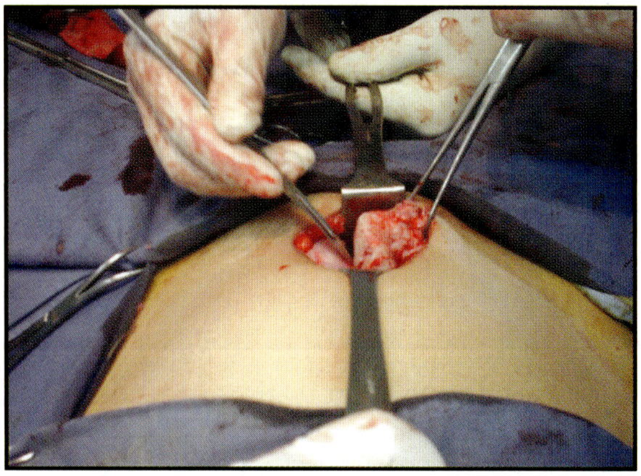

Figure 13.9C. Enucleation of the myoma

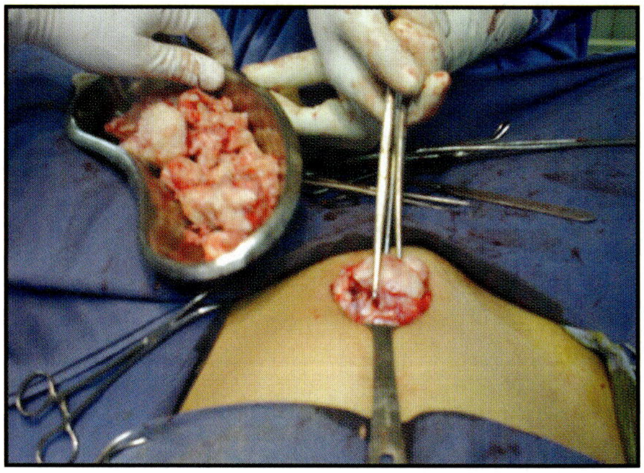

Figure 13.9D. Removing the myoma piecemeal

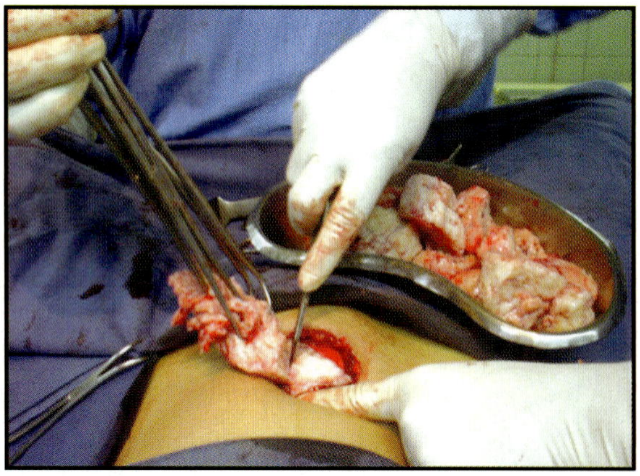

Figure 13.9E. Cutting chunks of myoma using conventional knife

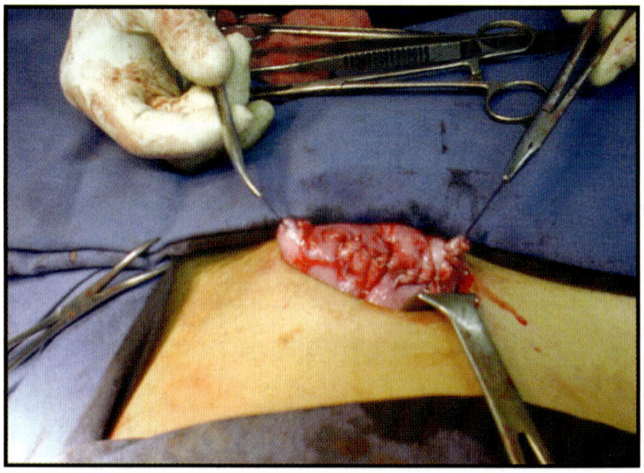

Figure 13.9F. Completed suturing of myoma bed

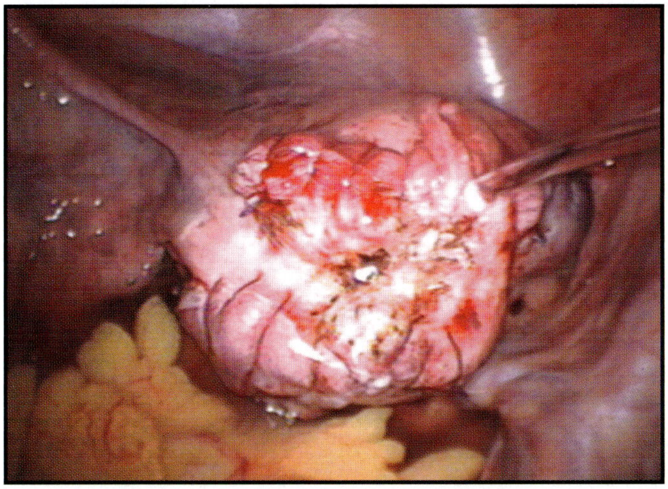

Figure 13.10A. Uterus after completed myomectomy

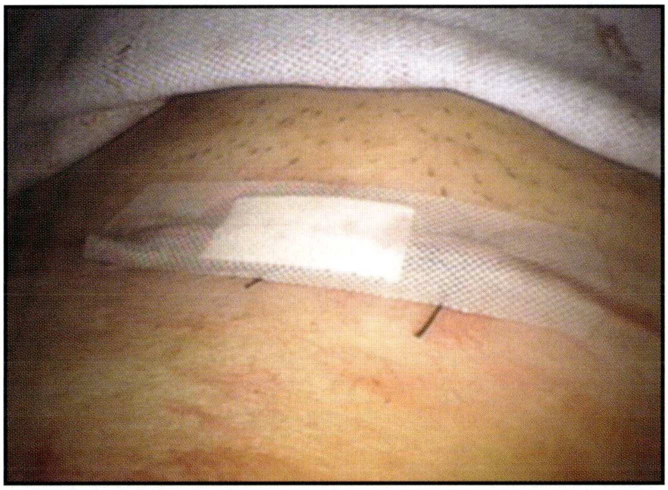

Figure 13.10B. Final appearance of minilap incision

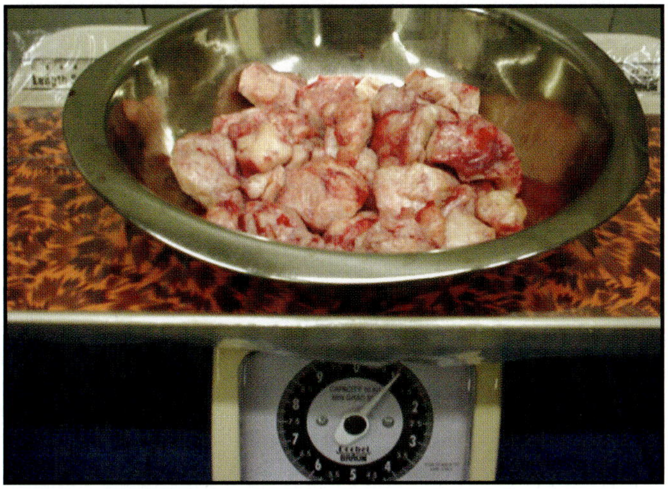

Figure 13.10C. Weight of the myoma

laparoscopic system available. They include the original Dexterity Pneumo Sleeve (Dexterity Surgical Inc., Rosewell, GA), Omniport (Advanced Surgical Concepts, Wicklow, Ireland), Gelport (Applied Medical, Randio Santa Margarita, CA) and the LAP DISC hand access device (Ethicon Endo-Surgery, Inc. Cincinnati, OH). The various systems available for hand-assisted laparoscopies are shown in Figure 13.12. They all provide extracorporeal extension of pneumoperitoneum and abdominal access for the surgeon during laparoscopic surgery, while maintaining constant peritoneal gas pressure.

Difficulties during Minilap Myomectomy

The most common problem that occurs lies in localizing the very deep posterior myomas. Due to the small incision the uterus cannot be hooked anteriorly to a great extent. In this situation, assistance can be taken from the vaginal manipulator but this may also not work at times. Once, I had to go back laparoscopically during a minilap myomectomy to make the incision over the deep posterior myoma. Enucleation and suturing was done by minilap incision. So the best technique is to localize all myomas laparoscopically and make an incision over them laparoscopically, before proceeding for minilap myomectomy, more so for posterior and deep myomas. Anterior myomas are very easily accessible even when situated deep in the myometrium. The second difficulty usually arises with big (15-20 cm) myomas is in their piecemeal removal. With adequate surgical technique and patience there will be no need to widen the incision. It is best to keep tractions on the myoma by stout tenaculums and to keep cutting with a surgical knife whatever myoma is presenting in the minilap incision. Hurrying up this step may unnecessarily widen the incision while pulling out a big myoma.

Another problem could be lost myomas. During the laparoscopic phase of the surgery it is advisable to restrict oneself to only superficially enucleating the myomas and not entirely so that they are not lying free in the pouch of Douglas. While changing the patient's positioning from steep Trendelenburg to routine minilap, the myomas may get lost. So, it is advisable to keep track of the exact

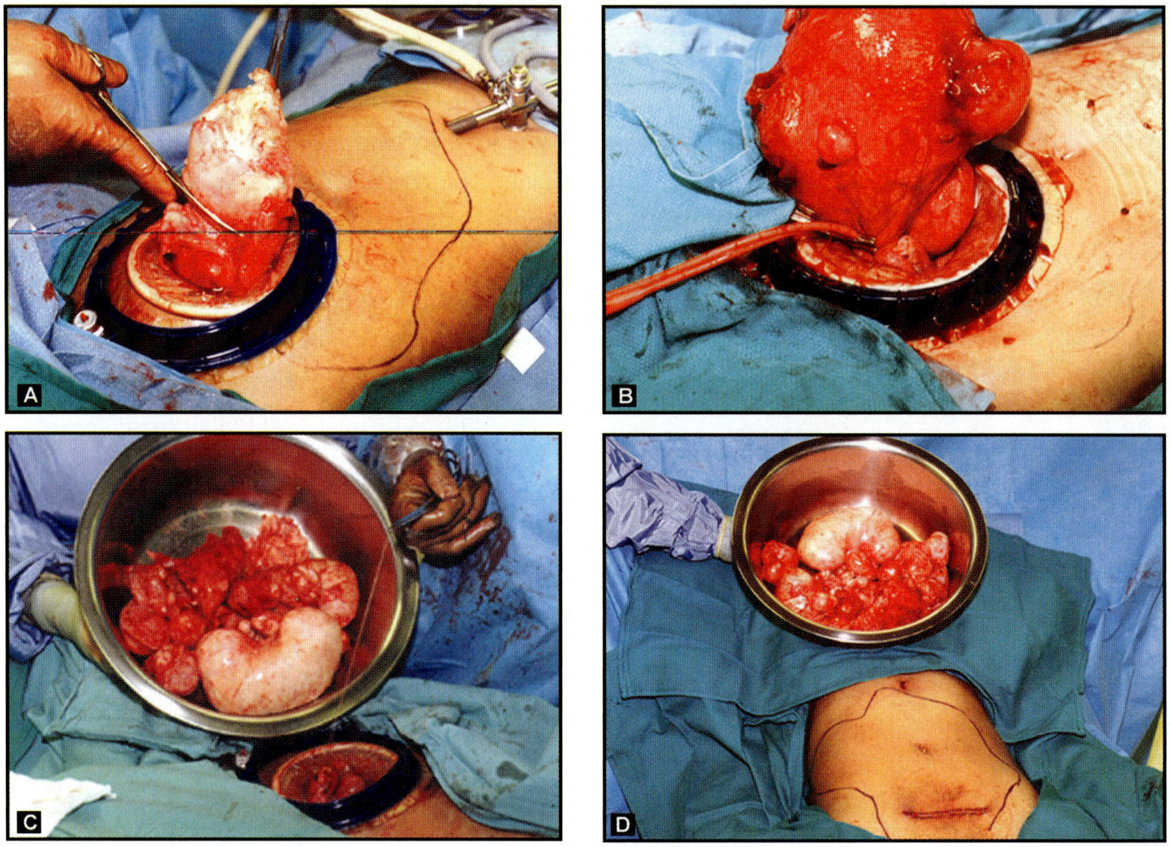

Figures 13.11A to D. Hand-assisted laparoscopic myomectomy. (A) Hand-assisted laparoscopic myomectomy results in a significant reduction in uterine size that allows partial exteriorization through the abdominal incision to continue the myomectomies. This creates a further decrease in uterine size, (B) The debulked uterus is then easily delivered through the incision to complete the myomectomies. A rubber hemostatic tourniquet is routinely used, (C) The uterus is reconstructed using a layered conventional suturing technique, (D) The laparoscopic and the hand-assisted laparoscopic incision are then closed. The total weight of the case example was 3,120 gm

number of myomas: those seen initially, during surgery and those enucleated and removed.

Another difficulty could be bleeding. It is usually not excessive, it is simply that when large myomas are removed and till they are sutured the myoma bed may bleed. Many of these patients could be having a low hematocrit preoperatively on account of prolonged spells of menorrhagia. So compounded with low hemoglobin and relatively more blood loss, these patients may require blood transfusion. Hence, it is always good to have the patient's blood cross-matched and extra units kept ready.

Time spent on such surgeries where large size and large number of myomas are removed in combination to the laparoscopic and abdominal route is usually about 120-150 minutes. So the anesthetist, surgeon and surgical team should be prepared for a prolonged procedure. Surgical time can be reduced by adopting the laparoscopic route for inspection, adhesiolysis, myoma mapping, and chromopertubation and injecting Pitressin. Making incision by monopolar cautery or harmonic scalpel over the biggest myoma and deep and posterior myomas and spending time only on more superficial enucleation which is enough to reach the definite plane of myoma, then attaching myoma screw on the myoma and quickly going over the minilap route rather than spending lot of time laparoscopically and then at the minilap. The end result is the same, so it is a better option to spend less time in enucleating the myoma during the

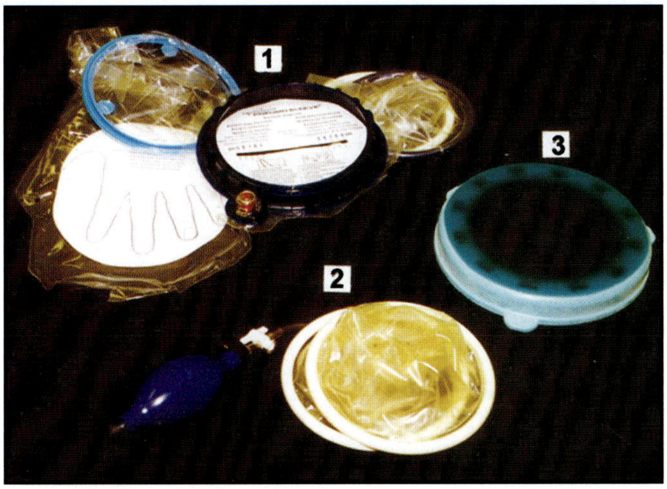

Figure 13.12. Current hand-assisted laparoscopy systems. (1) Dexterity® Pneumo Sleeve (Dexterity Surgical Inc. Rosewell, GA), (2) Omniport (Advanced Surgical Concepts, Wicklow, Ireland), (3) Gelport (Applied Medical–Rancho Santa Margarita, CA)

laparoscopic phase of the surgery as we are actually converting an open laparotomy into a more feasible minilap procedure which will ensure a good outcome.

COMPLICATIONS

We have not encountered any complications and as such there does not appear to be any complications which could arise during a minilap procedure. Hemorrhage and blood transfusion are taken as acceptable for large and multiple myomas. Infection could arise; so prophylactic antibiotics are given at induction of anesthesia and two doses thereafter of third generation cephalosporin.

RESULTS

Lap-assisted minilap myomectomy appears to be safer and relatively simpler procedure in the hands of experienced laparoscopists as well as novices since the much dreaded steps of myomectomy, i.e. suturing and morcellation can be completed by the minilap route. So, for the less experienced an 8 cm myoma can be dealt by minilap while an advanced endoscopist will resort to minilap for multiple and very big myomas. It appears to be a patient friendly procedure giving all the benefits of laparoscopy with the help of a small, 3-4 cm incision which heals well in the postoperative phase. We have done about 105 minilap-assisted lap myomectomies for myoma size ranging up to 23 cm and largest number of fibroids removed was 31 and weight of myomas ranging between 450-1100 gm. Mostly the indication is multiple 10-12 myomas and largest myoma being more than 15 cm. This is planned preoperatively, there is no sudden conversion on the table from laparoscopic myomectomy to laparoscopic assisted myomectomy. At least 10 patients required blood transfusion, which was anticipated preoperatively.

There has never been conversion to laparotomy and never a hysterectomy!. At our center, this procedure has been established with good surgical result in terms of reproductive outcome. Pregnancy rates are very encouraging. Second look scopies performed in three patients revealed moderate, flimsy adhesions, showing the procedure to be less adhesiogenic. Most patients are delivered by cesarean section as the uterine cavity is usually opened in the face of multiple myomas. There has been no incidence of scar dehiscence during pregnancy or labor. Similar results have been found and published by several other surgeons. Nezhat et al have compared all three groups, i.e. laparotomy, laparoscopic myomectomy (LM) and laparoscopic assisted myomectomy (LAM) and have found that adhesion score, postoperative recovery, hospital stay, blood loss and days for complete recovery are not statistically different in the groups of LM and LAM. Postoperative stay for LAM was 1.28 whilst .91 for LM, Blood loss was 267 ml in LAM and 143 ml in LM, days to resume normal activity were 12.2 in LAM and 12.2 in LM. All these compared to laparotomy were less, blood loss 245 ml, postoperative hospital stay 3.3, days to resume normal work 39 days. Thus, it appears that LAM compares favorably with LM and empowers the surgeon to avoid the full laparotomic approach thereby giving patient all the benefits of minimally invasive surgery and good reproductive outcome.

So, in conclusion, LAM operation is safe, feasible, offers easy to perform minimally invasive myomectomy for deep intramural and multiple fibroids with all the benefits of laparoscopic surgery and good reconstructive and reproductive outcome.

REFERENCES

1. Novak ER, Jones GS, Jones HW. Myomes uterins. In Novak ER, Jones GS, Jones HW (Eds): Gynecologic Pratiquue. Paris: Editions maloine.1970;309-22.
2. Novak ER, Woodruff JD. Myoma and other benign tumors of the uterus. Gynecologic and Obstetric Pathology (8th edn). Philadelphia: London, Toronto, WB Saunders Co. 1979;260-2.
3. Wallach EE. Myomectomy. In Thompson JD, Rock Ja (Eds): Telinde's Operative Gynecology (7th edn). JB Lippincott Company: Philadelphia 1992;647-60.
4. Thompson JD, Rock Ja. Leiomyomata uteri and myomectomy. In Rock Ja, Thompson JD (Eds): Te Linde's Operative Gynaecology. Philadelphia: Lipincott-Raen, 1992;371-9.
5. Reich H, Thompson KA, Nataupsky LG, Grabo TN, Sekel L. Laparoscopic myomectomy: An alternative to laparotomy myomectomy or hysterectomy? Gynecological Endoscopy 1997;6:7-12.
6. Goldfarb HA. Laparoscopic coagulation of myoma (myolysis). Obstet Gynecol Clin North Am 1995;22(4):807-19.
7. Philips DR, Milim SJ, Nathanson HG, Haselkorn JS. Experience with laparoscopic leiomyoma coagulation and concomitant operative laparoscopy. J Am Assoc Gynecol Laparosc 1997;4(14):425-33.
8. Goodwin SC, Vedanthan S, McLucas B, Forna AE, et al. Preliminary experience with uterine artery embolization for uterine fibroids. J Vasc Interv Radiol 1997;8(4):517-26.
9. Hutchins FL Jr, Worthington-Kirsch RL, Popky GL. Uterine arterial embolization for the management of leiomyomas: Quality of life assessment and clinical response. Radiology 1998.
10. Leroy Charles, Personal Communication.
11. Takeeuchi H, Kinoshita K. Evaluation of adhesion formation after laparoscopic myomectomy and systematic second-look microlaparoscopy. J Am Assoc Gynecol Laparosc 2002;9:442-6.
12. Dodson MG, Pache TD. In Dodson MG (Ed): The Uterus in Transvaginal Ultrasound (2nd edn); New York, Churchill Livingstone 1995;56-60.
13. Fedele L, Bianchi S, Dorta M, Arcaini L, Zanotti F, Carineli S. Transvaginal Sonography in the diagnosis of diffuse adenomyosis. Fertil Streil 1992;58:94-7.
14. Fedele L, Bianchi S, Dorta M, Zanotti F, Brioschi D, Carinelli S. Transvaginal ultrasonography in the differential diagnosis of adenomyoma versus leiomyoma. Am J Obstet Gynecol 1992;167:603-6.
15. Scoutt LM, McCarthy SM, Moss AA. Computed Tomography and Magnetic Resonance Imaging of the Pelvis in Computed Tomography of the Body edited by Moss AA, Gamsu G, Genant HK (2nd edn), Philadelphia: WB Saunders 1992;3:1233-4.
16. Dubuisson JB, Chapron C, Chavet X, et al. Laparoscopic myomectomy: Where do we stand? Gynaecol Endos 1995;4:83-6.
17. Tulandi T, Youseff H. Laparoscopy-assisted myomectomy of large uterine myomas. Gynaecol Endosc 1997;6:105-8.
18. Nezhat C, Nezhat F, Bess O. Laparoscopically assisted myomectomy: A report of a new technique in 57 cases. Int J Fertil 1994;39:39-44.
19. Nezhat C, Nezhat F, Luciano AA, et al. Uterine surgery. Operative gynecologic Laparoscopy: Principles and techniques. New York: McGraw Hill 1995;205-38.
20. Nezhat C, Nezhat F, Silfen S. Laparoscopic Myomectomy. Int J Fertil 1991;36,275-80.
21. Benedetti-Panici P, Maneschi F, Cutillo G. Surgery by minilaparotomy in benign gynecologic disease. Obstet Gynecol 1996;87:456-9.
22. Nezhat C, Nezhat F, Fess O. Laparoscopically assisted myomectomy: A report of a new technique in 57 cases Intl J Fertil & Menop Studies 1994;39:39-44.
23. Lethaby A, Vollenhoven B, Sowter M. Efficacy of preoperative gonadotropin releasing hormone analogues for women with uterine fibroids undergoing hysterectomy or myomectomy: A systematic review. BJOG 2002;109:1097-1108.
24. Fredrick J, Fletcher H, Simeon D. Intramyometrial vasopressin as a hemostatic agent during myomectomy. Br J Obstet and Gynecol 1994;101:435-7.
25. Fedele L, Bianchi S, Dorta M, Brioschi D, Zanotti F, Vercellini P. Transvaginal ultrasonography versus Hysteroscopy in the diagnosis of uterine submucous myoma. Obstet Gynecol 1991;77:745-8.
26. Kurjak A, Kupesic S, Zalud I, Predanic M. In Dodson MG (Ed): Transvaginal Color Doppler. Transvaginal ultrasound. New York: Churchill Livingstone 1995;325-39.
27. Flesicher AC, Kepple DM, Entman SS. Transvaginal Sonography of uterine disorder. In Timor-Tritsch IE, Rottam S (Eds): Transvaginal Sonography (2nd edn). New York; Elsevier, 1991:109-30.
28. Mark H. Glasser minilap myomectomy: A minimally invasive alternative for the large fibroid uterus Journal of Minimally Invasive Gynaecology 2005;12,275-83.
29. Pelosi MA III, Pelosi MA II. Laparoscopic-assisted transvaginal myomectomy. J Am Assoc Gynecol Laparosc 1997;4:241-6.
30. Pelosi MA II, Pelosi MA III. Hand-assisted Laparoscopy (handoscopy) for megamyomectomy. A case study. J Reprod Med 2000;45:519-25.

14 Endoscopic Myomectomy in Infertility: Current Scenario and Our Experience

Prakash Trivedi, Anil Chittake

INTRODUCTION

Leiomyomata uteri are extremely frequent and most common gynecological tumors, occurring in 20-25 percent of sexually active women (Novak et al,[1] 1970) and 30-35 percent of all women (of all age). They are perhaps one of the most talked about, benign tumors in women. Since the advent of better diagnostic modalities like ultrasonography, more and more fibroids are being detected incidentally even in asymptomatic women.

The symptomatology is quite variable ranging from asymptomatic, small to very large lump in abdomen, accidental detection with infertility or menorrhagia or pressure symptoms. Buttram et al[2] in 1981 suggested that upto 40 percent of patients with multiple fibroids had infertility (27%), repeated miscarriage (3%) and preterm labor (3 to 4%) as chief presenting complaints.

INCIDENCE AND OUR EXPERIENCE

In our experience of 1648 women with fibroids, single or multiple, seen over incidence of symptomatology was as follows:

In our study of 1648 cases of fibroids (Table 14.1) seen over a period of 14 years by the author for various indications specially in 49 percent for cases of Infertility. Overall 962 underwent laparoscopic myomectomies and the rest 301 required hysteroscopic myomectomies. In the remaining 385 cases (23.4%) the patients did not require any surgical management specifically for fibroids, as their complaints were insignificant. However, since ours is a referral Center for Advanced Endoscopic Surgery in Asia along with an Advanced Infertility Management (IVF – ICSI) Center, the actual incidence might be less. Moreover these data exclude cases with fibroids requiring hysterectomy, mainly for menorrhagia. This chapter is exclusively an attempt to deal with fibroid uterus endoscopically, still conserving the uterus and restoring normal anatomy, with analysis of various extirpative and minimally invasive methods in conservative management of this gynecological pathology.

Table 14.1. Symptomatology and incidence of fibroids

Symptoms	*Percentage*
Menorrhagia with or without infertility	42
Associated with infertility *	49
Asymptomatic lump/accidental finding	14
Pressure symptoms **	4

* Fibroids may or may not be the cause of infertility
** Symptoms like urinary retention, abdominal or pelvic pain, constipation, and heaviness in the abdomen.

Apart from other symptoms one of the most important areas of concern and debate is fibroid and its association with infertility. Pritts EA[3] (2001), and various other research teams (Bulletti et al[4] 1999) have found definite association of fibroids and infertility. Though the exact cause and effect relationship is debatable, there seems to be some convincing facts as some fibroids may be responsible for reduced fertility, if not infertility.

The very fact that significant number of women with fibroid uterus has enough number of successful pregnancies, yet we do not know that when these women were pregnant, fibroids where actually present or not. Nevertheless in our vast experience of laparoscopic and hysteroscopic removal of fibroids in patients with fibroids with long standing infertility, occurrence of many pregnancies is not anecdotal. We have sighted more specific situations where removal of these fibroids actually improved fertility.

Buttram and Reiter et al[2] (1981), Rubin[5] (1958) and Wallach[6] (1995) have suggested that fibroids may reduce fertility various mechanisms, but according to us the following are important:

1. Fibroids significantly distorting bilateral proximal tubo-ovarian anatomy.
2. Intracavitary or submucous fibroids of significant size.
3. Large intramural fibroids distorting the endometrial cavity.
4. Submucous fibroids with increased vascularity of to the uterus.
5. Submucous fibroid and intramural fibroid with larger cavitary component interfering with proper implantation thereby causing infertility or miscarriage.
6. Multiple fibroids of significant size and long duration of infertility.
7. Raised prolactin: This is a surprising clinical entity, which we encountered in our clinical practice that 36 percent of these women with fibroids and infertility had hyperprolactinemia (Prolactin levels–ranging between 45-60 u/ml) with or without galactorrhea. This association was corroborated as we found 29 percent pregnancy rate after laparoscopic myomectomy, with actual normalization of prolactin level, in these patients.

VARIOUS LOCATIONS OF FIBROIDS SEEN IN OUR SERIES (FIGURES 14.1 TO 14.2L)

Diagnosis and Evaluation

The need of the modern gynecological practice is not just the diagnosis, but having a deep insight of location, number and size of fibroids,wheter indenting the cavity, associated endometriosis, adnexal mass, hyperprolactinemia, etc.

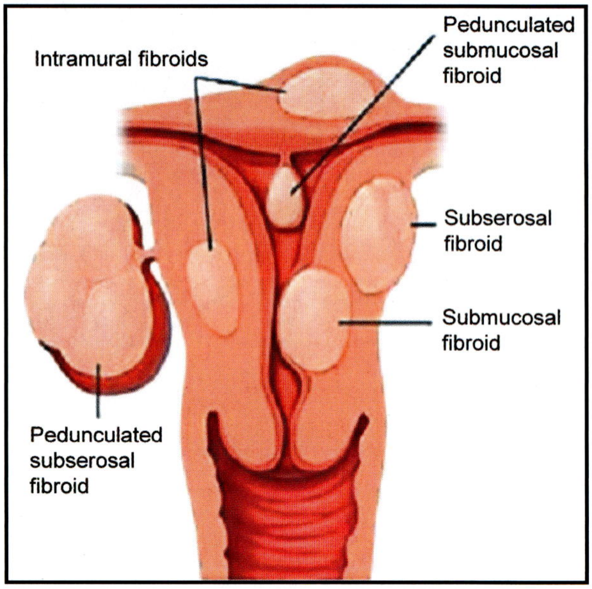

Figure 14.1. Schematic representation of various types and location of fibroids

A good bimanual and clinical examination, evaluation of fibroid, which can give the idea about size, fixity, number, location especially in sexually active women, per-rectal examination is truly informative in virgin women.

IMPORTANT INVESTIGATIONS

a. **Ultrasonography**: If considered individually the single most important investigation for evaluation of size, shape, echotexture, evidence of degenerative changes and exact distance from the endometrial cavity or serosal is an abdominal and especially transvaginal ultrasonography.

   The fibroids are visible as hypo-echoic areas and if they have dense hyperechoic areas then it suggests calcification of the fibroid/occasionally Dermoid. Further we had 26 cases of bulky uterus with hypoechoic circular area which was endometrioma of uterus since we incised drained chocolate colored thick fluid.

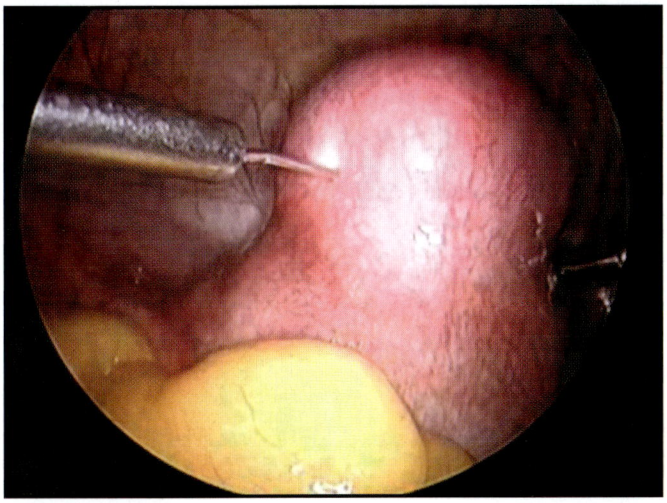

Figure 14.2A. Anterior fibroid

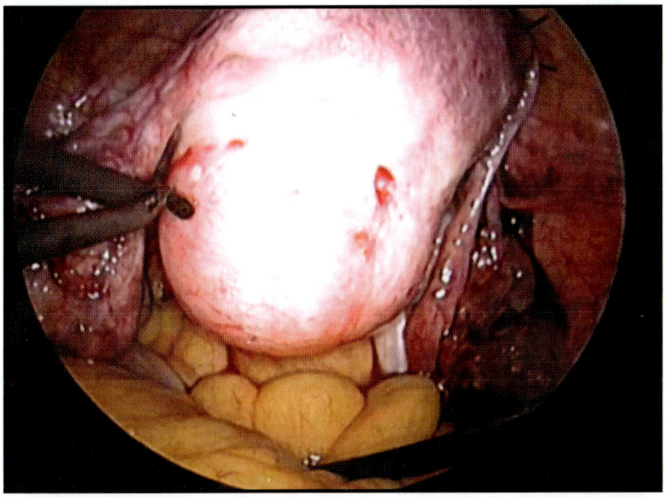

Figure 14.2B. Posterior fibroid

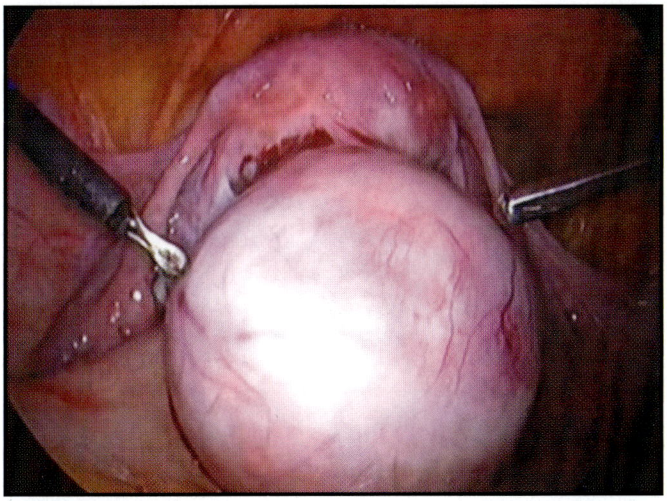

Figure 14.2C. Large posterior fibroid with smaller base

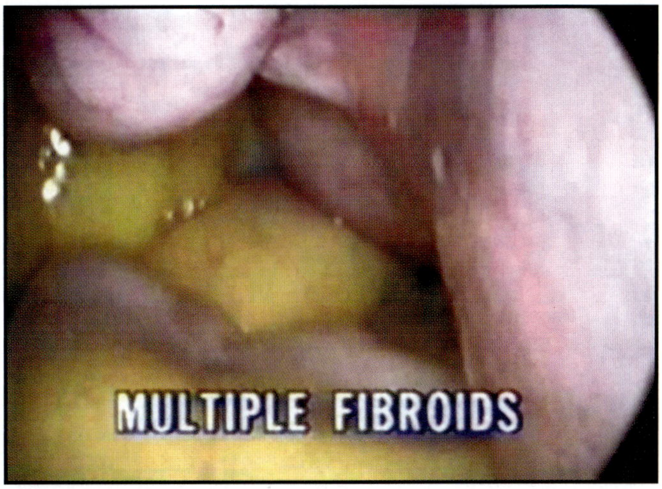

Figure 14.2D(i). Multiple fibroids

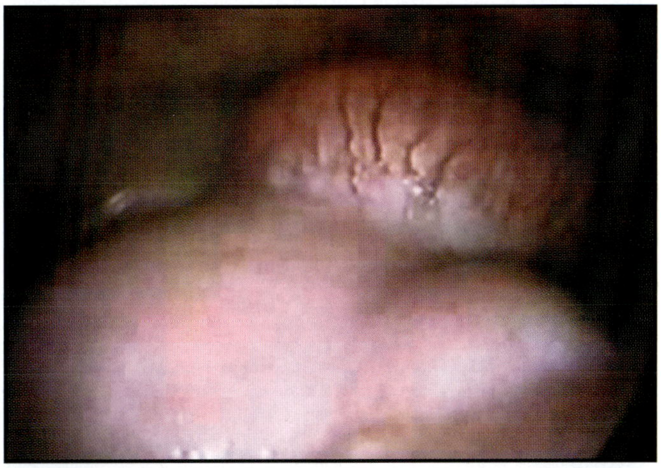

Figure 14.2D(ii). Multiple fibroids

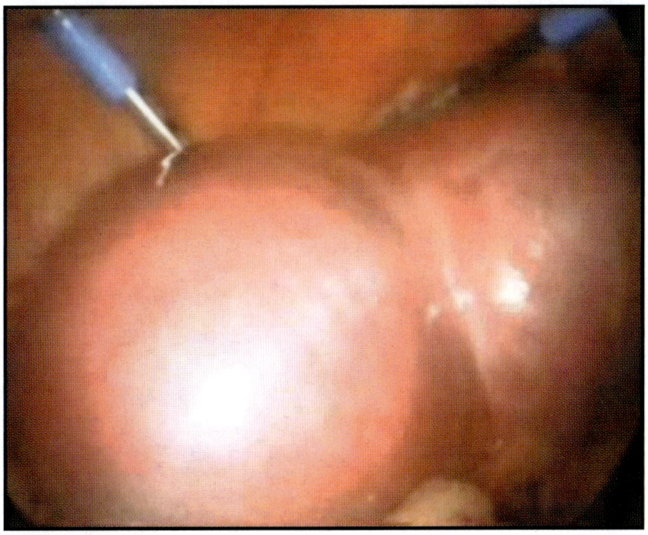

Figure 14.2D(iii). Multiple fibroids

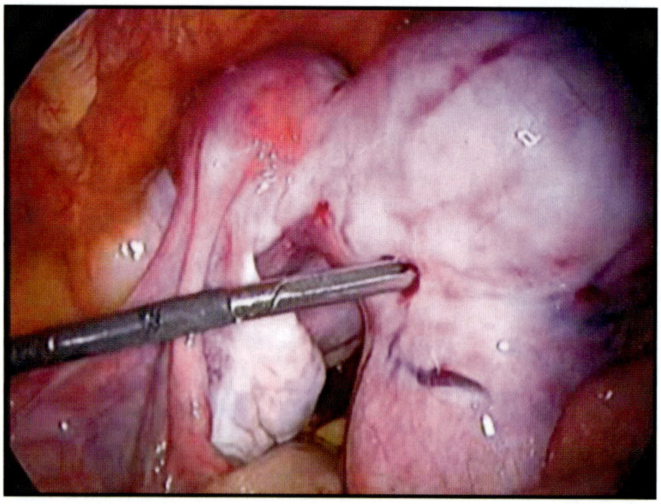

Figure 14.2D. Large pedunculated fibroids

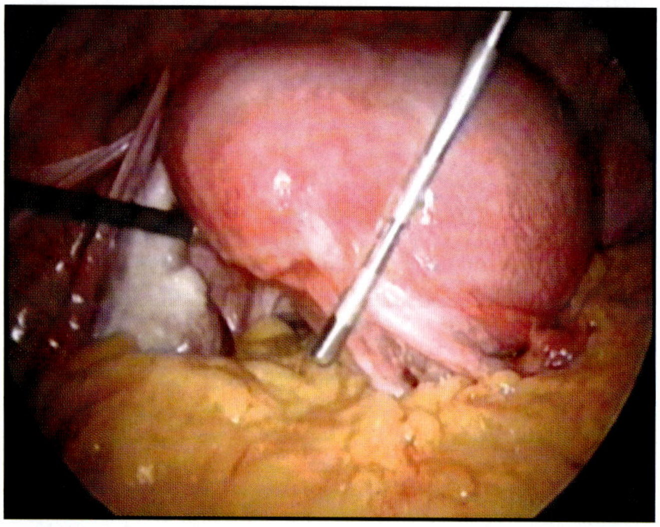

Figure 14.2E. Large antero-posterior fibroid

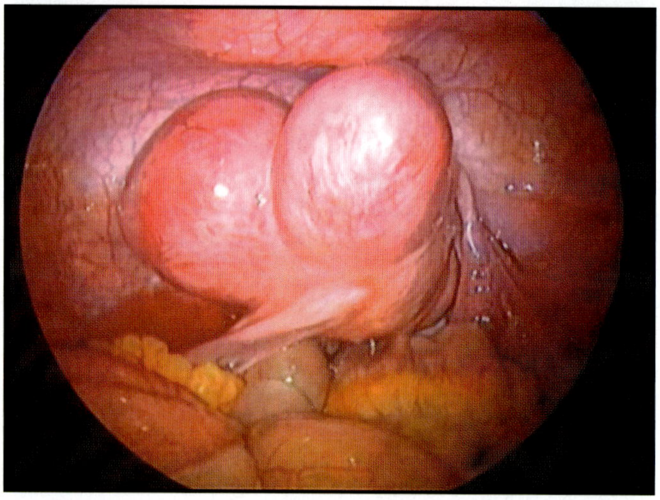

Figure 14.2F. Large multiple – Distorting the anatomy

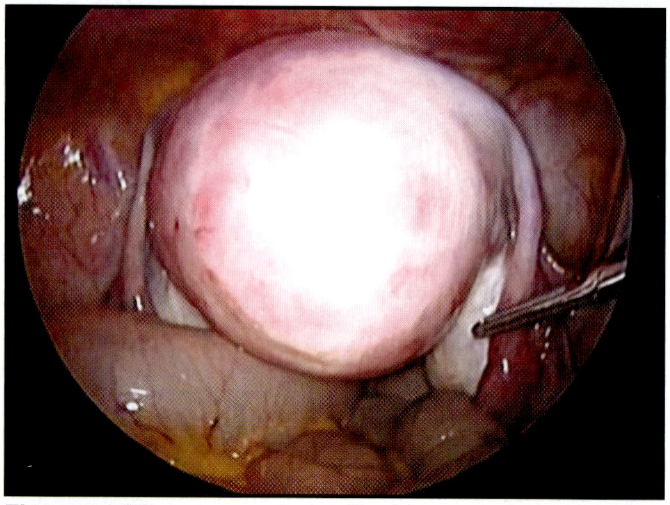

Figure 14.2G. Large posterior fibroid

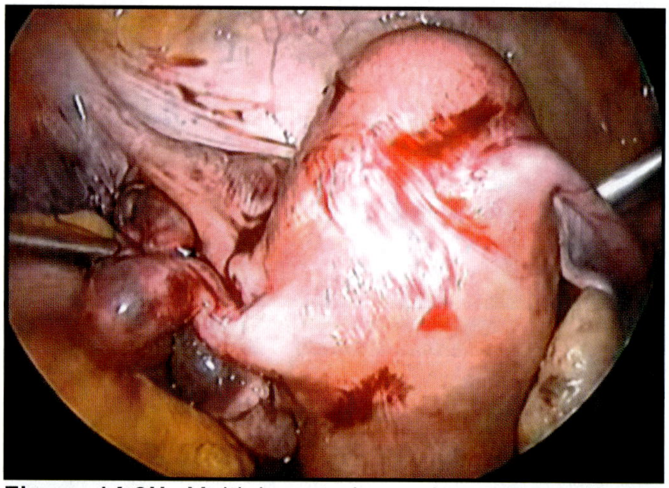

Figure 14.2H. Multiple anterior and posterior fibroids distorting uterine anatomy

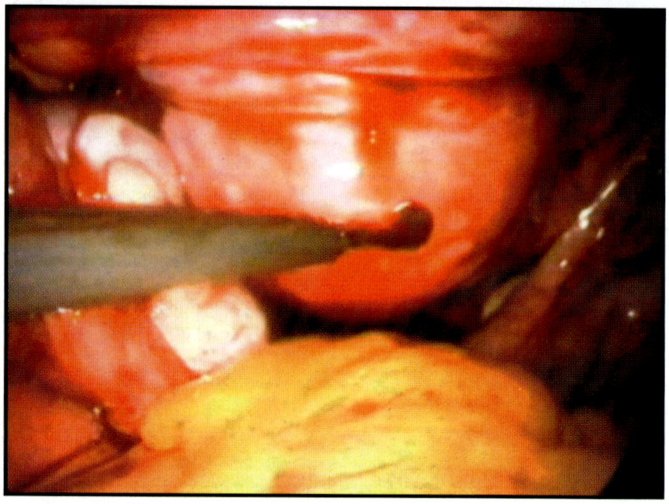

Figure 14.2I. Posterior cervical fibroid

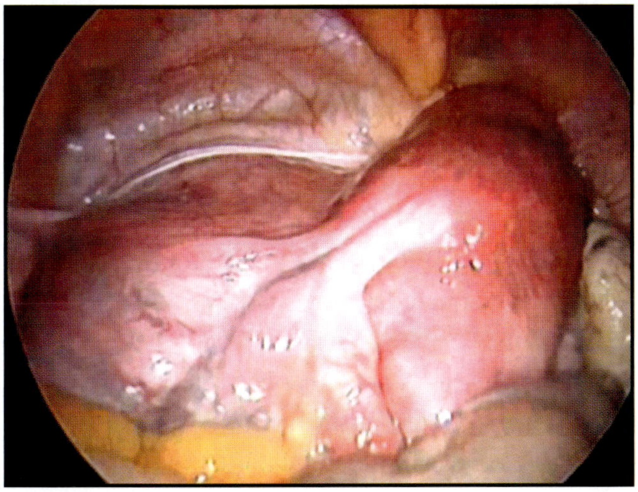

Figure 14.2J. Left large broad ligament fibroid totally distorting the anatomy

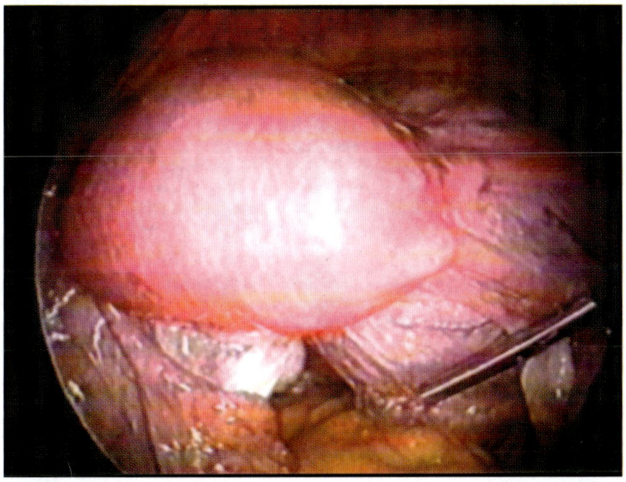

Figure 14.2K. Right large broad ligament fibroid

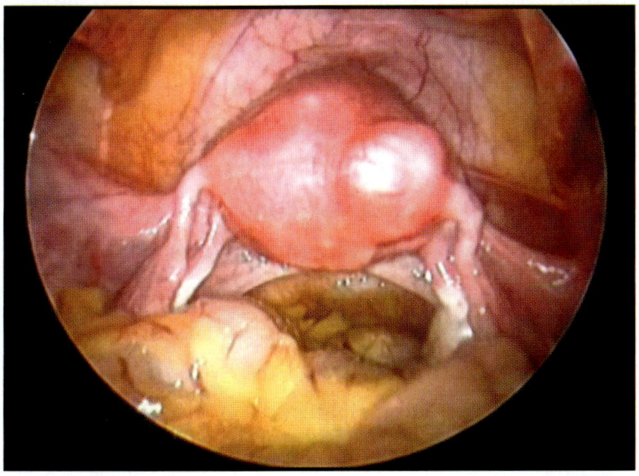

Figure 14.2L. Right cornual fibroid in a case of infertility (who subsequently conceived after laparoscopic myomectomy)

However, occasionally fundal fibroids can be still sometimes missed by a transvaginal ultrasound. Hence an abdominal ultrasound should always be performed with partially full bladder for complete evaluation.

b. **Color Doppler**: This diagnostic modality is of major significance, especially in high-risk situation for large size uterine malignancy or a sarcomatous fibroid. Another important fact is the ability of color Doppler to distinguish between a possible localized adenomyoma.
c. **Hysterosalpingography** for cavitary fibroid, the author doesn't prefer sonosalpingography due do possibility of infection, false positive results.
d. **MRI, CT scan and 3-D ultrasound:** Though costly, the role of these sophisticated modalities cannot be underrated in cases suspected to have extensive pathology like compression of ureters, urinary bladder and distal gastrointestinal tract. Rarely other solid tumor may mimic fibroids and it might be worthwhile to perform these investigations.

However, as far as a laparoscopic surgeon is concerned, apart from the size and location the single most criterion is to evaluate exact area of contact of fibroid with the uterus to decide the probable number of sutures to be placed after removal, if a laparoscopic route of removal of fibroid is contemplated.

MANAGEMENT

Unfortunately there is always a large personal bias in treating fibroid with infertility depending on the skill and knowledge of the consultant who may be an endoscopist or ART Specialist or a conventional gynecologists.

Apart from the actual need of removal of the fibroid, we will share our experience with laparoscopic and hysteroscopic myomectomy, role of GnRH analogues prior to the surgery (if any), situations in which laparotomy is necessary and a brief write-up of uterine artery embolization as probable alternative, though debatable.

Myomectomy is unnecessarily presumed to be a major open surgery, since according to us more than 90 percent of the fibroids can be removed laparoscopically. and many hysteroscopically. However, myomectomy is truly indicated in following cases mentioned above (60%). Whereas in 40 percent of the cases there is no indication to remove some fibroids, on the contrary it may lead to adhesions or other risks.

We at our Center NILES have a vast experience of endoscopic removal of leiomyoma over a period of 14 years. In our experience, we found laparoscopic removal of fibroids a very graceful, effective procedure in the hands of experts unless performed in inappropriately selected cases.

Laparoscopic Myomectomy

Many gynecological surgeons viz. Dubuisson et al[7] (1996), Nezhat et al[8] (1991); Hasson et al[9] (1992); Daniell and Gurley[10] (1991) have reported moderate to significantly high success of laparoscopic myomectomy as a procedure. Moreover they have reported significantly improved pregnancy rates in patients with associated infertility after laparoscopic removal of fibroids.

However, with improvised techniques, increasing expertise and skill, we found that conquering the technical difficulties of the procedure, which the above researchers referred to, was not beyond the reach of the hands of any gynecological surgeon with basic skills of operative laparoscopy. This is specifically with ipsilateral suturing and the availability of good morcellators, which render the removal of even larger fibroids effortless.

IMPORTANT ASPECTS OF OUR LAPAROSCOPIC TECHNIQUE

We prefer to give a thorough bowel preparation to the patient with Polyethylene glycol solution with electrolytes (viz. PEGLEC) a day prior to surgery. Appropriate preoperative evaluation, investigations; consent for surgery is taken prior to the procedure explaining the exact benefits and risks.

Prerequisite for laparoscopic myomectomy:

a. Skilled laparoscopic surgeon with a trained assistant, both conversant with the procedure, especially laparoscopic suturing and morcellation.
b. Anesthesiologist well experienced with endoscopic surgery and well used to advanced monitoring gadgetry.
c. Skilled and trained nursing staff and operation theater assistants.
d. A complete set of operative laparoscopy instruments and myomectomy instruments viz. myoma screw, electronic reusable morcellator.
e. Suitable cautery, both monopolar and bipolar with separate footswitches.
f. Operation table with double pelvic cut for good anteversion, modified lithotomy leg holders and a padded shoulder rest.
g. Irrigation and aspiration system.
h. Proper suturing set with needle holders, knot pushers for extracorporeal knots and intracorporeal suturing, good scissors.
i. Injection vasopressin or Pitressin – 20 units in 100 ml of normal saline.

Primary Procedure

The procedure is performed under general anesthesia with endotracheal intubation. If the fibroid is significantly large, we prefer to put a nasogastric tube for convenient introduction of a supraumbilical port for the camera and the telescope. The patient is catheterized with suitable Foley's catheter (14 or 16 G) after painting and draping. A Hulka's or Rumi's uterine manipulator is inserted to help suitable mechanical positioning of the uterus to aid proper visualization and simplify the steps of the laparoscopic removal of the fibroid and suturing of the defect. We prefer two monitors at comfortable distance and recording facilities for the purpose of documentation, always ensuring least deviation from the precise microsurgical principles.

Port Placement

We use one intraumbilical/supraumbilical primary port for a 10 mm 0° or occasionally a 30° telescope with camera, two 5 mm ports kept at left and right iliac fossa placed depending on the size of fibroid. The suprapubic port is given up by us since it hangs and comes in the way of the optics and is not efficient as our normal 3rd ipsilateral port which is placed at the intersection of imaginary line drawn vertically up from left lower port placed higher to the umbilical level depending on the size of fibroid, to ensure enough space to allow proper traction, tissue dissection and suturing. With 2 ports on the side of the surgeon the suturing and other operative movements are like open surgery for, e.g. the left (lower) hand using the bipolar and right (upper) hand using a monopolar spatula or scissor and similarly for suturing The assistant has to hold the camera and the instrument from the patient's right side. This method of advanced laparoscopic surgery totally avoids surgical fatigue associated with older technique were we cross the hand to opposite side, which leads to strain on the right deltoid muscle and affects the performance of the surgery (Figure 14.3A).

Surgical Procedure

Unlike the popular belief, fibroids of any size do not have stalk blood supply. They have a "parasitic" blood supply.

A 30° Trendelenburg's position is given to take the bowels away upwards to ensure proper visualization of the pouch of Douglas. This helps visualization of the fibroid in the best possible view. A 30° optics can be used for a low posterior cervical or low anterior fibroid. After thorough inspection of pathology, dilute vasopressin 1 ampoule (20 unit) in 100 ml of Ringer lactate is injected in the cleavage between fibroid capsule and uterine muscle (Figures 14.3B to D). Once the fibroid is seen as shown in the diagram a horizontal incision is made with a monopolar spatula, adequate to remove the fibroid (Figure 14.4A). We always prefer horizontal incision because spiral arteriols are circumferential and if vertical incision taken causes more bleeding and it will be similar to classical cesarean section. The current settings preferred by us are 100 watts of pure cutting current and 60 watts of coagulating current on monopolar instrument or 25-30 watts of bipolar current with separate footswitch and machine. A myoma screw is put in left upper port to fix the fibroid and gently pull it as spatula dissects the surrounding tissue of the fibroid (Figures 14.4B and C). Finally at the end due to effective traction on the fibroid, the base of fibroid with tissue attachment is seen, which is cut with spatula and current (Figures 14.4D to G). Care should be taken of using monopolar current, specially in terms of insulation of instrument, to prevent burns of important organs like bowel/bladder. We do not feel use of pure cutting current hampers tissue healing over scissors cutting with unnecessary bleeding.

The separated fibroid is parked in appendicular area since there are least instruments movement in that area and other fibroids are then removed in same way. After the removal of fibroids a thorough lavage is given, which is then aspirated and small area of bleeding are coagulated.

Suturing of the uterine flaps after the enucleation of the fibroid (Figures 14.5A to I) by ipsilateral ports is largely simplified by the author. The suturing can be successfully accomplished by following steps, with excellent results. In our experience, with this technique of suturing we had least incidence of adhesions and no reports of rupture or scar dehiscence. Hence, the author strongly recommends the following technique for suturing which makes laparoscopic myomectomy an enjoyable procedure, even more than an abdominal myomectomy, as it also does not compromise the safety and the treatment.

Step 1

The suture on curved needle is introduced through the left lower port (with flower valve) by H Reich and Clarke method. We commonly use polyglactin 910 no.1 for suturing the myometrial flaps. Adequate length of the suture is taken inside and this can be done by holding

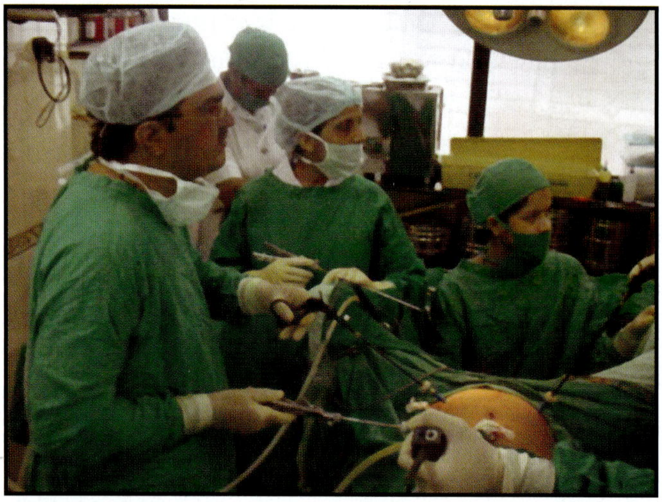
Figure 14.3A

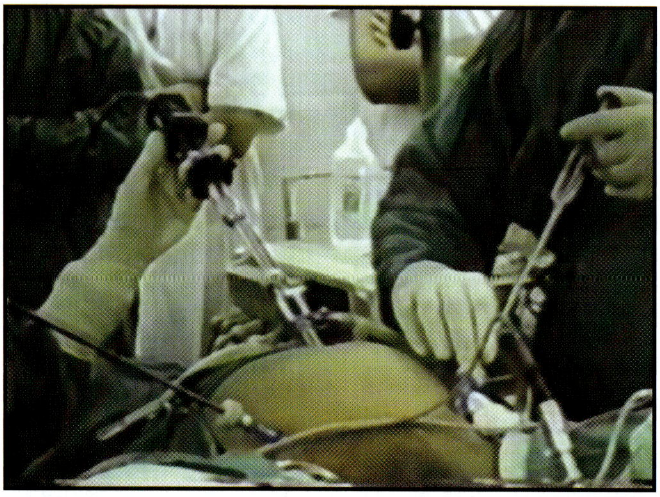
Figure 14.3B

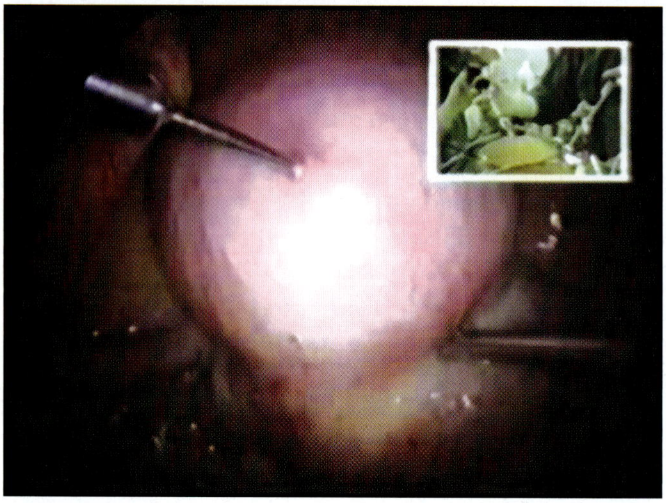
Figure 14.3C

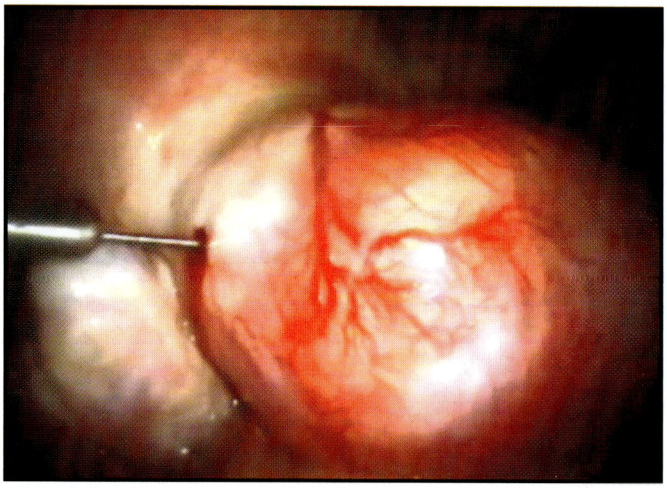
Figure 14.3D

Figures 14.3A to D. Injecting vasopressin in the subserosal plane

the thread and pulling vertically down. The first knot is essentially an extracorporeal knot, since the thread is too long and manipulation becomes difficult for an intracorporeal knot. The needle is held in perfect place and direction with the convexity downwards, by the dominant needle holder, while the assistant holds the thread with a flat grasper, 3 cm. away from the swage, preventing wobbling and slipping of the needle from the grip (Figure 14.5A).

Step 2

After the surgeon stabilizes the posterior uterine wall with a new Trivedi's curved needle holder cum toothed grasper through the left lower port (Figure 14.5B). The dominant needle holder (left upper port) then drives the needle along the curve through the posterior myometrial flap then the anterior flap, which is stabilized by the assistant. The movement is essentially in the "vertical zone" making it truly physiological and comfortable.

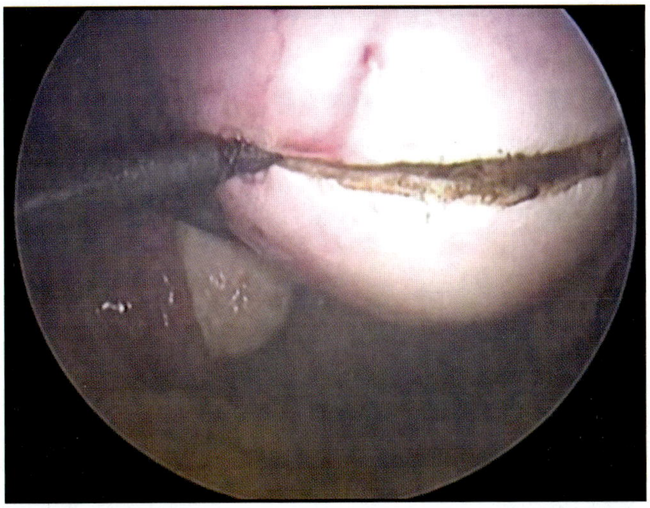

Figure 14.4A. Horizontal incision with a spatula with monopolar cautery

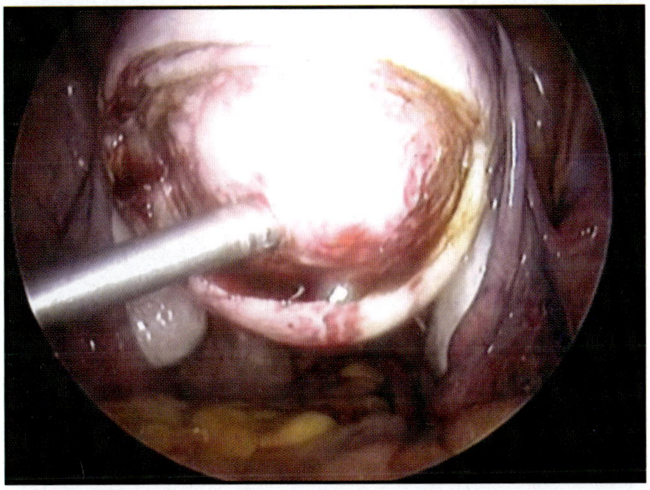

Figure 14.4B. Stabilizing the myoma with the myoma screw

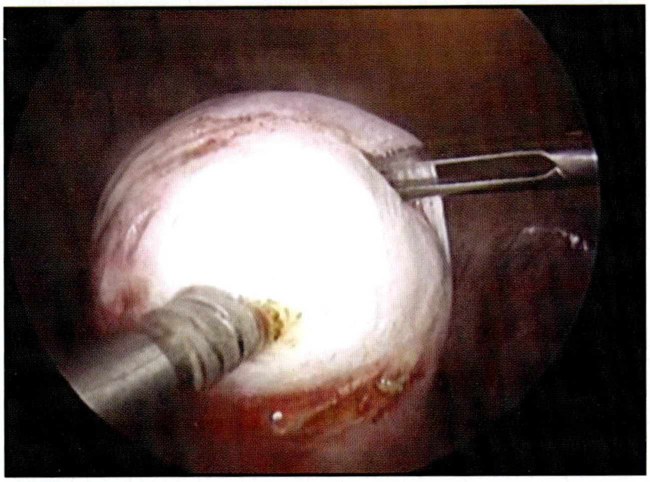

Figure 14.4C. Traction with the screw

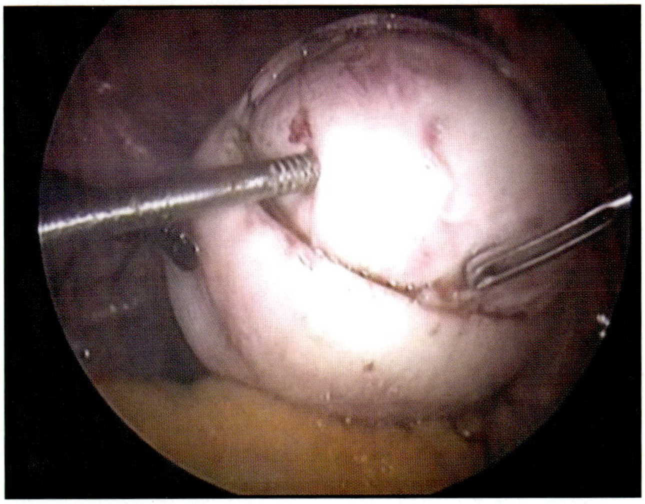

Figure 14.4D. Dissection of the myoma

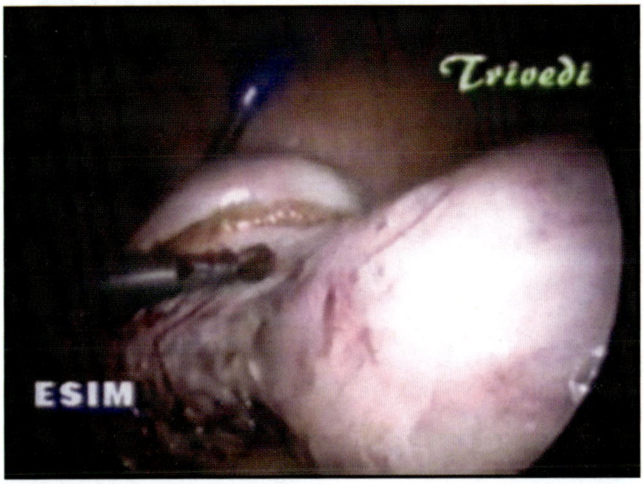

Figure 14.4E. Complete removal from the base

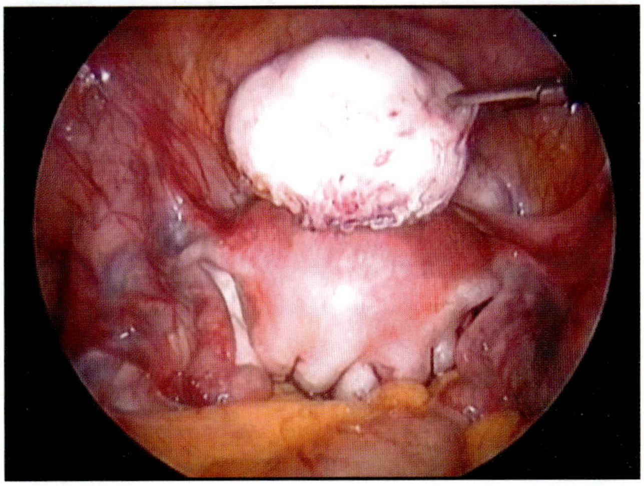

Figure 14.4F. Enucleated fibroid

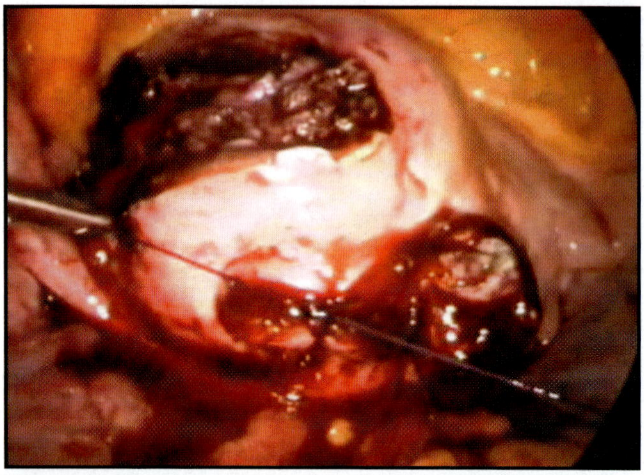

Figure 14.4G. Myoma bed after the removal of the fibroid
Figures 14.4A to G. Removal of the fibroid

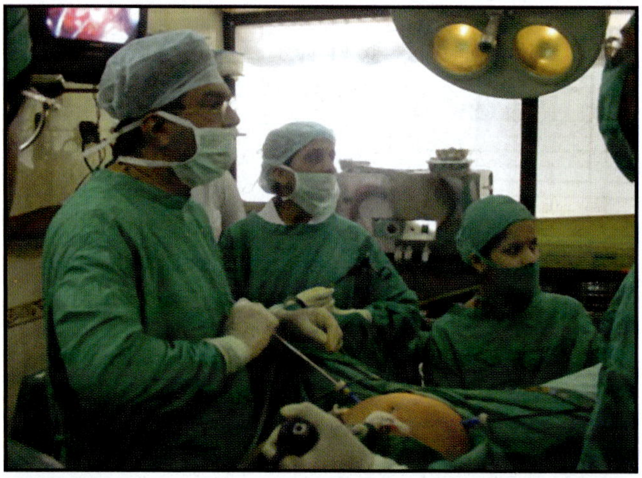

Figure 14.5A. Port placement and pushing extracorporeal knot

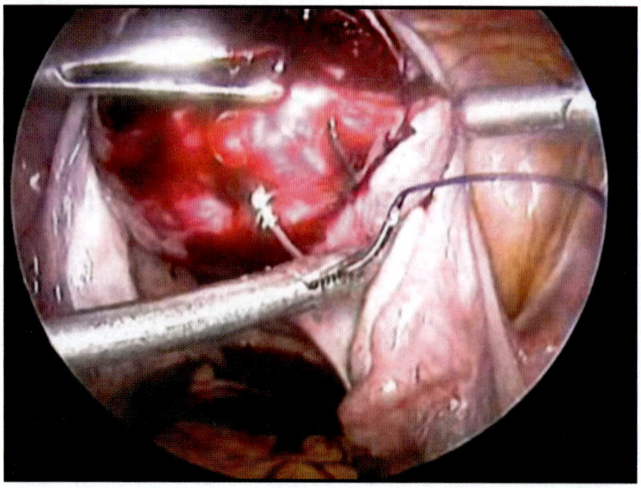

Figure 14.5B. Ipsilateral suturing—Ist suture

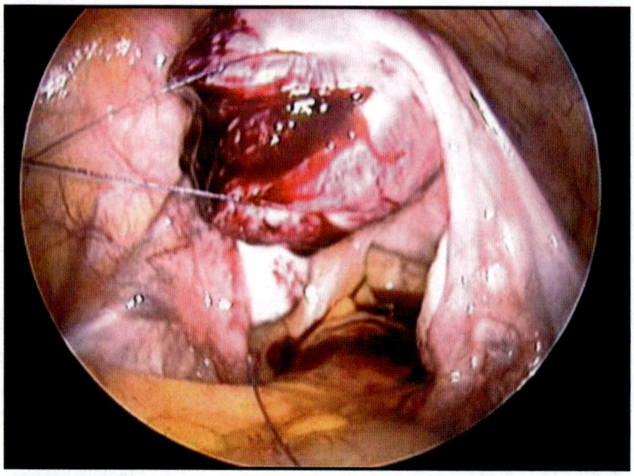

Figure 14.5C. Ist extracorporeal knot

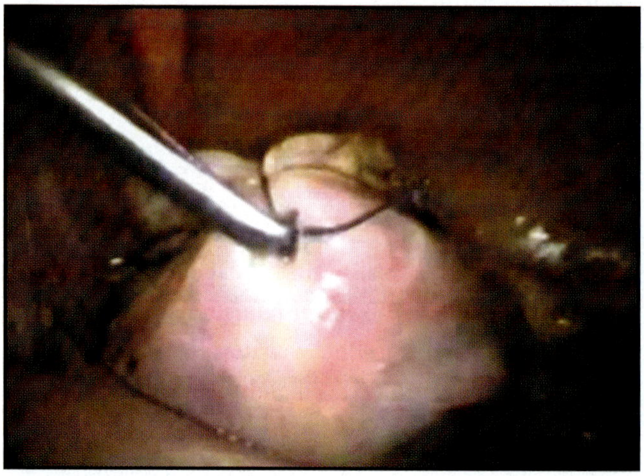

Figure 14.5D. Extracorporeal knot placement

Step 3

The first extracorporeal knot requires a significant length of the suture to draw both the ends out through the left lower port. The thread is cut keeping adequate length and the needle then is parked in the right iliac fossa. The free ends of the thread are then withdrawn through the left lower port and the extracorporeal knot is tied (Trivedi's simplified knot). The knot is then pushed by a special knot pusher designed by the author (Figure 14.5D). After the knot is placed, the thread is cut.

Step 4

Subsequent series of the knots are intracorporeal knots placed intermittently (Figures 14.5E to H). The ipsilateral

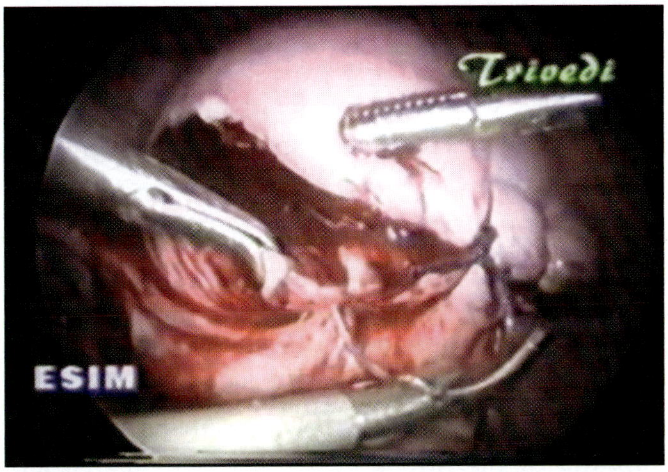

Figure 14.5E. Interrupted intracorporeal sutures

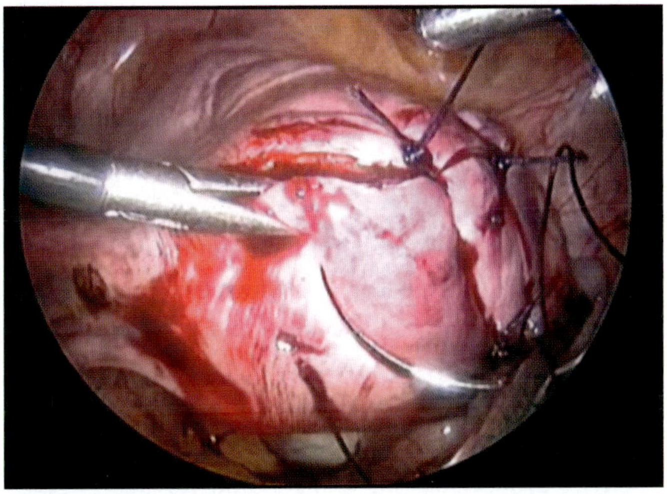

Figure 14.5F. Interrupted intracorporeal sutures

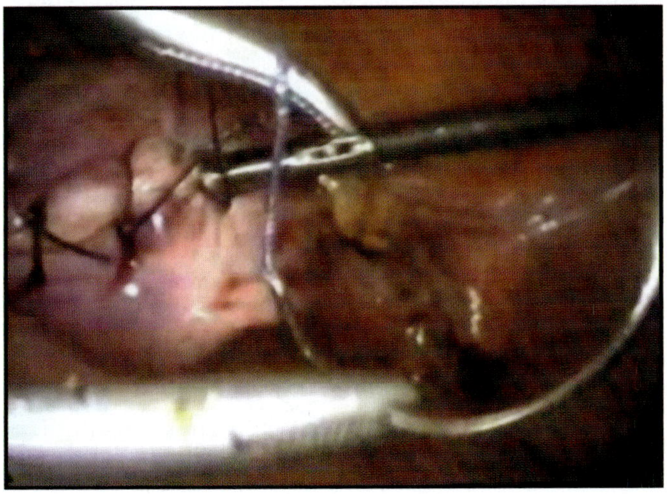

Figure 14.5G. "Smiling needle" technique

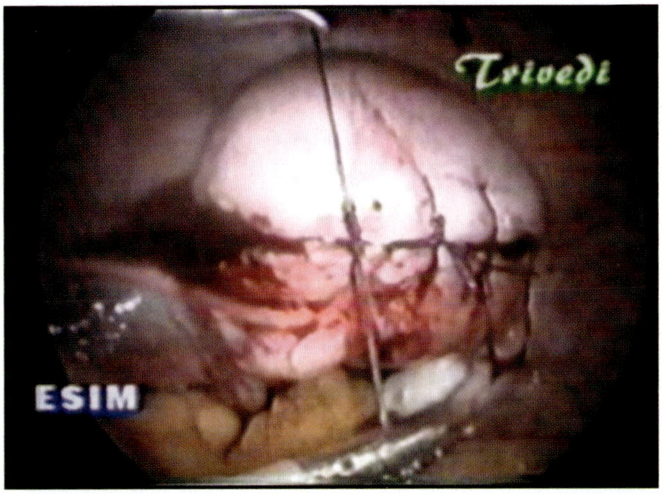

Figure 14.5H. Placement of subsequent intracorporeal knots

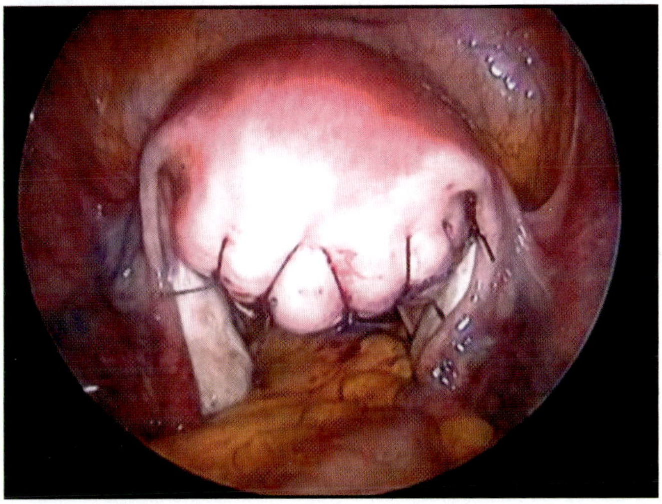

Figure 14.5I. Completely sutured uterine flaps

placement of two ports (left lower and left upper) makes the movements physiological and prevents fatigue even in the learning phase. The dominant needle holder again holds the needle in the similar way and the needle is again driven through the uterine wall from posterior to anterior in a vertical zone, piercing at a distance of 0.75 cm from the first knot. One should always keep in mind that since single layer suturing is done the needle should take deep bites of the uterine tissue, and make sure that the myometrial bed is obliterated completely. This ensures proper hemostasis and also approximates the free myometrial flaps. This second knot is then tied by the series of synchronized movements of the dominant and

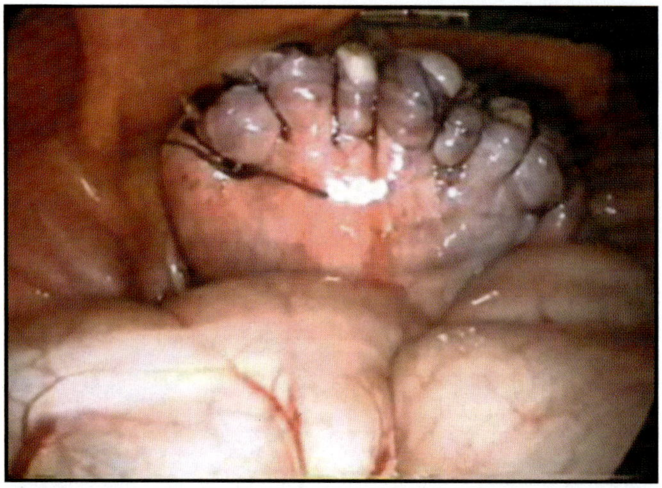

Figure 14.5J. Completely sutured uterine flaps

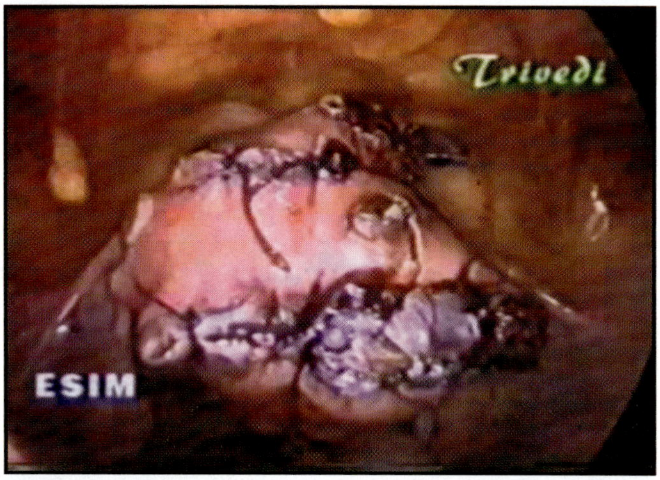

Figure 14.5K. Completely sutured uterine flaps

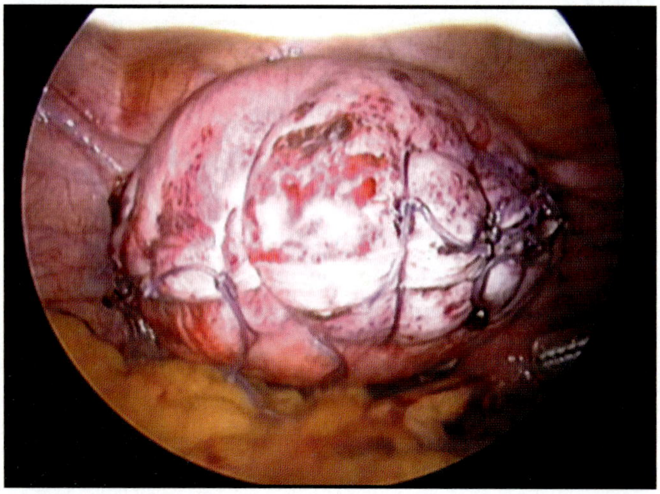

Figure 14.5L. Multiple fibroids (12) removed and sutured (requiring 25 sutures)

Figures 14.5A to L. Ipsilateral closure of the uterine flaps

non-dominant needle holders. Adequate length of the suture is pulled first and then a flamingo forceps is used to make the "C" with the convexity of the "C" towards the surgeon by holding the thread with the dominant needle holder at suitable position as to avoid strangulation of the knotting instrument.The curved needle holder from the left lower port remains stable, while the dominant straight needle holder is the active instrument for the most of the knot formation and placement. The dominant needle holder is rolled over the curved needle holder taking series of loops, avoiding slipping of the thread. The knot is then tied and subsequent throws are given after placing the knot properly. After three throws, the thread is cut and the remaining flap is sutured in the same fashion (Figures 14.5J to L). Normally, 5 to 6 sutures can be taken easily with the standard suture length.

Adequate hemostasis is achieved and the needle is removed by Reich's method.

We prefer to use deep interrupted sutures, which allow any exudate to come out freely, which can drain through an intraperitoneal drain, which is placed subsequently at the end of the procedure. Routine use of hemostatics like Surgicel is given up by us as nothing is important than a clean surgery.

After proper suturing a meticulous lavage is given and fibroids are removed by morcellation described later. We have found that in majority of cases suturing in single layer had no disadvantages over multiple layer suturing. In our experience, multiple layer suturing rather has associated risk of eversion of layers while suturing, which makes suturing difficult and adds to the risk of rupture due improper approximation. Nezhat et al have also reported that single layer suturing, if done by a skilled laparoscopic surgeon, does not compromise the integrity of the subsequent scar.

In situations of low cervical, an anterior or posterior fibroid, a 30° scope is preferred as suturing at such sites may not be easy without clear vision. In cases of broad ligament fibroid, we prefer a posterior incision. It is always to be borne in mind that the ureters are always lateral to such fibroids and their course is altered. Proper

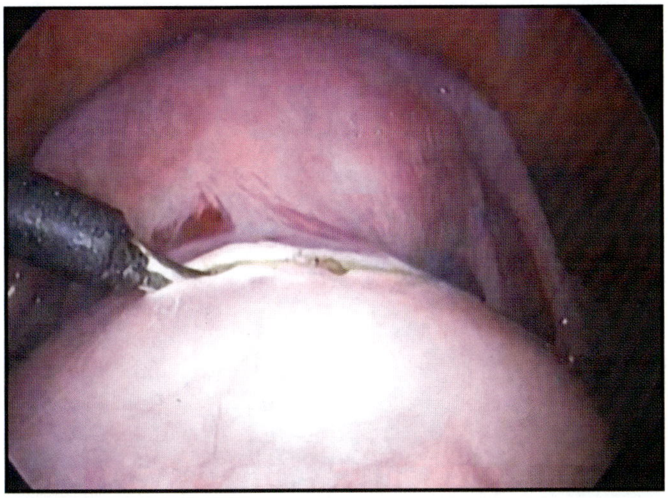

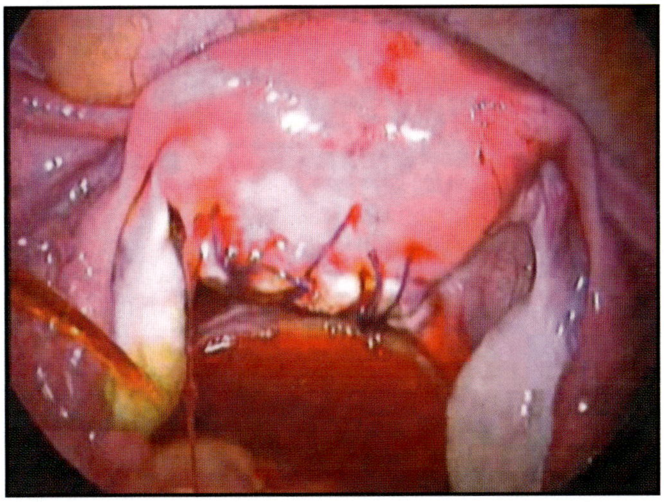

Figures 14.6A and B. A large fibroid with small base, removal and suturing

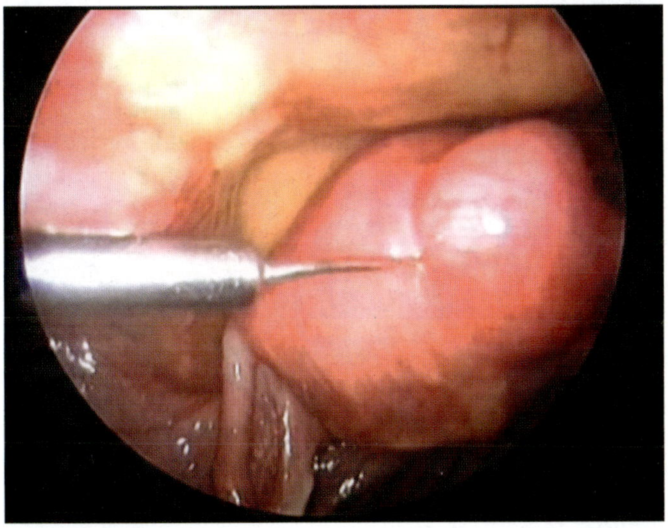

Figure 14.7A

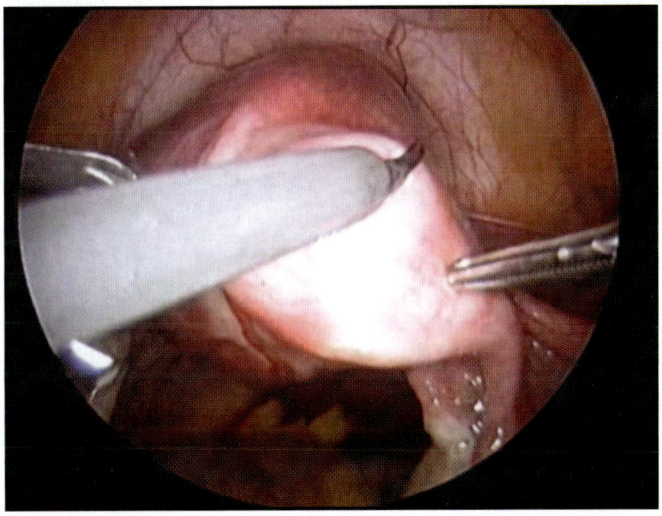

Figure 14.7B

visualization of ureters might be occasionally necessary in case of doubt or suspicion of injury. Most of the broad ligament fibroids might not require the suturing of the bed or dead space, as they do not involve a bulk of the myometrial tissue (Figures 14.6A and B). Hence they are less dangerous as far as the risk of dehiscence is negligibly less. Drainage in such cases are always posterior. In cases of multiple fibroids it is always prudent to remove the fibroids from the most prominent area. The fibroids sitting on each other can be removed from the same incision.

After the procedure the anatomy of the fallopian tube and ovary are invariably checked, their normalcy ensured (Figures 14.7A to G).

Removal of Fibroid by Morcellation (Figures 14.8A to I)

Morcellation is done with a 10/12/15 mm morcellator. We normally prefer a reusable morcellator – Rotocut, Sawalhe's morcellator (Karl Storz, Gmbh Germany) (Figures 14.8A and B), however, a claw forceps 10 mm or 15 mm size is used with a 8/12 mm grasping tip to take

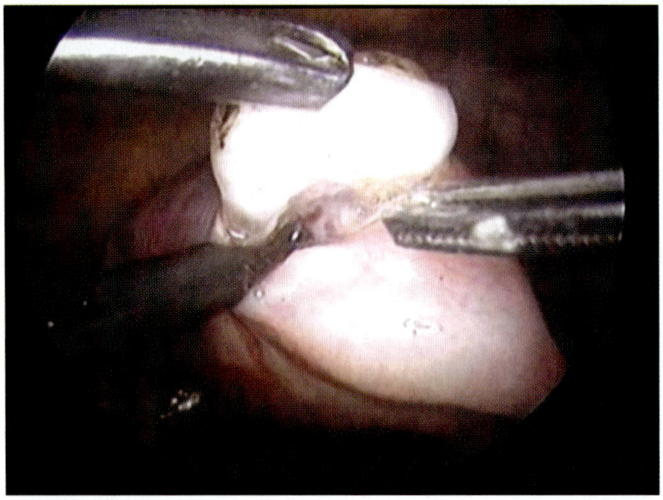

Figure 14.7C

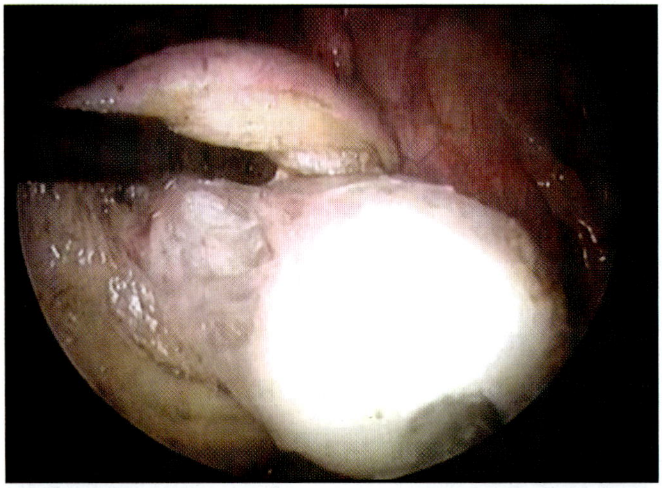

Figure 14.7D

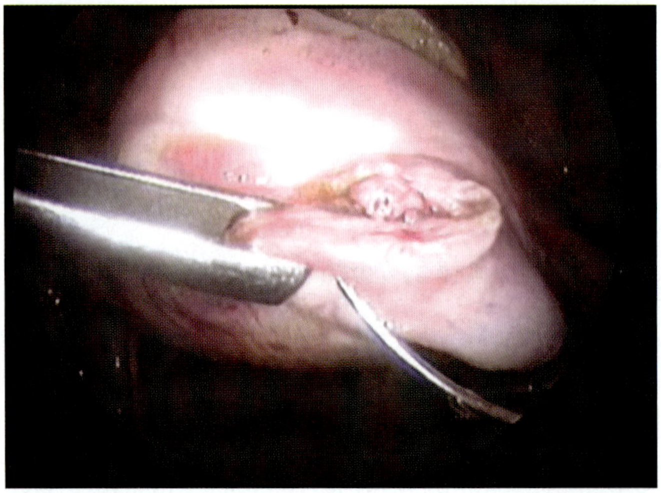

Figure 14.7E

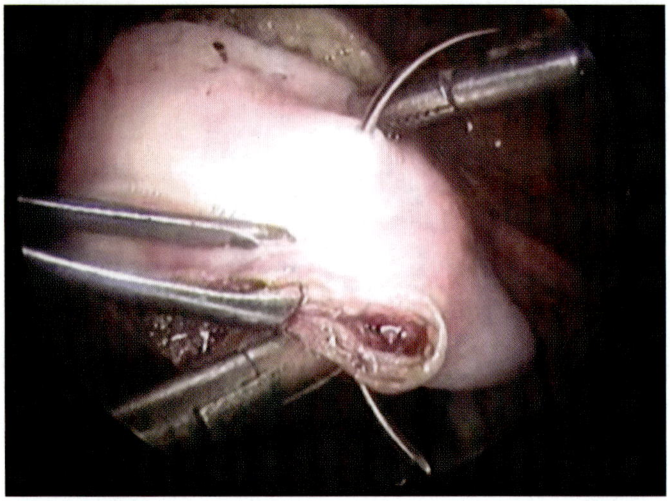

Figure 14.7F

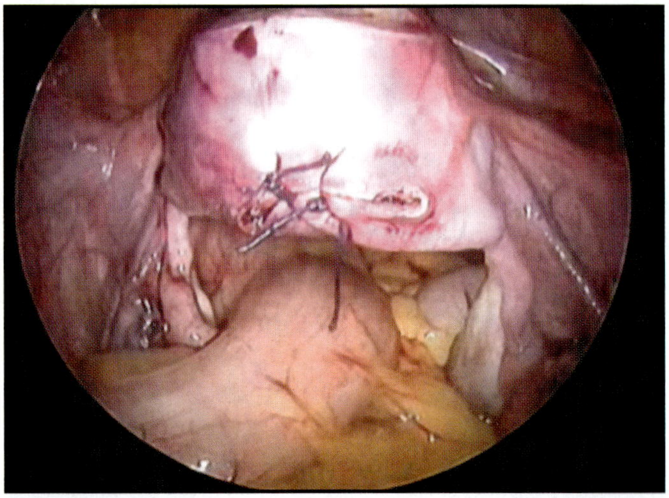

Figure 14.7G

Figures 14.7A to G. Removal of the right cornual fibroid and suturing

out the myoma in long strips. The left lower port is the preferred port wherein the 5 mm incision is widened to 15 mm after infiltrating injection sensorcaine. Prior to insertion of the morcellator, the pneumoperitonium pressure is elevated to 20 mm of Hg to allow safe entry of sharp morcellator. Once the morcellator is introduced the trocar is removed, and care is taken to prevent gas leakage. Morcellator has a foot switch, which is used only after ensuring proper grip of the myoma in the claw forceps. Morcellation is done in a horizontal direction with left hand holding the claw to pull the fibroid and

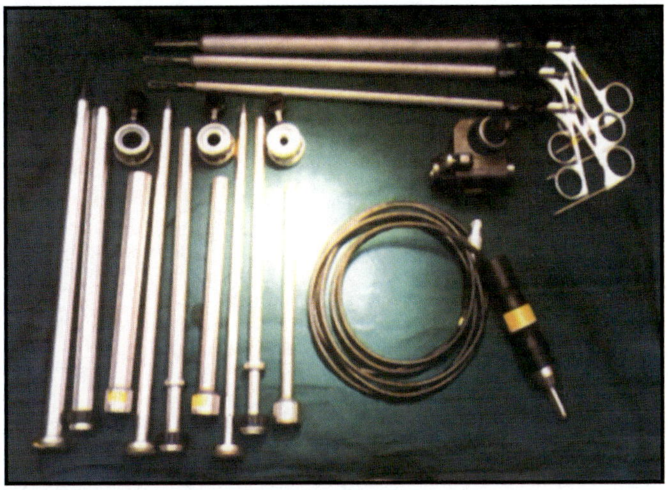

Figure 14.8A. Sawalhe's morcellator

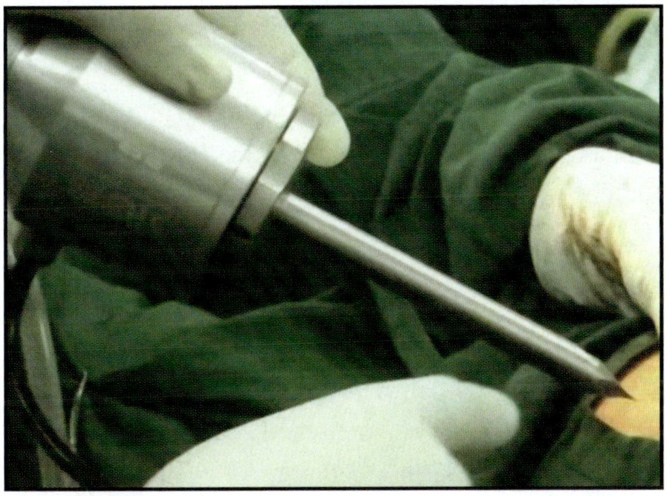

Figure 14.8B. Rotocut morcellator

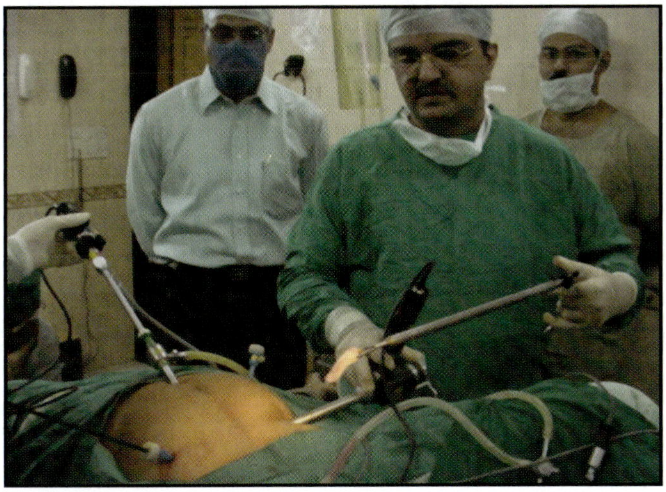

Figure 14.8C

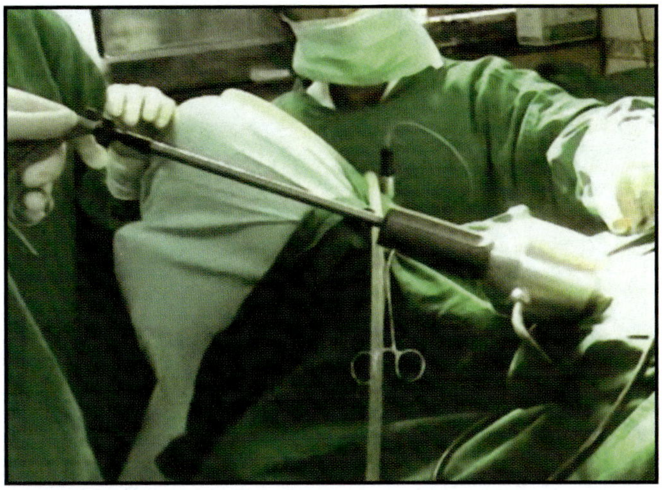

Figure 14.8D

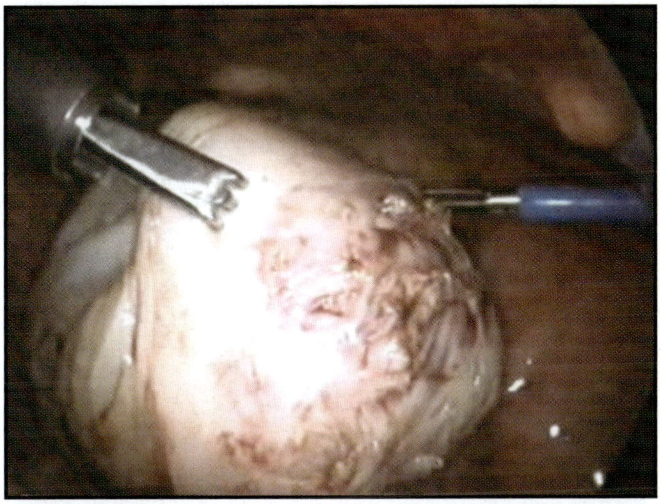

Figure 14.8E

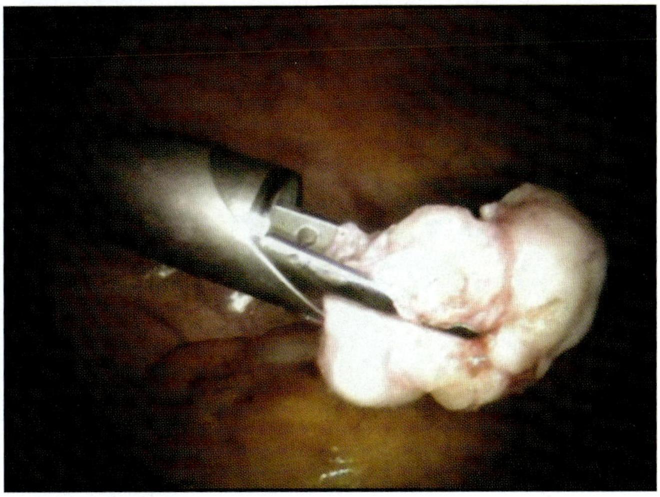

Figure 14.8F

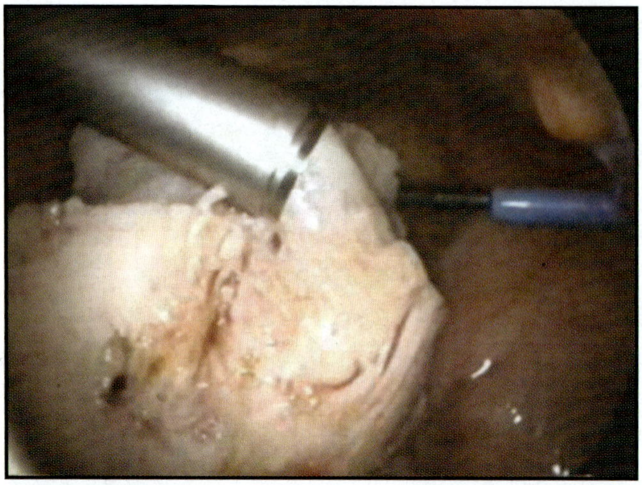

Figure 14.8G

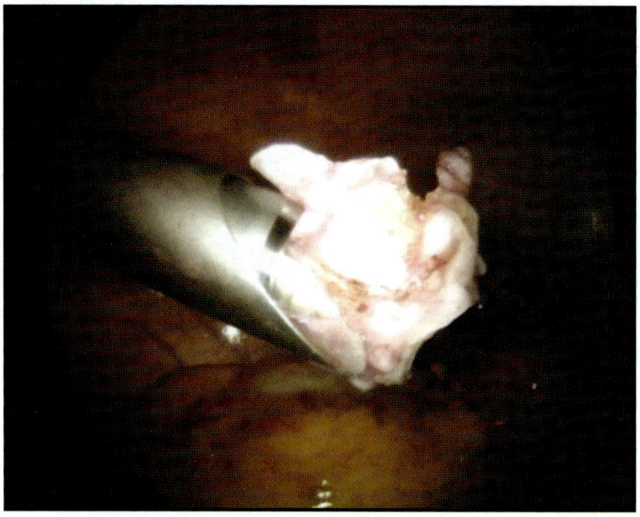

Figure 14.8H

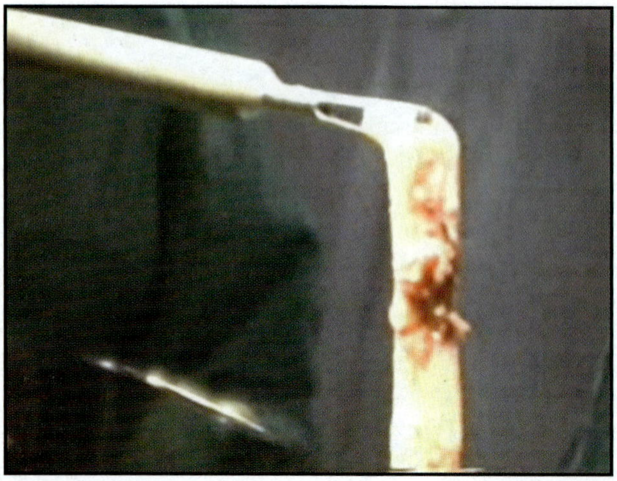

Figure 14.8I

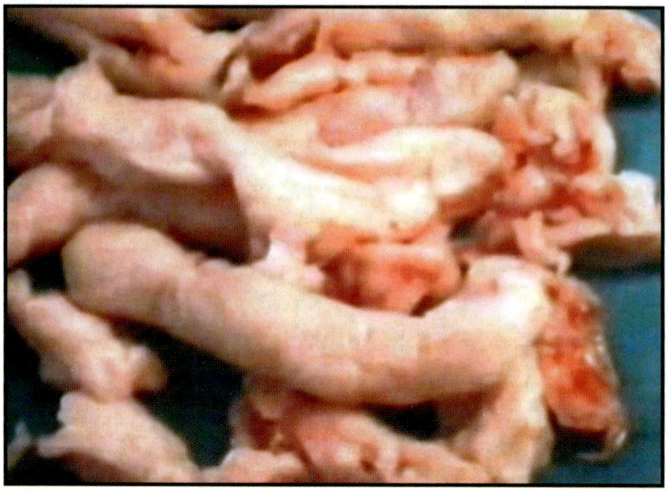

Figure 14.8J

Figures 14.8A to J. The electronic morcellator, steps of morcellation and morcellated fibroid

the right hand stabilizing the morcellator (Figure 14.8C). The assistant feeds and stabilizes the fibroid by a claw forceps. After ensuring the entry of the sharp rotating blade, the fibroid is pulled by the claw forceps (held in the left hand). Pressing the foot switch then commences the morcellation. The fibroid can be successfully extracted in the form of morcellated strips (Figure 14.8J). We have been fortunate to have used all types of morcellators during our series of laparoscopic myomectomy viz. Steiner's morcellator,[12] Sawalhe's, Rotocut (Karl Storz), Wisap's, Gynecare, Wolf's morcellator, etc. It is worth mentioning that morcellator should never be used if vision is hampered or if the grip of the claw is wider than the diameter of the morcellator. If this is not avoided it may cause malfunction of the morcellator. The Rotocut morcellator with possibility of use of all 3 Karl Storz morcellator is the best at present.

We have removed significantly large fibroids – upto 18 cms and multiple fibroids upto maximum of 16 in a single case successfully. However, the whole procedure is finished within 150-200 minutes. All these are demonstrated in the photographs in detail. We do not prefer mechanical morcellators. Similarly, we also do not prefer to use morcellators from other ports, as they are unphysiological and prone to accidental injuries.

Using a 10 mm / 5 mm spring action retractable knife entering through the 5 mm port and morcellating the fibroid freely in the peritoneal cavity could be dangerous and looks very crude though showed by experts. In the absence or malfunction of morcellator, if the patient is sexually active, I feel colpotomy is a "poor man's morcellator" is acceptable by many endoscopists. It is done using CCL trocar (Colpo-Chirurgie Lausuane, Karl Storz, Tuttlingen, Germany). Colpotomy is performed by a spatula with monopolar cautery, incising over the protruding CCL. Fibroids are fed from above to the claw forceps in the vagina. The stretchability of the vagina is remarkable and hence even the large fibroid can be removed. The wound is closed from below using polyglactin no. 1 or 1-0. After removal of all pieces of fibroid and giving a meticulous lavage with dilute Betadine solution in the pelvis and pelvic gutter, an intraperitoneal drain, usually 14 or 16 G Ryle's tube is placed through the right port, surprisingly we get 100-150 ml of drainage in the first 24 hours as this is a normal tissue. Unlike endometriosis, which is fibrotic disease, drainage is removed within 36 hours.

Port incisions are approximated using glue (Nectacryl or Adhihist) and the 15 mm incision (for the morcellator) is sutured in two layers viz. the rectus sheath by polyglactin no.1 and the skin by nonabsorbable no. 2-0 or 3-0.

Postoperative analgesia is ensured by administering a rectal suppository or injectable opioid analgesics. Parental antibiotics are given as routine. Patients are usually discharged by 48 hours.

Risks of Laparoscopic Myomectomy

Any endoscopic surgery procedure whether laparoscopic hysterectomy, laparoscopic myomectomy or advanced endometriosis, will have common risk related to pneumoperitonium. Trocar entry and certain risks with anesthesia, which are not elaborated as they are covered in a separate section.

Specific Risks of Laparoscopic Myomectomy[7]

1. Time taken for surgery and hence anesthesia is longer than abdominal myomectomy. If the monitoring of the parameters is judicious, prolonged anesthesia may not be worrisome. A good laparoscopic surgeon consistently takes little longer time for laparoscopic myomectomy even after sufficient experience.
2. Major risk imagined after a laparoscopic myomectomy is the future rupture of the uterus in pregnancy[13-18]—in antenatal period or during labor. This is due to the popular belief, rather misconception, that laparoscopic suturing is inferior to that during an open surgery. David's[13] (1953) and Brown et al[14] (1956) initially reported that incidence of uterine scar dehiscence or rupture was relatively rare in an abdominal myomectomy. However, Golan et al[15] (1990) found the incidence significantly reduced though still higher as compared to abdominal myomectomy. It is our experience after performing 968 laparoscopic myomectomies that laparoscopic suturing and myomectomy is superior, specially in an infertile patient, in the hands of an expert, skilled surgeon. We feel that rupture of uterus after myomectomy is viewed with a microscope only after the advent of laparoscopic method. It is not that in abdominal myomectomy, rupture uterus is unknown. However, important word of caution is (since we do ipsilateral) if a laparoscopic surgeon is not conversant with more than optimum suturing technique or gets fatigued with the number of sutures placed, as quite often noticed with contralateral suturing, or for unknown reasons becomes a little lazy to do proper suturing, then there is a strong possibility of rupture uterus in such cases which unnecessarily tarnishes the benefits of laparoscopic myomectomy. It is our observation that vertical scars are more prone to rupture, and hence we do not prefer the use of

vertical incision for the removal of myoma since the spiral arterioles are horizontal in distribution (Farrer-Brown et al[17]). We are also eager to wait and watch our patients who have undergone laparoscopic myomectomy, especially for significantly large or multiple fibroids with regards to their obstetric outcome. Since so far we have not come across a single case of uterine rupture, though, of approximately 30 percent of cases who became pregnant subsequently, few have delivered vaginally and the rest by cesarean section. In certain specific patients we, however, advise an elective cesarean section like those conceiving after a laparoscopic myomectomy for significantly large fibroids or those located posteriorly or on the fundus, as this is the area, which is stretched to the maximum during pregnancy.

3. Hemorrhage is a significant risk factor. There is an increased risk if we do not use dilute vasopressin or we are in the wrong plane of dissection, which causes prolonged surgery and thereby increasing the blood loss. In our series, we found that the blood loss was higher in the early phase, and was on the decrease because of improvement in the suturing time over the period. We strongly recommend that one should abstain from the temptation to use GnRH analogues prior to removal of large fibroid, though literature reviews suggest probable benefit. The advantage of reducing vascularity is lost by merging of tissue planes making the actual dissection and complete removal of fibroid more difficult and time consuming, sometimes even impossible, increasing the risk of hemorrhage indirectly by increasing the duration of surgery. H Reich[11] also reported the disadvantage of GnRH analogues prior to surgery enough since the tissue planes merge and surgery is rendered more difficult. We firmly believe that if the surgeon were skilled, the removal of large myomas using above technique would always circumvent the risk of hemorrhage. In our clinical experience, GnRH analogues can definitely offer significant benefit, only in severely anemic patients, in whom immediate surgery would otherwise be contraindicated. We can buy sometime before surgery can be contemplated, simultaneously preventing their growth and reducing the amount of menorrhagia in such patients. Various researchers have reported upto 50 percent reduction in the actual size of the fibroid after 4-6 months of therapy. GnRH analogues may also be useful in reducing the size of a submucous myoma or an intracavitary myoma > 5 cm, thereby making a hysteroscopic myomectomy feasible.[19-21]

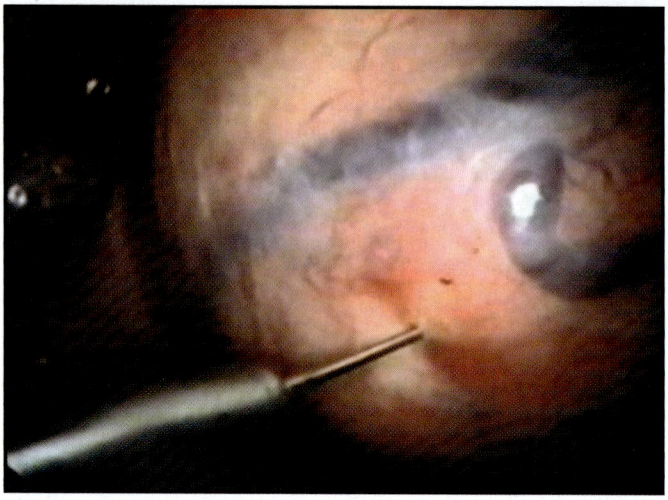

Figure 14.9. A highly vascular fibroid

In an unusual case one may come across a very vascular fibroid (Figure 14.9). In these cases the possibility of the malignancy should be always considered and a frozen section should be performed intraoperatively. The risk of hemorrhage is higher in such vascular fibroids, even if malignancy is ruled out or vasopressin is employed for minimizing the blood loss. In such cases it is solely dependent on the surgeon's surgical skill and expertise to proceed with a laparoscopic myomectomy or sometimes a laparotomy is indicated even if the surgeon is skilled, which may be a prudent decision and as safety is the prime concern.

4. This usually happens in inappropriately selected cases in whom otherwise an abdominal myomectomy is the method of choice. Hence this risk factor can be significantly taken care of and is avoidable.
5. We have noticed a little higher incidence of postoperative residual small fibroid unnoticed during a laparoscopic myomectomy, which could be otherwise detected by direct palpation during an abdominal myomectomy. However, the sizes of such fibroid are usually small, the significance of residual fibroid or recurrence cannot be exaggerated.
6. *Conversion to laparotomy:* It is worth mentioning that conversion of a laparoscopic myomectomy to a laparotomy, in our study we had 1.85 percent (18 cases) of conversion to a laparotomy. In retrospection it was clearly evident that these were mainly due to inappropriate patient selection. The risk of conversion is definitely higher, nearly three times more, when the size of the fibroid is >11 cm, or are anterior in location. Dubuisson et al[40] (1996) reported a three times higher conversion rate when fibroids measured > 8 cm or located anteriorly. Conversion to a laparotomy is actually a prudent judgment on the part of the surgeon to do at an appropriate time in the interest and welfare of the patient, rather than unnecessarily deferred.
7. *Postoperative adhesions:*[22,23] In any surgery, whether even operative laparoscopy, especially when fibroids are large and multiple, the defects are repaired by sutures and hence the possibility of adhesions always arises. However, it may be interesting to note that at the adhesions after laparoscopic myomectomy, which is a remote control surgery usually done without any close approximation of the tissue on the abdomen, chances of adhesions are much lesser than that of an open surgery. Some researchers have advocated the use of products like Interceed, which are thought to prevent or significantly reduce the incidence of formation of postoperative adhesions. However, we do not prefer to use such foreign material as they might interfere with healing, and their actual benefit is still a matter of debate.
8. *Accidental adenomyoma/adenomyosis:* (16 cases) may surprise us during laparoscopic myomectomy. This can be avoided by proper sonography. This does not have any specific laparoscopic treatment.
9. *Accidental opening of endometrial cavity during a laparoscopic myomectomy:* We find it unnecessary to suture the endometrial cavity or do a multilayer closure in laparoscopic myomectomy, since approximation of myometrium and healing is more controlled by muscular element of uterine wall by secondary healing. In our experience, multiple layer suturing leads to eversion of layers, making it difficult to suture and also exposing it to risk of rupture due to faulty and difficult suturing.
10. Accidental finding of sarcomatous or malignant change in a fibroid or large uterus can be very often differentiated by a proper color Doppler. A frozen section in such a case can be very useful.

Complications of Laparoscopic Myomectomy and Prevention

Most of the complications are covered in the subject of risks of laparoscopic myomectomy, viz.

1. Longer operative time, longer anesthesia
2. Hemorrhage
3. Rupture of scar
4. Adhesions
5. Technical problems

Few of the complications are worth mention:

a. *Breakage of myoma screw:* A not so rare complication during a laparoscopic myomectomy is the breakage of myoma screw while pulling the myoma with the screw out of the uterus, which can be dissected out by the spatula. This can be minimized by ipsilateral placement of the myoma screw in the left upper port with the spatula in the left lower port. Proper stabilization of the uterus should be done by a uterine

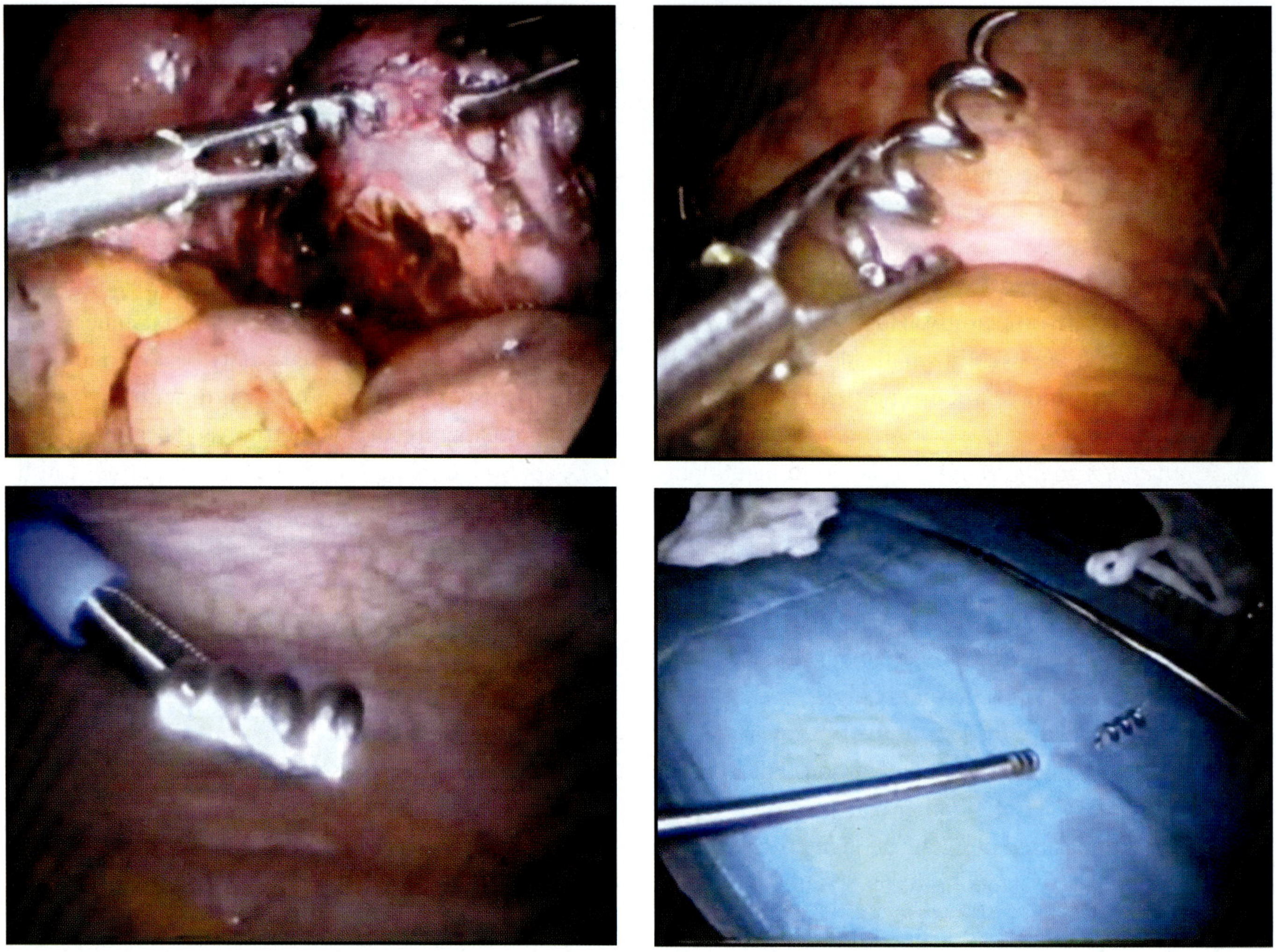

Figures 14.10A to D. Breakage of the myoma screw and removal of the piece

manipulator, which is placed vaginally. Additionally, the incision made to enucleate the fibroid should never be less than optimum. The surgeon should ensure that the myoma screw is made up of more dense revolution and should be mandatory single-piece and not welded or soldered. One should ensure that removal of the broken piece is always done before the conclusion of the procedure, taking care of not slipping suddenly when it can get lost in the peritoneal cavity (Figures 14.10 A to D).

b. *Endometrial serosal fistula:* In patients who have large intramural fibroids or deep uterine wall defects, there is a risk of formation of endometrial serosal fistula. This late complication may result in an occasional case. However, the exact cause of this is not known but is probably thought to be inadequate or improper suturing of the uterine wall after the removal of the fibroids. However, fortunately we have not yet come across this entity in our series. When the surgeon is not well-conversant with laparoscopic suturing, specially in cases of large fibroids, one must consider laparoscopic assisted myomectomy (mentioned below) for better suturing to avoid occurrence of such sequelae.

When to do Abdominal Myomectomy ?[45]

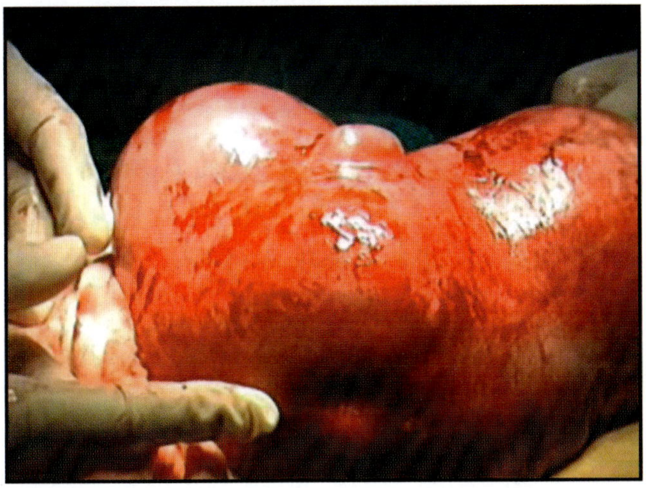

Figure 14.11. A case of large multiple fibroids (28-30 weeks size)

Indications

At this moment we find that in an infertile patient or a patient with menorrhagia (keen to conserve her uterus), abdominal myomectomy is indicated in the following situations:

1. Uterus size comparable to > 22 weeks pregnancy (Figure 14.11).
2. Fibroids >14 cm in size, with broad base (pedunclated fibroids of this size or even greater can be successfully removed laparoscopically).
3. Previous history of extensive abdominal surgery, e.g. for endometriosis, adnexal pathology or suspected to have severe adhesions involving gastrointestinal tract may be due to abdominal tuberculosis.
4. Laparoscopist not well-trained or poor in laparoscopic suturing.
5. Strong suspicion of malignancy, even if the surgeon is experienced, because we believe that laparoscopic surgery for malignancy is still in experimental stages and may be incomplete or increase spread.
6. High-risk medical conditions not permitting pneumoperitoneum required for laparoscopic surgery warrant abdominal myomectomy.

Last but not the least, we strongly feel that endoscopic enthusiasm should not merge into endoscopic fanaticism.

Place of Laparoscopic Assisted Myomectomy[24, 25]

Any laparoscopic myomectomy involves three major steps, viz.

1. Dissecting the fibroid out of the uterine serosa.
2. Removal of the fibroid from the peritoneal cavity by morcellation or colpotomy.
3. Reconstruction of the uterine defect.

Nezhat et al[24,25] had come across few cases of utero-peritoneal fistula following a laparoscopic myomectomy. Hence, he suggested that laparoscopic assisted myomectomy may replace laparoscopic myomectomy in such the high-risk cases, thereby offering the benefit of obviating the need of performing laparotomy and simultaneously preventing the formation of uteroperitoneal fistula by ensuring meticulous suturing through a minilaparotomy incision. Thus minilaparotomy for good suturing may be tried by gynecologists not well-trained for laparoscopic suturing or a high medicolegal scenario.

After the insertion of regular ports, a corkscrew manipulator or a myoma screw is introduced through the suprapubic port and inserted into the myoma. The myoma is then pulled towards the anterior abdominal wall with the trocar and screw attached; this 5 mm incision is further increased transversely to 4-5 cm. The abdominal wall is then opened as in minilaparotomy. The myoma is then brought to the incision and then shelled out and morcellated. The resulting defect is clearly visualized and sutured in layers by no. 1 or 1-0 polyglactin suture after elevating the uterus upto the incision. The incision may be temporarily closed in single layer to visualize residual myomas if not seen through the minilaparotomy incision and the laparoscope is reintroduced. After identifying them they are brought to the incision as before. In cases of posterior myomas, a complete laparoscopic removal is done followed by suturing of the defect through the incision. Nezhat et al[24, 25] did not prefer to suture the serosa. After suturing, uterus is thoroughly palpated for any small intramural myomas. Then, it is returned to the peritoneal cavity. The minilaparotomy incision is closed in layers as routine using no. 1 and 1-0 polyglactin 910 sutures.

In today's era of hostile medicolegal environment, laparoscopic assisted myomectomy may be considered. We however, feel that instead of only suturing by minilaparotomy, an abdominal myomectomy is preferred, as it does not serve the purpose of 'button-hole' surgery. But we acknowledge that Nezhat et al were proficient in laparoscopic suturing, and hence this thought must be pondered by budding endoscopists in a non-compromising patient population.

ALTERNATIVE MINIMALLY INVASIVE METHODS

Uterine Artery Embolization (Figures 14.12A and B)

McLucas et al[26] have advocated uterine artery embolization as a non-surgical, though minimally invasive procedure, which has proven benefit in reducing the size of fibroids and thereby significantly relieving the symptoms like menorrhagia and pressure symptoms (Spies et al[27]) and extended to even infertility patients.

Injection of tiny polyvinylglycol particles of the size of grains of sand into the uterine artery on both sides through a properly placed catheter. This causes blockade of the feeding vessel to the fibroid thereby causing ischemic necrosis, reducing the size.

McLucas et al[26] (Int Journal Gyn Obst, 2001) suggested that the radiation exposure was quite minimal. Further, he opined that the risk of infertility following uterine artery embolization is negligibly less. Moreover, patients conceiving after this procedure had completely uneventful antenatal as well as intrapartum course. Hence, he concluded that associated infertility does not really contraindicate uterine artery embolization and some patients can be selectively offered this therapeutic modality with definite success.

Complications

1. Radiation exposure
2. Premature menopause
3. Infertility
4. Severe postoperative pain.

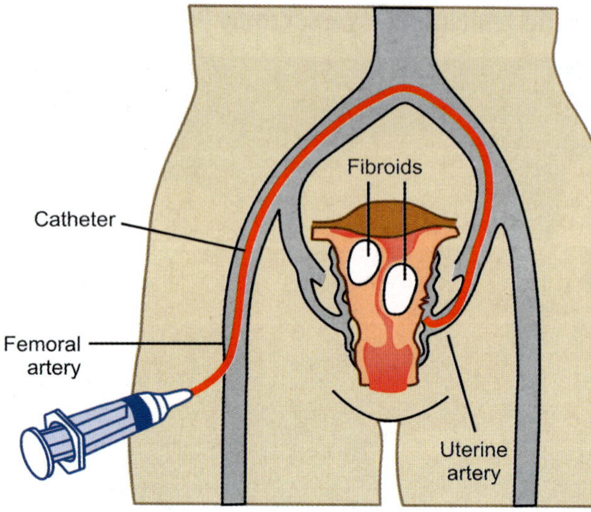

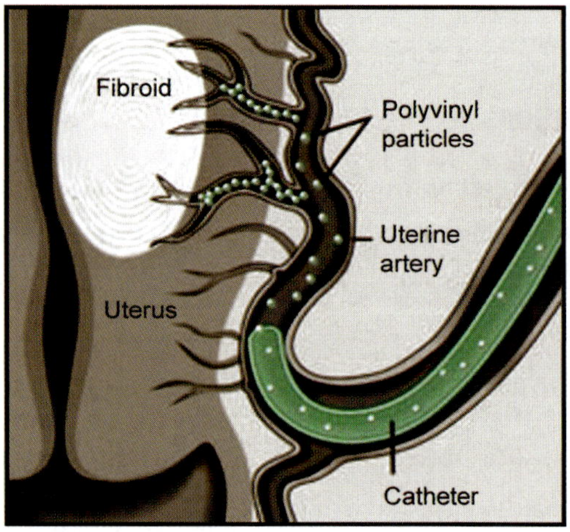

Figures 14.12A and B. Uterine artery embolization

Author believes that fibroids are parasites in uterus, hence only blocking uterine arteries will reduce fibroids dependent on uterine blood supply.

Laparoscopic Myolysis

Laparoscopic myoma coagulation, termed as myolysis was developed in Germany in 1986 (Gallinat and Leuken,[28] 1993). However, Goldfarb[29] (1992) first performed this procedure and reported it in the literature. The procedure employs the use of bipolar needle or other energy source to pierce the myoma and coagulate the feeding blood vessels at multiple places. Various modes are used by different researchers to destroy the stroma and vascular supply of the targeted leiomyoma, e.g.

1. Nd: YAG (neodymium:yttrium-aluminum-garnet) Laser bare fiber by Goldfarb[29] 1992; Nisolle[32] 1953; Philip[33] 1997.
2. Monopolar needle – Wood et al[34] 1994.
3. Bipolar coagulation needle – Goldfarb 1995[30]; 1996; Phillip[33] 1997.
4. Hyperthermia electrode – (diathermy) Chapman[35] 1993.
5. Recently cryomyo probe – Zreik[36] 1998.

Goldfarb and Chapman[30,35] report 50-70 percent shrinkage of the volume of fibroids following this procedure, with no recurrence over a follow-up period of 12 months. They used preprocedure GnRH analogue in the form of leuprolide acetate Depot (3.75 mg) or Goserelin 3.6 mg for 3 months before the procedure.

They recommended not to perform myolysis in patients:

1. Who have < 25 percent shrinkage of total uterine volume following GnRH analogue therapy
2. Who remain symptomatic even after 3 months of GnRH therapy.

Major disadvantage of this procedure was missing or delaying the diagnosis of sarcomatous degeneration in occasional fibroid, which can occur in 0.04 to 0.29 percent of leiomyomas (Corsacaden and Singh[37] 1958, Montague et al[38] 1965). Hence the actual benefit cost effectiveness of myolysis is still under question. An experienced laparoscopic surgeon may not prefer myolysis to myomectomy.

Our Experience with Laparoscopic Myomectomy

From March 1993 to 2005 we have carried out laparoscopic myomectomy in 962 patients removing over 1264 fibroids altogether. Average age of patients was 34.5 ± 3.2 years (Range 21-53 years). Many patients with fibroids beyond this age group required hysterectomy and hence are not included.

The common indications were (Table 14.2):

Table 14.2. Common indications for laparoscopic myomectomy

Incidence of symptoms	*Trivedi et al (2005)*	*Dubuisson et al (1996)*
1. Menorrhagia	42%	18.8%
2. Lump in abdomen with pain or accidental detection	14%	31.9%
3. Associated with Infertility	49%	32.9%
4 Pressure symptoms	4%	—

There was a considerable overlap of symptoms as some patients had mixed complaints.

Apart from laparoscopic myomectomy in these patients, other laparoscopic procedure done simultaneously were (Table 14.3).

Table 14.3. Additional procedures done with laparoscopic myomectomy

Associated surgery	*Trivedi et al*	*Dubuisson et al*
1. Laparoscopic adhesiolysis	118	4
2. Salpingoovariolysis	51	24
3. PCO drilling	37	—
4. Tubal ligation	12	15
5. Fulguration of endometriosis	68	24
6. Salpingectomy	—	—
7. Ovarian cystectomy	18	23

Our Observation

In our series the average duration of surgery was about 150 minutes. We observed that with increasing skill the operating time decreased significantly. The minimum time required was 22 minutes. The average blood loss was 65 ml. In one case there was significant blood loss of upto 750-800 ml. Three patients in our series required blood transfusion. The mean hemoglobin drop was 0.9 gm percent. The maximum number of fibroids removed from a single patient was 12. The largest fibroid removed laparoscopically was 18 cm. Most of our patients were discharged within 24 hours of the surgery, the average duration of stay being 26 hours (Table 14.4).

The pattern of distribution of fibroids in our series was as follows (Table 14.5):

Table 14.4. Our observations and comparison

Laparoscopic myomectomy (details)	*Trivedi et al (2005)*	*Dubuisson et al (1996)*
1. Average duration	150 ± 42 min (22-255 min)	130 ± 56.1(range – 30-300)
2. Average blood loss	65 ml (20-800 ml)	——
3. Average hemoglobin drop	0.9 ± 1.48 (range – 0-5 gm/dl)	1.4±1.18 (range – 0-6gm/dl)
4. Average no. of myomas removed per patients	2.85 ± 1.9 (range – 1-12)	2.05 ±1.5 (range –1-10)
5. Maximum no. removed in one patient	16	——
6. Size of the myomas	5.7 ± 3.18 cm (range – 1-18 cm is largest so far)	5.3 ± 2.2 cm (range – 1-12 cm)
7. Maximum size removed	18 cm	12 cm
8. Average duration of hospital stay	26 ± 6.34 hours (range –16-96 hours)	——

Table 14.5. Pattern of distribution of fibroids

	Trivedi et al	*Dubuisson et al*
1. Multiple fibroids	371 (62%)	108 (50.7%)
2. Posterior	348 (58%)	99 (46.5%)
3. Anterior	312 (51%)	61 (28.6%)
4. Fundal	152 (24%)	46 (21.6%)
5. Broad ligament	41 (6 %)	7 (3.3%)
6. Cervical	16 (3%)	—
7. Pedunculated	64 (10%)	11.8%

Role of Hysteroscopic Myomectomy

In our experience, we have found that 13 to 15 percent of fibroids were submucous fibroids or intramural fibroids with significant intracavitary component. To firmly say that how many of this actually caused infertility is difficult, but 85 percent of them were done in patients presenting with infertility (Garcia et al).[50] We found that the pregnancy rates were phenomenally improved giving approximately upto 85 percent of pregnancy rate (Ubaldi et al). [51]

However, hysteroscopic myomectomy is a very technically demanding procedure (Vercellini et al),[52] the efficacy of this procedure is proven to be far superior to open or laparoscopic myomectomy due to the inherent advantage of bypassing the need of incising and suturing the uterine musculature for removal of fibroid. Nevertheless, there are some technical issues before one contemplates a hysteroscopic removal for a patient with an intracavitary fibroid or polyp, especially in a patient of infertility.

Prerequisites for Safe Hysteroscopic Myomectomy (Figures 14.13A to D)

1. The fibroid should be intracavitary, confirmed by a thorough ultrasound and if necessary Doppler study.
2. At least 30 percent or more of the fibroid should project into the cavity (fibroids upto 6 cm have been successfully resected hysteroscopically at our center), higher risk of fluid overload than TCRE, etc.
3. Thorough knowledge of fluid dynamics and glycine metabolism, as there are chances of glycine absorption, especially if fibroid is large.
4. Adequately trained, experienced and skilled surgeon.
5. Anesthetist well-conversant with endoscopic procedures.

Hysteroscopic myomectomy can be performed using a resectoscope (Brook et al,[53] Corson et al),[54] or versapoint or the vaportrode (Which vaporizes the fibroid due to high wattage) and laser. We at our center have performed 301 hysteroscopic myomectomies till date. We prefer to use resectoscope with the forward and backward loops alternately, at 110 watts of pure cutting current for the resection (Figures 14.13E to I) . The main advantage with the resectoscope is that the chips of the fibroids can be obtained. After resection of fibroid

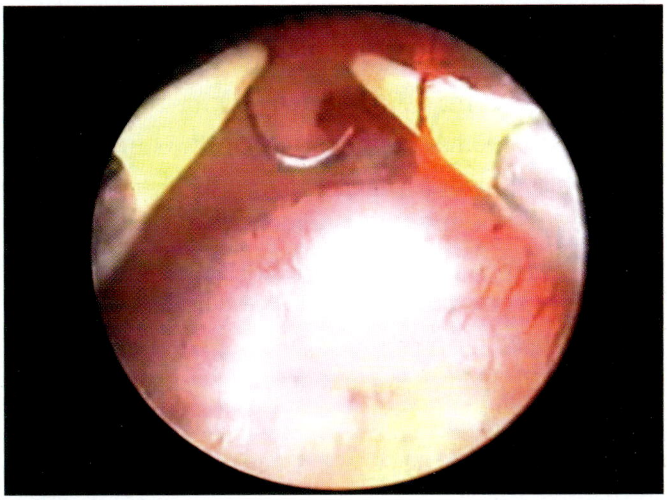
Figure 14.13A. Posterior wall fibroid

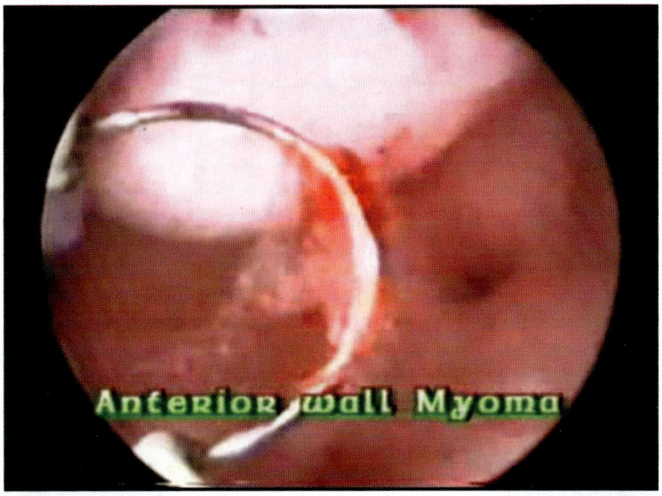

Figure 14.13B. Anterior wall fibroid

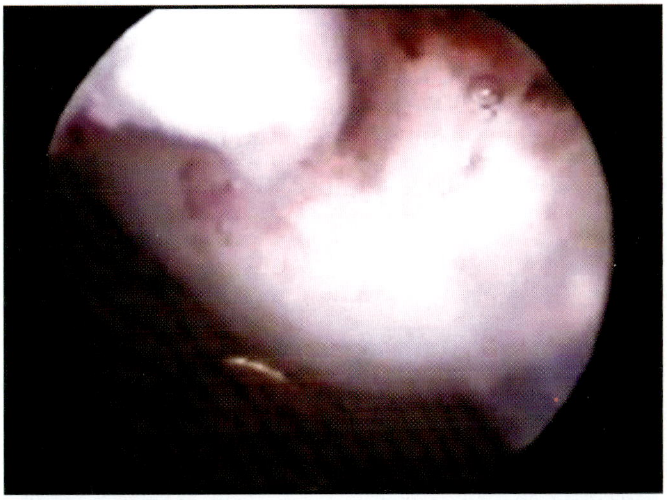
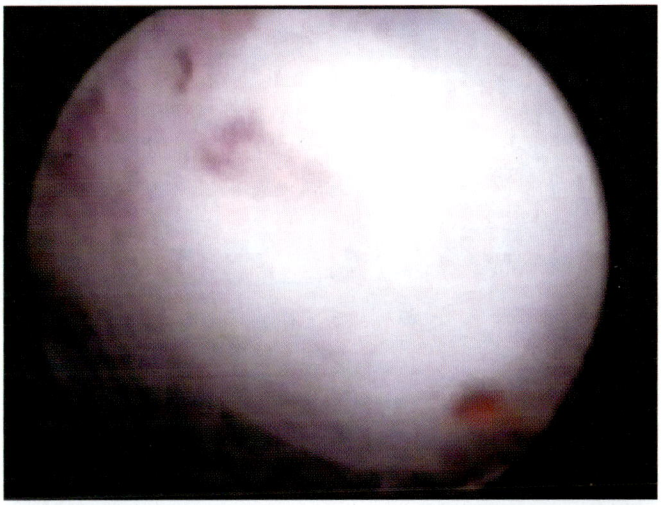
Figures 14.13C and D. Large anterior wall submucous fibroid

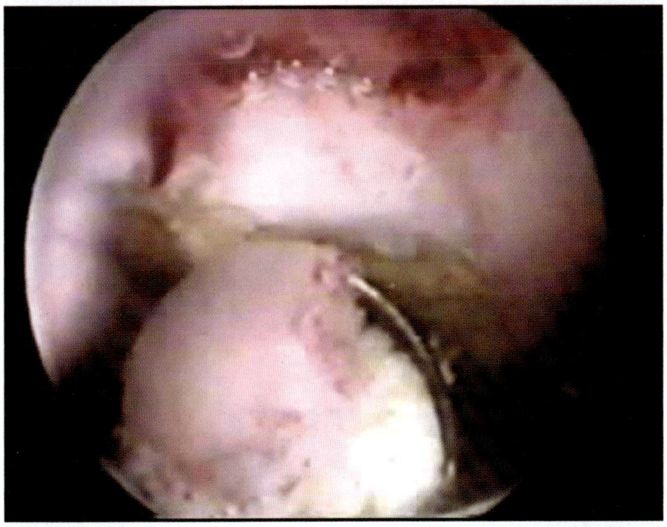
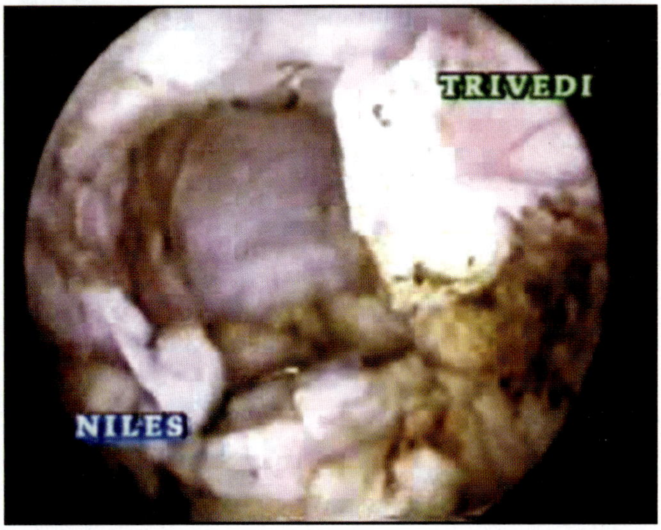

Figures 14.13E and F. Resection of anterior wall fibroid

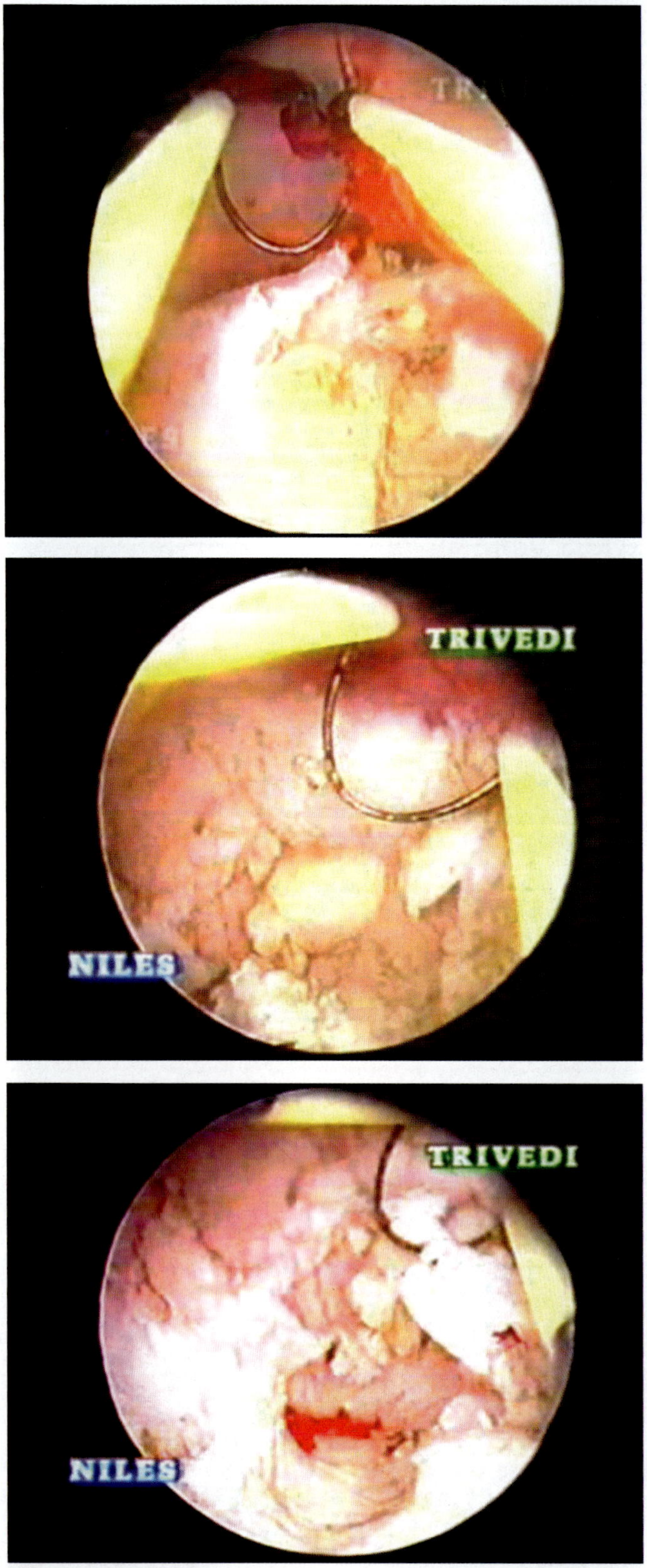

Figures 14.13G to I. Resection of posterior wall fibroid

hemostasis is achieved with cylinder or roller ball monopolar loop (Figure 14.13J). The vaportrode vaporizes the fibroid and may not be effective for fibroids more than 3 cm. Another major factor as far as infertility is concerned is, since vaportrode employs a very high wattage, it is destructive to endometrium and hence is not recommended for the fibroids presenting with infertility. Versapoint has the disadvantage, as it is a pointed tipped electrode, may not be effective for larger fibroids. We have abandoned laser for hysteroscopic myomectomy as it only achieves superficial destruction of the fibroid and hence is not effective for larger fibroids or fibroids with large intracavitary component.

Precautions during Hysteroscopic Myomectomy

The main area of concern in any major operative hysteroscopic surgery is fluid overload. Hence, one should be vigilant of the volume of glycine used and the volume in the output jar. In case of major discrepancy (more than 600-800 ml), one should withhold the procedure and consider administration of diuretics and wait for adequate urine output. Pulmonary examination should reveal clear airway and absence of adventitious sounds. The procedure can be continued only when one is sure that the discrepancy has been taken care of. Another important issue is to what depth one has to resect

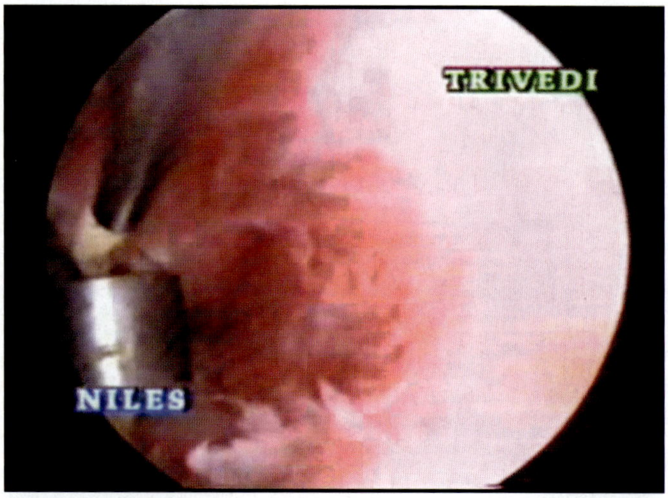

Figure 14.13J

the fibroid. It may be some time difficult to judge the completion of the procedure and in such situations there are chances of perforating the uterus. At such occasions it is prudent to abandon the procedure at that stage and do the second stage completion procedure after 8 weeks or later. However, with increasing experience and skill, one can master the procedure and resect a fibroid upto 5 to 6 cm successfully without any untoward sequelae.

Role of Preoperative GnRH Agonists[19-21]

We have found that preoperative administration of GnRH agonists to be effective and can be considered to reduce the size of a large intracavitary fibroid. However, with increasing expertise the feasibility of hysteroscopic myomectomy increases and fibroids upto 5 to 6 cm can be resected successfully. But till a surgeon achieves skill and is well-conversant with the procedure, administration of GnRH agonists for 4 to 6 months (Depot preparation of 3.6 mg of goserelin, once a month for 4-6 months) can reduce the size of fibroid to make a hysteroscopic myomectomy feasible. The major concern in administration of Gnrh analogues is its cost, while the other significant issue is adverse effects like osteoporosis.

Some researchers have tried danazol preoperatively. However, there is no role of danazol in cases where a hysteroscopic myomectomy is planned. GnRH analogues can offer a better advantage, by reducing the size by up to 40 percent of original size, if given for longer periods.

Postoperatively, one can contradictorily administer low-dose estrogens in cases where there has been large fibroid and a large area was denuded during the resection. This ensures formation of a good endometrial lining on the operative area and reduces the chances of fibrosis.

REVIEW OF RESULTS AND FERTILITY OUTCOME

The success of fertility after laparoscopic myomectomy in our experience was 45 percent in patients having no other cause of infertility and upto 29 percent in patients with other associated factors contributing to their infertility, e.g. polycystic ovaries, hyperprolactinemia, endometriosis after concurrent surgical management with active fertility treatment. Our results were in accordance with the observations of several International studies. Buttram and Reiter[2] reported a 40 percent rate of pregnancy, while Verkaufe et al[39] had a higher pregnancy rate of 59.4 percent. Dubuisson[16, 40] and Dessolle et al[41] reported pregnancy rates of more than 40 percent after laparoscopic myomectomy. They however, stressed upon proper patient selection. Rossetti et al[42] found that pregnancy rates were as high as 65 percent after a laparoscopic myomectomy.

It is surprising to note that the actual pregnancy rates reported in the international data ranged between as low as 16.7 percent (Berkeley et al)[43] to as high as 88.9 percent (Frederick et al).[44]

CONCLUSION

We have come to believe, after a few hundred laparoscopic myomectomies, that laparoscopic myomectomy if judiciously employed in properly selected cases definitely offers significant advantages over an abdominal myomectomy. Withholding cases of large and multiple fibroids with no other cause for infertility is the route cause for getting same patients later with larger and difficult myomectomy.This can be minimized by timely interaction and removal of the same by good endoscopists. However, we still maintain that the surgeon should be well-trained and skilled in the procedure, while still not converting his endoscopic enthusiasm into endoscopic fanaticism. In skilled and experienced hands laparoscopic myomectomy is a very graceful, effective surgical modality, especially for women with infertility due to or associated with fibroids. The safety of the procedure and early postoperative recovery was suggesting that laparoscopic route of removal of fibroids offers a minimally invasive method without compromising the surgical therapy for the patient. However, laparoscopic myomectomy in unindicated or inappropriately selected cases may be detrimental. Acquiring excellence in skill of laparoscopic suturing is necessary. Nevertheless inspite of improved pregnancy rates after myomectomy

Table 14.6. Comparison with abdominal myomectomy[45-47]

Sr No	*Abdominal myomectomy*	*Laparoscopic myomectomy*
1. Type of surgery	Routine major surgery	Truly microsurgery
2. Requirement of skill	Average surgical skill	High skill, experience and expertise
3. Age of patient	Variable	More for younger age group
4. Average blood loss	250-300 ml (max-1200 ml)	80-150 ml (Occ. 1000 ml)
5. Postoperative hospital stay	72-12hours (avg- 82 hours)	16-96 hours (avg. 26 hours)
6. Risk of recurrence	Lesser	Marginally high, due to missing of small myomas
7. Postoperative adhesions	Dense and thereby reducing fertility by disturbing tubo-ovarian anatomy	Significantly less, not affecting fertility
8. Risk of uterine rupture	Apparently less, mainly due to lower pregnancy rates	Not reported in our series (*)

* In Dubuisson's[16] series among 34 cases of pregnancy following laparoscopic myomectomy, there was one case of uterine rupture.

evidence based data has yet to establish the actual benefit and improvement in fertility after laparoscopic or abdominal myomectomy (Table 14.6).[48]

TAKE HOME MESSAGE

1. Though the role of myomas in infertility and habitual abortion is unproven, we have found out in our series that if laparoscopic myomectomy is done for properly selected indications for infertility as mentioned in the chapter the pregnancy rate improved by 40 percent.
2. Reluctance of infertility consultants to operate a significant size fibroid or multiple fibroids just because it is not indenting the cavity should be weighed with the results of endoscopist who prefers myomectomy in such cases.
3. Best result of endoscopic myomectomy are found in cavitary fibroids, multiple fibroids distorting the cavity, fibroids indenting the cavity, fibroids with raised prolactin, fibroids with long-standing (5-7 years or more) infertility with no other obvious or proven cause for infertility.
4. Ipsilateral port placement and laparoscopic suturing with horizontal incision over fibroid for myomectomy makes laparoscopic myomectomy easy and allows laparoscopic suturing in vertical zone preventing fatigue and frustration of operating team with excellent restoration of anatomy.
5. Hysteroscopic removal of cavitary fibroids gives phenomenal improvement in pregnancy rate. In our study pregnancy rate improved upto 65 percent after hysteroscopic myomectomy.
6. Definitely there are limitations for laparoscopic myomectomy. Excessively large fibroid with size of more than 20-22 weeks size are difficult by laparoscopic route.
7. Risk of uterine rupture in pregnancy following laparoscopic myomectomy is a myth. Out of 129 pregnancies following laparoscoic myomectomy we had 69 percent delivered by LSCS and 31 percent by normal vaginal delivery with not a single incidence of uterine rupture.
8. Laparoscopic or hysteroscopic myomectomy is far superior to the open myomectomy not only in terms of infertility management but also in patient recovery, and less adhesion formation.

REFERENCES

1. Novak ER, Jones GS, Jones HW. Myomes uterins. In: Novak ER, Jones GS, Jones HW (Eds): Gynecologie Pratiquue. Paris: Editions maloine 1970;309-22.
2. Buttram VC, Reiter RC. Uterine leiomyomata: Etiology symptomatology and management. Fertil Steril, 1981;36:433.

3. Pritts EA. Fibroids and infertility: A systematic review of the evidence. Obstet Gynecol Surv 2001;56:483-91.
4. Bulletti C, De Zeigler D, Polli V, Flamigni C. Role of Leiomyoma in Infertility. J Am Assoc Gynecol Laparosc 1999;6:441-5.
5. Rubin IC. Uterine fibromyomas and sterility. Clin Obstet Gynecol 1958;1:50.
6. Wallach EE. Evaluation and management of uterine causes of infertility. Clin Obstet Gynecol 1979;22:43-60.
7. Dubuisson JB, Chapron C, Levy L. Difficulties and complications of laparoscopic myomectomy. Journal of Gynecologic Surgery 1996a;12:159-65.
8. Nezhat C, Nezhat F, Silfer SL, et al. Lap Mymectomy. Int J Fertil 1991;36:275-80.
9. Hasson HM, Rotman C, Rana N, Sistos F, Dmowski WP. Laparoscopic myomectomy. Obstetrics and Gynecology 1992;80:884-8.
10. Daniell JF, Gurley LD. Laparoscopic treatment of clinically significant symptomatic uterine fibroids. Journal of Gynecologic Surgery 1991;7:37-40.
11. Reich H. Laparoscopic myomectomy. Obstetrics and Gynecology Clinics of North America 1995;2(4):757-80.
12. Steiner RA, Wight E, Tadir Y, Haller U. Electrical device for laparoscopic removal of tissue from the abdominal cavity. Obstetrics and Gynecology 1993;81:471-4.
13. Davids A. Myomectomy: Surgical technique and results in a series of 1150 cases. American Journal of Obstetrics and Gynecology 1952;63:592-604.
14. Brown AB, Chamberlain R, Te Linde RW. Myomectomy. American Journal of Obstetrics and Gynecology 1956;71: 759-63.
15. Golan D, Aharoni A, Gonon R, et al. Early spontaneous rupture of the post myomectomy gravid uterus. International Journal of Gynecology and Obstetrics 1990; 31:167-70.
16. Dubuisson JB, Chapron C, Chavat X, Morice P. Uterine rupture during pregnancy after laparoscopic myomectomy. Human Reproduction 1995;10:1475-77.
17. Farrer-Brown G, Beilby JOW, Tarbit MH. The vascular patterns in myomatous uteri. The Journal of Obstetrics and Gynaecology of the British Commonwealth 1970;77:967-75.
18. Harris WJ. Uterine dehiscence following laparoscopic myomectomy. Obstet Gynecol 1992;80:545-6.
19. Freidman AJ, Barbieri RL. Leuprolide acetate: applications in gynecology. Curr Probl Obstet Gynecol Fertil 1988; 11:207-44.
20. Freidman AJ, Hoffman DI, Comite F, Browneller RW, Miller JD. (Leuprolide Study Group). Treatment of leiomyomata uteri with leuprolide acetate depot: A double blind, placebo-controlled, multicenter study. Obstet Gynecol 1991;77:720-5.
21. Friedman AJ, Daly M, Juneau-Norcross M, Rein MS. Predictors of uterine volume reduction in women with myomas treated with a gonadotropin-releasing hormone agonist. Fertil Steril 1992;58:413-5.
22. diZerega GS. Contemporary adhesion prevention. Fertil Steril 1994;61:219-35.
23. Farquhar C, Vandekerckhove P, Watson A, Vail A, Wiseman D. Barrier agents for preventing adhesions after surgery for subfertility. Cochrane Database Syst. Rev 2000;2: CD000475.
24. Nezhat CR, Nezhat F, Bess O, et al. Laparoscopically assisted myomectomy: a comparison of a new technique to myomectomy by laparotomy and laparoscopy. Int J Fertil 1994;39:39.
25. Seidman DS, Nezhat CH, Nezhat FR, Nezhat C. Spontaneous uterine rupture in pregnancy 8 years after laparoscopic myomectomy. J Am Assoc Gynecol Laparosc 2001;8:333-5.
26. McLucas B, Goodwin S, Adler L, Rappaport A, Reed R, Perrella R. Pregnancy following uterine fibroid embolization. Int J Gynecol Obstet 2001;74(1):1-7.
27. Spies JB, Ascher SA, Roth AR, Kim J, Levy EB, Gomez-Jorge. Uterine artery for fibroid. J Obstet Gynecol 2001; 98(1):29-39.
28. Gallinat A. Current trends in the therapy of myomata. In: Endoscopic Surgery in Gynecology. Lueken RP, Gallinat A (Eds): Demeter Verlag GMBH 1992;69-71.
29. Goldfarb HA. Nd: YAG laser laparoscopic coagulation of symptomatic myomas. Journal of Reproductive Medicine 1992;36:636-8.
30. Goldfarb HA. Laparoscopic coagulation of myoma (myolysis). In: Hutchins FL, Greenberg MD (Eds): Obstetrics and Gynecology Clinics of North America. Uterine Fibroids. Philadelphia: WB Saunders 1995b;807-19.
31. Goldfarb HA. Laparoscopic coagulation of myoma (myolysis). In: Tolandi T (Ed): Infertility and Reproductive Medicine Clinics of North America. Uterine Myomas. Philadelphia: WB Saunders 1996;129-41.
32. Nisolle M, Smets M, Malvaux V, et al. Laparoscopic myolysis with Nd-YAG laser. Journal of Gynaecology 1993;9:95-9.
33. Phillips DR, Nathanson HG, Milim SJ, et al. Experience with laparoscopic leiomyoma coagulation and concomitant operative hysteroscopy. Journal of the American Association of Gynecologic Laparoscopists 1997b;4:425-33.
34. Wood C, Maher P, Hill D. Myoma reduction by electrocautery. Gynaecological Endoscopy 1994;3:163-5.
35. Chapman R. Treatment of uterine myomas by Interstitial hyperthermia. Gynecological Endoscopy 1993;2:227-34.

36. Zreik TG, Rutherford T, et al. Cryomyolysis: A new procedure for the conservative treatment of uterine fibroids. Journal of American Association of Gynecologic Laparoscopist 1998.
37. Corscaden JF, Singh BP. Leiomyosarcoma of the uterus. American Journal of Obstetrics and Gynecology 1958;75: 149-55.
38. Montague A, Schwartz A, Woodruff J. Sarcoma arising in a leiomyoma of the uterus. American Journal of Obstetrics and Gynecology 1965;92:421-7.
39. Verkauf BS. Myomectomy for fertility enhancement and preservation. Fertility and Sterility 1992;58:1-15.
40. Dubuisson JB, Chapron C, Chavat X, Gregorakis SS. Fertility after laparoscopic myomectomy of large intramural myomas: preliminary results. Human Reproduction 1996; 11(3):518-22.
41. Dessolle L, Soriano D, Poncelet C, Benifla JL, Madelenat P, Darai E. Determinates of pregnancy rate and obstetric outcome after laparoscopic myomectomy for infertility. Fertil Steril 2001;76:370-4.
42. Rossetti A, Sizzi O, Soranna L, Mancuso S, Lanzone A. Fertility outcome: long-term results after laparoscopic myomectomy. Gynecol Endocrinol 2001;15:129-34.
43. Berkeley AS, DeCherney AH, Polan ML. Abdominal myomectomy and subsequent fertility. Surg Gynecol Obstet 1983 ;156:319-22.
44. Ranney B, Frederick I. The occasional need for myomectomy. Obstetrics and Gynecology 1979;53:437-41.
45. Darai E, Deval B, Darles C, Benifla JL, Guglielmina JN, Madelenat P. Myomectomie: coelioscopie ou laparotomie?. Contraception, Fertilite, Sexualite 1996;24(10):751-6.
46. Mais V, Ajossa S, Guerreiro S, Mascia M, Solla E, Melis GB. Laparoscopic versus abdominal myomectomy: a prospective, randomized trial to evaluate benefits in early outcome. American Journal of Obstetrics and Gynecology. 1996;174:654-8.
47. Rossetti A, Sizzi O, Soranna L, Cucinelli F, Mancuso S, Lanzone A. Long-term results of laparoscopic myomectomy: recurrence rate in comparison with abdominal myomectomy. Hum Reprod 2001;16:770-4.
48. Haney AF. Duke University Medical Center North Carolina, USA: Clinical decision making regarding leiomyomata: What we need in the next millennium.
49. Gar CR, Tureck RW. Submucosal leiomyomas and infertility. Fertil Steril 1984;42(1):16-19.
50. Ubalandi F, Tournaye H, Camus M. Fertility after hysteroscopic myomectomy. Hum reprod Update 1995; 1(1):81-90.
51. Vercellini P, Zaina B, Yaylayan L. Hysteroscopic myomectomy: Long-term effects on menstrual pattern and fertility. Obstet Gynecol 1999;94(3):341-7.
52. Brooks PG. Resectoscopic myoma vaporizer. J Reprod Med 1995;40(11):791-5.
53. Corson SL, Brooks PG. Resectoscopic myomectomy. Fertil Steril 1991;55(6):1041-4.

15 Hysteroscopic Management of Intrauterine Adhesions

Nozer Sheriar, Nagendra Sardeshpande

"Occasionally the whole cavity of the body of the uterus is obliterated from the os internum to the fundus and yet the cavity of the cervix continues patent..."

INTRODUCTION

Thus wrote James Simpson, that master obstetrician and gynecologist in 1844 in what is possibly one of the earliest descriptions of intrauterine adhesions. Fifty years later in 1894, Heinrich Fritsch published the first case report associating uterine curettage with intrauterine adhesions. In 1946 Henry Byford recognized trauma by curettage or cauterization as a possible cause of cicatrical contraction of the uterine walls with obliteration of the uterine cavity.

However, intrauterine adhesions and their clinical implications became widely recognized and accepted when Joseph Asherman of Tel Aviv's Hadassah Hospital published the most comprehensive analysis and evaluation of the etiology, pathogenesis, diagnosis and treatment of this condition. His initial series of adhesions in the cervical canal and cervical stenosis published in 1948 was later expanded to include both intracervical and intrauterine adhesions resulting in the partial or complete obliteration of the cervical canal and the uterine cavity. These cases all followed curettage for postpartum hemorrhage, incomplete abortion or missed abortion. Labeled by him as *uterine atresia* or *amenorrhea traumatica*, this clinical entity is now commonly recognized as the *Asherman's syndrome.*[1-3]

Intrauterine adhesions are now recognized as a cause of not just menstrual disorders (amenorrhea and hypomenorrhea) as hitherto believed, but also a potentially correctable anatomical cause of infertility and recurrent pregnancy loss.[4] With the developments in modern imaging techniques and diagnostic and operative hysteroscopy and their widespread availability and application, the definitive diagnosis and accurate targeted management of intrauterine adhesions is now a reality, resulting in significantly superior clinical outcomes. Hysteroscopy is the accepted new standard and benchmark in the diagnosis and treatment of intrauterine adhesions. This chapter presents an overview of the etiology, classification, diagnosis and management of intrauterine adhesions, highlighting the role of hysteroscopy in making optimum correction of this pathology possible.

ETIOLOGY AND CONTRIBUTING FACTORS

The primary cause for intrauterine adhesions is trauma to the uterine endometrium, especially damage to the basal layer and at times the myometrium, with failure of regeneration allowing adhesion formation between the denuded areas.

The most frequent cause of endometrial trauma triggering intrauterine adhesions is uterine curettage or evacuation undertaken for obstetric conditions. These range from incomplete or missed abortions, therapeutic surgical termination of first and second trimester pregnancies or puerperal curettage for postpartum hemorrhage due to partially or completely retained placentae. This factor accounts for almost 90 percent of all cases.[5,6] Other surgical events known to cause intrauterine adhesions are conventional or laparoscopic myomectomy accessing the endometrial cavity, wedge resection of adenomyosis or excision of adenomyotic nodules, abdominal metroplasty and cesarean delivery, though the extent of contribution of each individual operation and other underlying pathogenic factors is unclear.

Hysteroscopic surgery such as polypectomy, myomectomy, septal incision and metroplasty, by the intrauterine surgical dissection and inevitable endometrial denudation may itself occasionally contribute to the development of adhesions. While these could be related to the extent of dissection or excision, the energy source used and the quantum of energy applied and the resultant area of traumatized denuded endometrium (particularly on contralateral walls), intrauterine adhesions are an uncommon complication of hysteroscopic procedures performed well.

Endometrial infections may cause intrauterine adhesions. Tuberculosis is the commonest of these infections with a high incidence in developing countries causing significant endometrial damage and distortion of the uterine cavity.[7] Other uncommon infections are schistosomiasis or toxoplasmosis. Malacoplakia is a rare form of endometritis characterized by presence histocytes containing iron and calcium rich bodies (Michaelis-Gutmann bodies) in the endometrium. This condition is thought to be an abnormal and inadequate histiocytic response to *E.coli*. Fungal infections such as blastomycosis, Cryptococcus, Aspergillus and Coccidioides as a cause of intrauterine adhesions are extremely rare and are associated with disseminated disease in immunocompromised women.[8]

Intrauterine adhesions secondary to IUCD use are rare and may be due to a secondary bacterial infection, especially actinomycosis.

Rarely, even simple uterine manual exploration, manual removal of the placenta or gentle such as evacuation may induce adhesion formation.[9]

PATHOGENIC PROCESSES

The actual mechanism by which intrauterine adhesions form, be it a juxtaposition of denuded myometrium, constitutional factors in a given individual or vascular changes in the endomyometrium predisposing to fibrosis still remains to be determined.

The repair of endometrium is estrogen-dependent and may be compromised by low estrogen states. A delay in endometrial regeneration due to a hypoestrogenic state may predispose to adhesion formation between contiguous denuded walls of the uterine cavity. Iatrogenic hypoestrogenism induced by GnRH analogue therapy used preoperatively or immediately postoperatively for uterine polyps and myomas may increase such predisposition.

The presence of congenital anomalies is believed to be associated with a predisposition to the formation of adhesions. Occult infection, retained degenerating products of conception and lactational amenorrhea, itself, with its associated hypoestrogenic state may be contributing factors. However, it is now accepted that intrauterine adhesions can occur in the absence of postoperative or postpartum infections that had been previously thought to be necessary trigger events.

CLINICAL MANIFESTATIONS

Changes in menstrual pattern resulting in hypomenorrhea or complete amenorrhea occur in approximately 75 percent of women with Asherman's syndrome. However, this incidence varies from 6-80 percent depending on the severity of adhesions.[5,7] Menstrual changes are not an inevitable consequence of intrauterine adhesions. Sugimoto reported that 39 percent of patients with intrauterine adhesions detected by hysteroscopy had no significant menstrual complaints.[10]

Paradoxically the extent of intrauterine adhesions does not necessarily correlate with the severity of menstrual disturbance. Patients with severe adhesions may have normal menstrual patterns while mild adhesions may cause considerable disturbance. This is attributed to a change in the function and responsiveness of endometrium adjacent to adhesions. MRI studies reveal low intensity endometrial and junctional signals, a pattern persisting even with high-dose estrogen stimulation, suggesting dysfunctional endometrium.[4]

The most important reproductive consequences of intrauterine adhesions include infertility and recurrent spontaneous abortions. Infertility is seen in 20-25 percent of all women with intrauterine adhesions with 40 percent of associated pregnancies ending in abortion or preterm delivery. Overall, only about 30 percent of women with intrauterine adhesions achieve a full-term pregnancy.[11,12] An evaluation of the incidence of intrauterine adhesions by indication for hysteroscopy found the highest frequency with secondary infertility (23.5%), previous reproductive wastage (21.4%) and primary infertility (20.4%).[13] These reproductive implications are probably related to a distortion and decrease in uterine cavity space and capacity, poor distensibility of the uterine walls, mechanical obstruction of the cervical canal or ostia and endometrial vascular and receptor dysfunction.

CLASSIFICATION OF INTRAUTERINE ADHESIONS

Most clinical classifications rely on hysteroscopic appearances of intrauterine adhesions and their response to division to grade them by their severity. *Hunt and Siegler* classify intrauterine adhesions by their gross histological appearance and perceived vascularity (Table 15.1).[14]

Hamou using the microhysteroscopic technique classified intrauterine adhesions based on histology, cellular make-up and ease of hysteroscopic surgery (Table 15.2).[16]

At times, pathological evaluation may suggest a diagnosis of the underlying disease, such as tuberculosis which shows shaggy, yellow-white uterine walls with caseous material in the lumen and multiple granulomata,

Table 15.1. Classification of intrauterine adhesions by histology according to Hunt and Seigler

Mild adhesions
Filmy avascular adhesions, which can be easily disrupted
Moderate adhesions
Thick fibromuscular adhesions, that may be covered by endometrium and may bleed on division
Severe adhesions
Connective tissue adhesions without an endometrial lining and which do not bleed on touch
All the three degrees of adhesions may involve either part or whole of the uterine cavity. Most adhesions traverse the cavity antero-posteriorly although transverse bands have been described. Although adhesions are usually avascular, exaggerated vascularity and adenoma formation may occasionally occur.[15]

Table 15.2. Classification of intrauterine adhesions by cellular make-up according to Hamou

Type I: Endometrial adhesions (65%)
White with some glandular and vascular pattern, can be easily dissected, of less than a year's duration and often centrally placed
Type II: Fibrous or connective tissue adhesions (25%)
Thin, transparent bridge-like and poorly vascularized; usually central or isthmic and form stumps after lysis
Type III: Myometrial adhesions (10%)
Often extensive, older adhesions, limited uterine distention and required general anesthesia for lysis

caseation and fibrosis on microscopy. It is thought that connective tissue synechiae, with multiple areas of involvement and those involving at least one-third of the uterine cavity have the worst prognosis.

Diagnosis of Intrauterine Adhesions

While clinical presentation may suggest intrauterine adhesions, definitive diagnosis and assessment of severity requires the application of imaging techniques or direct visualization by hysteroscopy.

Hysterosalpingography (HSG)

HSG remains the most widely used modality to identify and evaluate intrauterine adhesions. It provides a 2D mapping of the type, location and extent and guides the performance of surgical correction. Comparison of preoperative and postoperative images helps determine the completeness of the surgery and the occasional need for a repeat procedure.

Approximately 50 percent of all HSG performed on women with recurrent abortions show evidence of filling defects suggestive of intrauterine adhesions. However, in as many as 40 percent of all cases, the interpretation of the HSG may be vague or incorrect.[12] Use of insufficient or excessive dye and failure to correct uterine displacement may lead to misleading results.

Intrauterine adhesions appear on HSG as sharply outlined central or marginal constant filling defects. Associated intravascular and lymphatic intravasation of dye may be noted. The uterine cavity may appear irregular and ragged, and the fallopian tubes may be difficult to outline.[15]

A prospective study identified intrauterine abnormalities on HSG in 286 patients and confirmed these at hysteroscopy in 200. Intrauterine lesions were also detected by hysteroscopy in 4 out of 50 patients in whom HSG were normal and were the most common finding on hysteroscopy. Statistical analysis revealed that HSG in the detection of intrauterine pathology had a sensitivity of 98.0 percent, specificity of 34.9 percent, positive predictive value of 69.9 percent, negative predictive value of 92.0 percent, and accuracy rate of 73.2 percent. A frequent incorrect diagnosis at HSG was the misdiagnosis of cervical stenosis as severe intrauterine adhesions.[17]

Siegler and Kontopoulas classify intrauterine adhesions based on HSG appearances and extent of cavity involvement (Table 15.3).[18]

Table 15.3. Classification of intrauterine adhesions by HSG appearance according to Siegler and Kontopoulas

Mild adhesions
Multiple, mostly central, linear defects with minimal uterine cavity distortion, involving less than a third of the cavity
Moderate adhesions
Irregular uterine cavity border with multiple lacunar defects, involving between a third to two-thirds of the uterine cavity
Severe adhesions
Completely distorted cavity especially at the fundus, vascular intravasation, with tubal occlusion often seen

Ultrasonography

Pelvic ultrasound may be useful in identifying endometrial distortion to diagnose intrauterine adhesions.[19] Intrauterine adhesions may be better visualized by transvaginal USG during menses or if the endometrial cavity contains fluid.[20] Sonohysterography may demonstrate the presence of adhesions appearing as thin, undulating membranes or broad brands crossing the fluid filled cavity. In case of dense adhesions, it may be difficult to distend the uterine cavity.[21] Ultrasound may occasionally demonstrate hematometra where adhesions interfere with the drainage of menstrual flow.

Three-dimensional ultrasonography allows the visualization of intrauterine adhesions in different planes and the determination of spatial orientation and relation of adhesions to the uterine walls.[22]

Magnetic Resonance Imaging

Though MRI can occasionally demonstrate intrauterine, it has no definitive advantage over ultrasound or HSG and its prohibitive cost makes if more of an experimental modality for this purpose.[23]

Hysteroscopy

Diagnostic hysteroscopy provides a direct visualization of the uterine cavity and is a more sensitive diagnostic technique for intracavitary pathologies than either HSG or USG. Today hysteroscopy is hence the gold standard for diagnosis as well as treatment of intrauterine adhesions.

Diagnostic hysteroscopy is performed using a conventional hysteroscope (4 mm 30° fore oblique telescope) or a microhysteroscope (Hamou) in a diagnostic sheath, using either carbon dioxide or a fluid (crystalloid) for distension. For diagnosing intrauterine adhesions, Sugimoto's criteria, that the adhesion be attached to the uterine wall at two points, either central or marginal, need to be fulfilled.[10]

Typical intrauterine adhesions following postpregnancy trauma are generally central, but may also be scattered throughout the cavity or obstructing the cornu or the cervix. They become fibrous and avascular with time. Postoperative intrauterine adhesions are localized to the site of surgical insult. Initially vascular the tend to become dense and rigid. The intrauterine adhesions associated with chronic inflammatory diseases such as tuberculosis are peripheral involving the fundus and lateral walls. They tend to be columnar with intervening alveolar pockets, initially vascular with hyperplastic overlying endometrium. With progression the endometrium becomes atrophic and the cavity shrunken, distorted and irregular with a tendency for distension media or intracavitary dye injected for HSG or chromopertubation to intravasate.

Pseudosynechiae are endometrial bridges occurring due to increased mucous content in the second half of the menstrual cycle. These bridges can be lysed by simple pressure with the edge of the hysteroscope.

March and Israel have graded adhesions by the extent of involved endometrial cavity as visualized on hysteroscopy (Table 15.4).[24,25]

Table 15.4. Classification of intrauterine adhesions by hysteroscopic visualization according to March and Israel

Minimal adhesions
Filmy adhesions involving less than half of the uterine cavity with none or minimal adhesions near the tubal ostia and upper fundus
Moderate adhesions
Adhesions involving half to three-fourth of the uterine cavity with walls not agglutinated and partial occlusion of the tubal ostial areas and upper fundus
Severe adhesions
Thick bands involving more than three-fourth of the uterine cavity with agglutination of the walls and tubal ostial areas and upper uterine cavity involved

Treatment Options

The traditional management of suspected intrauterine adhesions relied upon tactile probing of the uterine cavity by a uterine sound or dilators and disruption of the adhesions by a curette. These procedures were effective to a limited extent in achieving menses with mild and moderate adhesions, with improved though compromised resultant reproductive outcomes. However, with the application of available imaging techniques and diagnostic hysteroscopy in diagnosing and mapping intrauterine adhesions and visual hysteroscopic surgical treatment, there is no longer place or justification for the traditional blind procedures. Hysteroscopic adhesiolysis is now the method of choice for the treatment of Asherman's syndrome.

Hysteroscopic Adhesiolysis

The standard instrumentation used is a 4 mm hysteroscope in a 5 mm diagnostic or a 7.5 mm operating channel. The Versapoint 2.9 mm hysteroscope in a 4 mm operating channel requires minimal or no cervical dilatation. Minimal flimsy and central adhesions can be lysed either with a standard diagnostic hysteroscope or with the Versapoint as an outpatient procedure with minimal anesthesia or sedation. However, moderate to severe adhesions and lateral and fundal adhesions should be divided in a well-equipped OT set-up under general anesthesia and may require concomitant laparoscopy to guide dissection.[26]

Technical Nuances

Hysteroscopic adhesiolysis for severe adhesions is technically the most challenging hysteroscopic procedure associated with the highest risk of complication. The key to safe successful adhesiolysis is orientation, patience and a willingness to stop if undue risk is perceived.

At the very outset uterine entry may be difficult particularly in the presence of dense cervical or severe intrauterine adhesions. A preoperative HSG may help decide the direction and depth of entry while simultaneous transabdominal USG can visualize instrument entry and safely guide dilators and the hysteroscope into the uterine cavity. Uterine entry must be made under vision wherever possible, with the distension medium guiding the scope into the spaces between the adhesions.

Surgical Modalities and Techniques

A variety of hysteroscopic techniques can be used for adhesiolysis depending on the type, vascularity, extent and location of adhesions. The leading edge of a fore oblique scope is often used to disrupt flimsy adhesions and pseudoadhesions. However, using such blunt dissection is crude and damaging when dealing with fibrous adhesions and fraught with risk when used at the fundus. Wherever possible adhesiolysis must be achieved under adequate visualization and dissection performed at the midpoint between the anterior and posterior walls. Most adhesions retract with the few that persist may need focal excision.

Most adhesions are usually avascular and bleeding following adhesiolysis is rare almost always stops spontaneously when it occurs. Hence flexible or semirigid microscissors or an optical scissors are preferred for mild and moderate disease since they avoid thermal damage to already devitalized tissue. Scissors are most suitable for central and fundal adhesions and can be used to create an initial entry into a severely contracted uterine cavity to allow the passage of larger instruments such as the resectoscope.

Fibromuscular adhesions in contrast bleed on division and obscure the operative field. These adhesions are easily divided by high frequency electrosurgery using a resectoscope with a hook electrode (Collin's knife). By using a pure cutting current and the point electrode there is minimal thermal damage to contiguous tissues. Occasionally areas of extensive fibrosis need superficial excision with a loop electrode to allow endometrial regrowth from adjacent endometrium.

The argon, KTP 532 or the Nd:YAG lasers can be utilized for adhesiolysis. The fiberoptic laser allows precise destruction of adhesions while preserving surrounding endometrial tissue. The Nd: YAG laser with an attached sapphire probe can be used to photovaporize adhesions with limited scattering of energy. However, in practice, the laser has little benefit to offer as compared to a scissors or a resectoscope. In addition, it is cumbersome, expensive and is associated with various hazards requiring personnel protection.

Adjunctive Procedures

Postoperatively interposition devices such as an IUD, preferably after removing the copper wire, or an 8 or 10 Fr Foley's catheter with the balloon distended to 3 ml may be placed in the uterine cavity to prevent apposition of the uterine walls and readhesion of the dissected areas. They may be removed 48 hrs to 7 days later. A comparative study of IUD use (51) with Foley catheter (59) use, reported restoration of normal menstruation in 62.7 percent and 81.4 percent of the patients respectively ($p < 0.05$). Persistent post-treatment amenorrhea and hypomenorrhea occurred less frequently in the Foley' catheter group (18.6% vs 37.3%) ($p < 0.03$) and the conception rate was 33.9 percent compared with 22.5 percent. The Foley's catheter is hence a safer and more effective adjunctive method of treatment of intrauterine adhesions.[27]

A prospective, randomized study undertaken to assess the efficacy of auto-cross-linked hyaluronic acid gel in preventing the development of intrauterine adhesions following hysteroscopic adhesiolysis found a significant decrease in intrauterine adhesions at 3 months follow-up.[28]

Postoperative estrogens (ethinyl estradiol 50 mg, conjugated estrogens 1.25 mg or estradiol valerate 2 mg) have been prescribed after the procedure to stimulate endometrial growth over the raw areas created by adhesiolysis, though its benefit is uncertain. Estrogen may be administered for 30-60 days with progesterone being administered finally to induce withdrawal bleeding.

A hysterosalpingography may be performed in the subsequent cycle to confirm completeness or the anatomical results of surgery. A repeat hysteroscopy need only be considered in case of a suspicious HSG.

Procedure Related Complications

A prospective evaluation of over 1400 hysteroscopies, including 650 operative hysteroscopies was undertaken.[29] Hysteroscopic adhesiolysis was performed in 142 cases most of which were for moderate to sever adhesions. There were 12 perforations almost all being managed conservatively. A laparotomy was undertaken in one case at the time of a repeat hysteroscopy for an embedded IUD placed earlier as a uterine stent, fixed to the serosa of the small bowel. In a case where adhesiolysis was successful in achieving menstruation and pregnancy in a completely obliterated cavity, an obstetric hysterectomy had to be performed due to a placenta increta.

Adhesiolysis of severe intrauterine adhesions probably carries the highest risk of mechanical and thermal injury of all operative hysteroscopic procedures. Mechanical injury causing uterine perforation is reported in 2-3 percent of all hysteroscopies. Predisposing factors include poor visualization and lack of adequate uterine distension. Endomyometritis is a rare complication occurring in less than 1 in 1000 procedures.

Development of a false passage and perforation is one of the commonest complications of hysteroscopic adhesions. It may be seen in 1-2 percent of cases.[30] The highest risk of perforation is associated with fundal and lateral adhesiolysis in severe Asherman's syndrome. Obliterated cavities and dense adhesions demand the greatest skill. It is best to begin dissection with the narrowest scope and use mechanical dissection with the leading edge of the diagnostic sheath proceed to a semirigid or flexible scissors in a 7 mm operative sheath before finally introducing a resectoscope. Mechanical dissection may be resorted to begin with but on no account must blind fundal or cornual blunt dissection be attempted as this negates the visual advantage of operative hysteroscopy.

Safety Recommendations

Recognizing the risk of complications allows the institution of measures to prevent these. In cases with anticipated difficulty, ultrasound or laparoscopic guidance may assist dissection in a distorted cavity especially early in the learning curve. Concomitant laparoscopy may help direct hysteroscopic surgery in an obliterated cavity or deep in the myometrium by eliciting bright spots on transillumination or detecting serosal blanching prior to perforation. However, ultrasound guidance by allowing a more accurate measurement of the residual myometrial thickness may be more effective for serosal protection. Thermal energy is best avoided and sharp dissection preferred in doubtful situations. To minimize risk incision, dissection or resection should be carried downwards from the fundus wherever possible.

Management of Perforations

Sudden loss of distension or an unexplained endometrial or myometrial defect should alert the endoscopist to the possibility of perforation. Most perforations are benign and can be managed by observation or placing a simple suture by laparoscopy, though undetected electrical burns may involve the bowel or bladder and warrant exploratory laparotomy.

Mechanical perforation with the leading edge of the scope or semirigid instruments only requires diagnostic laparoscopy and close monitoring in most cases. If the perforation involves thermal or electrical energy a confirmatory laparoscopy with an adequate repair of the uterine defect by endosuturing is appropriate and preferred over coagulation. The egress of distension fluid hitherto under pressure, may offer some protection to peritoneal structures. Tracing the length of the intestine and repairing trauma at laparotomy is the best approach to manage suspected bowel injury.

Outcomes and Prognosis

Most series of hysteroscopic adhesiolysis have been retrospective and based on historic data. Full-term viable pregnancy rates are reported to vary from 67-94 percent.[31,32] Spontaneous abortions are reported in 7-8 percent, premature delivery in about 2 percent and obstetric complications such as placenta accreta, increta or percreta 3 percent of pregnancies following hysteroscopic adhesiolysis.

In a series of 75 patients undergoing hysteroscopic adhesiolysis 94.6 percent had functional restoration of menses. After two months 93.3 percent had anatomic resolution the uterine cavity being completely regular, a second surgical correction performed in the remainder.[33]

Donnez and Nissolle classified adhesions based on location and correlated them with outcome of surgery (Table 15.5).[34]

Table 15.5. Classification of intrauterine adhesions by location according to Donnez and Nissolle

I.	***Central adhesions*** (Bridge-like adhesions)	
	a.	Thin/filmy endometrial adhesions
	b.	Myofibrous/connective adhesions
II.	***Marginal adhesions*** (Myofibrous/connective adhesions)	
	a.	Ledge-like projections
	b.	Obliteration of one horn
III.	***Uterine cavity obliterated*** (Uterine cavity not seen on HSG)	
	a.	Occlusion of the internal os (pseudo-Asherman's syndrome)
	b.	Extensive coaptation of the uterine walls with absence of uterine cavity (true Asherman's syndrome)

According to this classification type I and IIa adhesions have an excellent postoperative prognosis. Type II b and III b adhesions usually tend recur and often have poor prognosis with regards to fertility and pregnancy outcome. Type III a adhesions may seem difficult to deal with, but once the uterine cavity is successfully accessed the end result and prognosis is favorable (Figures 15.1 to 15.6).

CONCLUSION

Intrauterine adhesions or Asherman's syndrome are an important cause of recurrent pregnancy loss and subfertility. Although the clinical features of

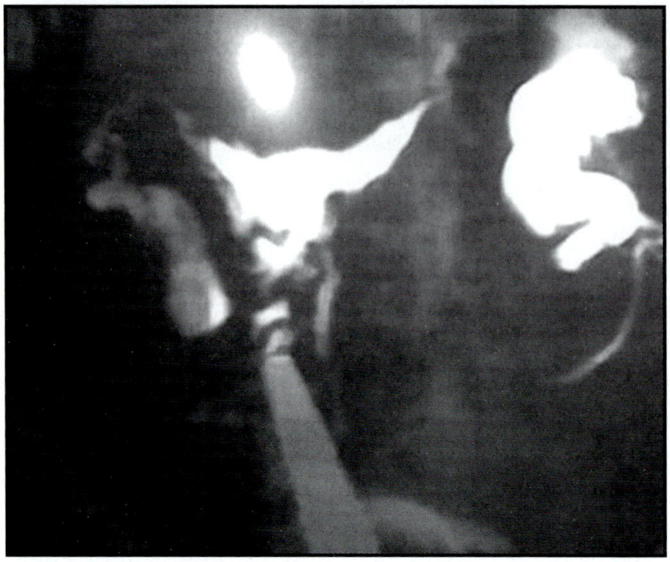

Figure 15.1. Moderate type IIa marginal adhesions

Irregular uterine cavity border with ledge-like projections involving between a third to two-thirds of the uterine cavity. History of a previous second trimester-induced abortion followed by suction evacuation for a first trimester missed abortion. Hysteroscopic adhesiolysis for a thick lateral columnar fibrous adhesion by electrosurgical incision with a resectoscope. Normal cavity achieved

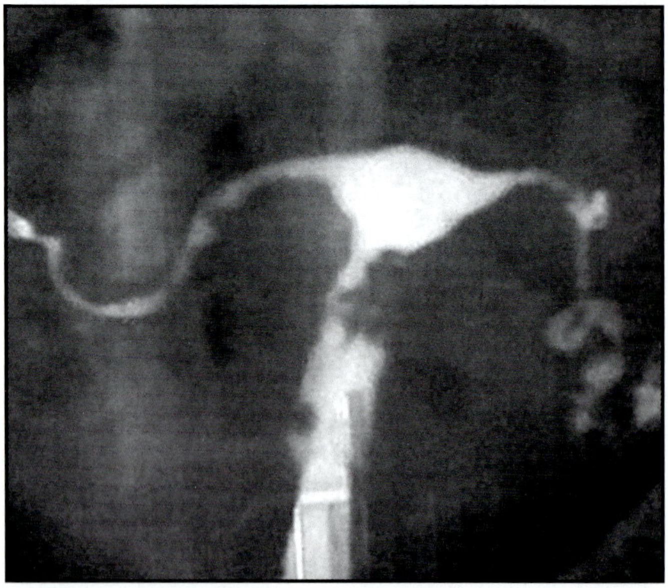

Figure 15.2. Intrauterine adhesions following hysteroscopic surgery.

Unilateral isthmic adhesions following hysteroscopic metroplasty for a triradiate hypoplastic uterine cavity. Hysteroscopic incisions and partial excision revealed adenomyotic elements

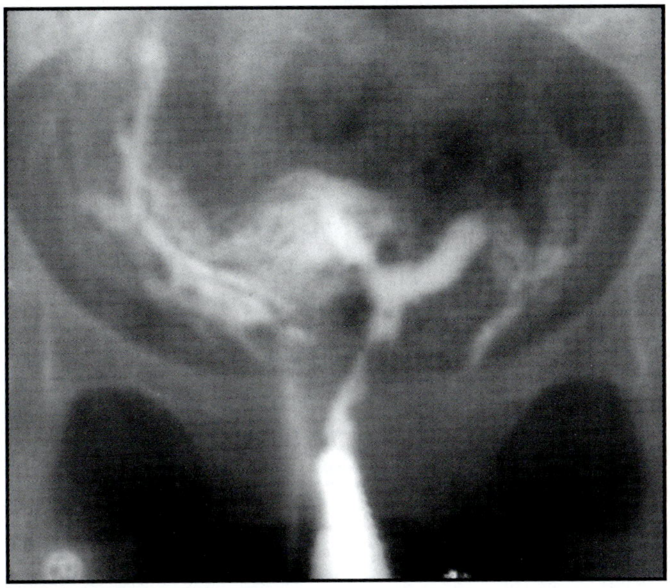

Figure 15.3. Intrauterine adhesions associated genital tuberculosis.

Peripheral adhesions involving the fundus and lateral walls. Initially columnar with intervening alveolar pockets with hyperplastic overlying endometrium. With progression endometrium becomes atrophic and the cavity shrunken, distorted and irregular with intravasation of injected dye

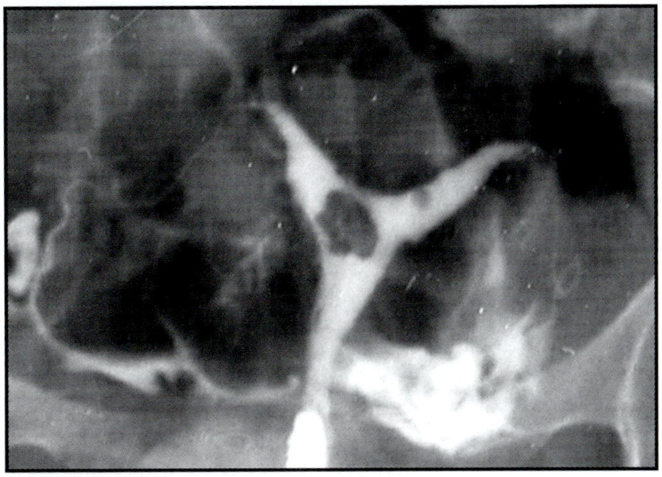

A. Preoperative HSG

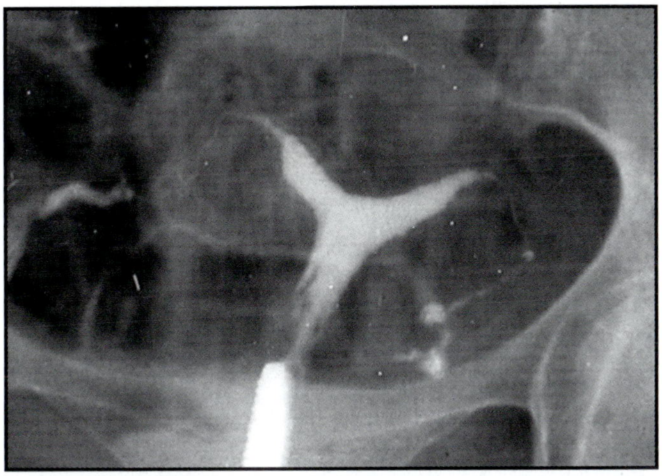

B. Postoperative HSG

Figures 15.4A and B. Mild type Ib central adhesion central defect with minimal uterine cavity distortion involving less than a third of the cavity. History of a previous first trimester abortion and a second trimester hysterotomy. Hysteroscopic adhesiolysis for a thick columnar fibrous adhesion with a semirigid scissors. Normal cavity achieved with a resultant normal pregnancy and delivery

hypomenorrhea, amenorrhea and recurrent pregnancy loss and the findings of a hysterosalpingogram can suggest their presence, hysteroscopy remains the only modality and hence the gold standard for definitively diagnosing intrauterine adhesions. Operative hysteroscopy now allows correction of this problem with minimum morbidity, achieving an excellent reproductive outcome. Questions do remain regarding the etiopathogenesis of Asherman's syndrome, its prevention, best instrumentation, energy source and technique for optimum outcome and the problem of surgical failures.

REFERENCES

1. Asherman JG. Traumatic intrauterine adhesions. J Obstet Gynecol Br Commonw 1948;55:23-7.
2. Soferman N, Professor Joseph G Asherman. An outline of his scientific medical Image. Harefuah 1969;76:32-5.
3. Speert H. Obstetrics and Gynecologic Milestones: Essays in Eponymy. The MacMillan Company, New York, 1958.
4. Letterie GS. Intrauterine Adhesions. In: Surgery, Assisted Reproductive Technology and Infertility, 2nd edition. Taylor and Francis, London and New York, 2000.
5. Patton PE. Anatomic uterine defects. Clin Obstet Gynecol 1994;37(3):705-21.
6. Westendrop IC, Ankum WM, Mol BM, Vonk J. Prevalence of Asherman's syndrome after secondary removal of placental remnants or a repeat curettage for incomplete abortion. Hum Reprod 1998;13:3347-50.
7. Lancet M, Kessler I. A review of Asherman's syndrome and results of modern treatment. Int J Fertil 1988;33:14-24.

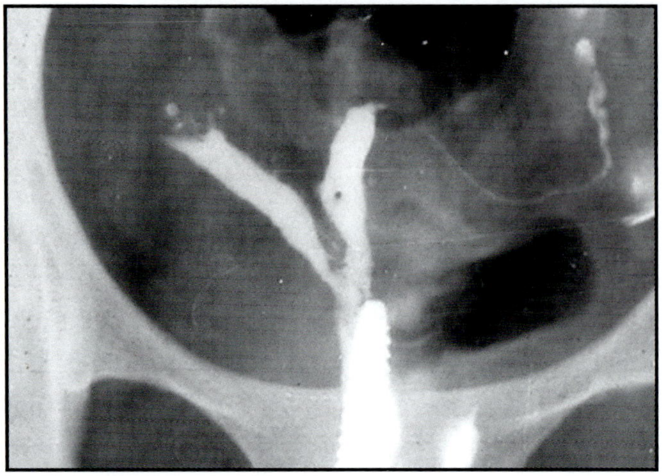

A. Preoperative HSG

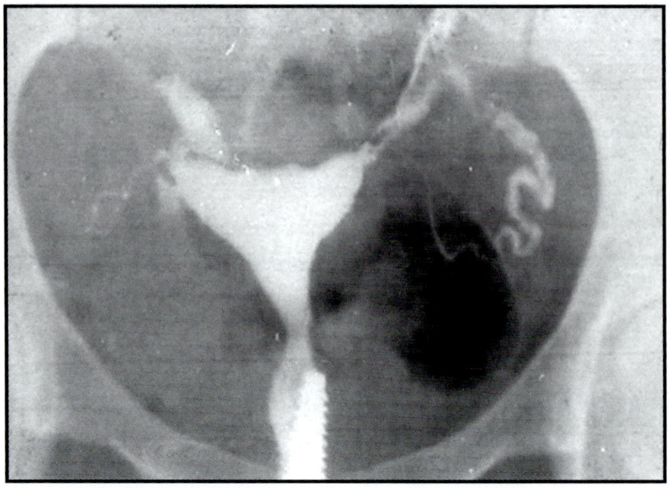

B. Postoperative HSG

Figures 15.5A and B. Moderate type IIa marginal adhesions. Irregular uterine cavity border involving between a third to two-thirds of the uterine cavity. Differentiated from a Mullerian defect by irregular linear margins. History of two previous first trimester abortions. Hysteroscopic adhesiolysis for a thick columnar fibrous adhesion by electrosurgical incision with a resectoscope. Normal cavity achieved with a resultant normal pregnancy and delivery

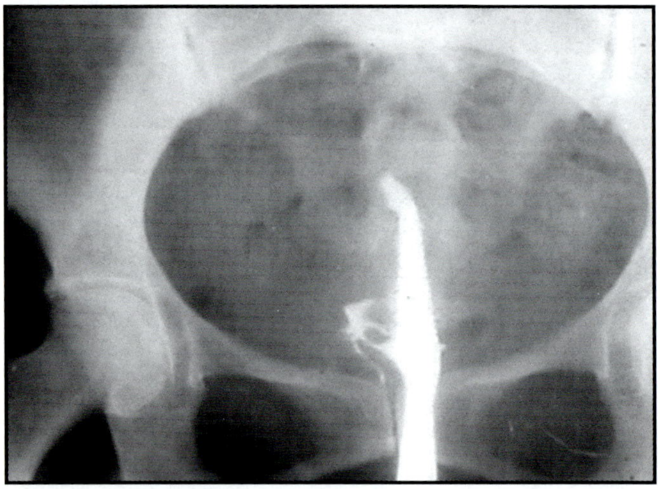

A. Preoperative HSG

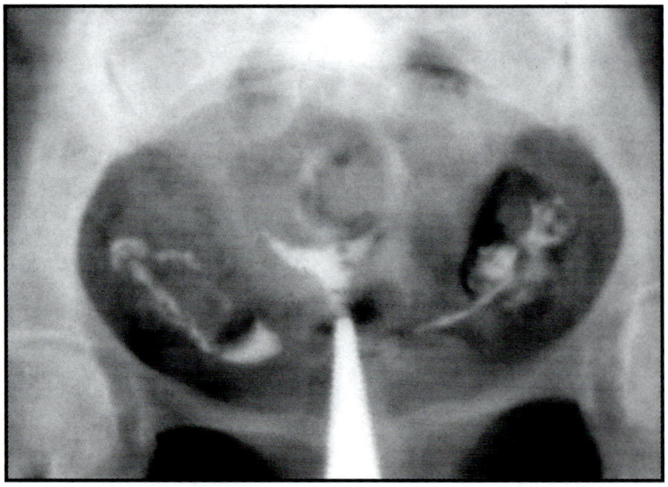

B. Postoperative HSG

Figures 15.6A and B. Severe type IIIa adhesions with uterine cavity obliterated. Occlusion of the internal os with obliterated cavity. History of three previous first trimester abortions. Hysteroscopic adhesiolysis for a thick cervical and isthmic adhesions by semirigid scissors followed by a resectoscope. Normal slightly hypoplastic cavity achieved. Resultant pregnancy requiring cerclage for premature opening of the cervix. Preterm delivery at 32 weeks with successful outcome after neonatal intensive care

8. Fox H, Buckley CH. Inflammatory disease. In Pathology for Gynecologists, 2nd edition. Edward Arnold, London, 1991.
9. Klein SM, Garcia CR. Asherman's syndrome: A critique and current view. Fertil Steril 1973;244:722-35.
10. Sugimoto O. Diagnostic and therapeutic hysteroscopic for traumatic intrauterine adhesions. Am J Obstet Gynecol 1978;131:539.
11. Schenker JG, Margalioth EJ. Intrauterine adhesions: An updated appraisal. Fertil Steril 1982;37:593.

12. Mencaglia L, Hamou JE. Treatment of intrauterine adhesions. In: Manual of Hysteroscopy. Straub Druck Medien GmBH, Germany, 2004.
13. Sheriar NK, Bharucha AR. The uterine factor in reproductive wastage. In: Krishna U, Tank DK, Daftary SN (Eds): Pregnancy at Risk, 4th edition. FOGSI and Jaypee Brothers, New Delhi, 2001.
14. Hunt RB, Siegler AM. Intrauterine adhesions. In: Hysterosalpingography: Techniques and Interpretation, 1st edition. Year Book Medical Publishers, Chicago, 1990.
15. Glezerman M, Levin S, Bernstein D. Asherman's syndrome: A self-limiting disease? Int J Obstet Gynecol 1978;15:522.
16. Hamou J, Salat-Baroux J, Siegler AM. Diagnosis and treatment of intrauterine adhesions by microhysteroscopy. Fertil Steril 1983;39:321.
17. Preutthipan S, Linasmita V. A prospective comparative study between hysterosalpingography and hysteroscopy in the detection of intrauterine pathology in patients with infertility. J Obstet Gynaecol Res 2003;29(1):33.
18. Siegler AM, Kontopoulas VG. Lysis of intrauterine adhesions under hysteroscopic control: A report of 25 operations. J Reprod Med 1981;26:372.
19. Confino E, Friberg J, Giglia RV, Gleicher N. Sonographic imaging of intrauterine adhesions. Obstet Gynecol 1985;66:596.
20. Carter JR, Carlson LF, Twiggs LB. Gynecologic Oncology. In: Nyberg PA, Hill LM, Bohm-Velez M, Mendelson BB (Eds): Transvaginal Ultrasound. Mosby Year Book, Chicago, 1992.
21. Gaucherand P, Pizcenza JM, Salle B, Rudriges RC. Sonohysterography of the uterine cavity: Preliminary investigations. J Clin Ultrasound 1995;23:339.
22. Weinraub Z, Herman A. Three-dimensional hysterosonography. In: Merz E (Ed): 3-D Ultrasonography in Obstetrics and Gynecology. Lippincott Williams and Wilkins, Philadelphia, 1998.
23. Letterie GS, Haggerty MF. Magnetic resonance imaging of intrauterine synechiae. Gynecol Obstet Invest 1994; 37:66.
24. March CM. Uterine surgical approach to reduce prematurity. Clin Perinatol 1992;19:319-31.
25. March CM, Israel R. Gestational outcome following hysteroscopic lysis of adhesions. Fertil Steril 1981;36:458.
26. Gimpelson RJ. Operative hysteroscopy – Myomas, septums and synechiae. In: Sammarco MJ, Stovall TG, Steege JF (Eds): Gynecologic Endoscopy–Principles in Practice. Williams and Wilkins, Baltimore, 1996.
27. Orhue AA, Aziken ME, Igbefoh JO. A comparison of two adjunctive treatments for intrauterine adhesions following lysis. Int J Gynecol Obstet 2003;82(1):49.
28. Acunzo G, Guida M, Pellicano M, et al. Effectiveness of auto-cross-linked hyaluronic acid gel in the prevention of intrauterine adhesions after hysteroscopic adhesiolysis: a prospective, randomized, controlled study. Hum Reprod 2003;18(9):1918.
29. Sheriar NK. Complications of hysteroscopy – Prevention and management. In: Desai SV, Joseph K (Eds): Gynecological Endoscopic Surgery: Current Concepts. FOGSI and Jaypee Brothers, New Delhi, 2002.
30. Neis KJ, Brandner P, Hepp H. Complications and side effects. In: Hysteroscopy – Textbook and Atlas. Thieme Med Publishers, New York, 1994.
31. Valle RF, Sciarra JJ. Intrauterine adhesions. Hysteroscopic diagnosis, classification, treatment and reproductive outcome. Am J Obstet Gynecol 1988;158:1459.
32. Shaffer W. Role of uterine adhesions in the cause of multiple pregnancy losses. Clin Obstet Gynecol 1986; 29:912.
33. Pace S, Stentella P, Catania R, Palazzetti PL, Frega A. Endoscopic treatment of intrauterine adhesions. Clin Exp Obstet Gynecol 2003;30(1):26.
34. Donnez J, Nisolle M. Hysteroscopic lysis of intrauterine adhesions (Asherman's syndrome). In: Donnez J, Nisolle M (Eds): An Atlas of Laser Operative Laparoscopy and Hysteroscopy, Parthenon, New York, 1994.

16 Role of Hysteroscopy in the Management of Infertility

Rakesh Sinha, Shweta Raje

INTRODUCTION

The traditional role of hysteroscopy in the management of infertility has changed in recent times as the capabilities of the procedure are increased while other diagnostic modalities replace some of its former uses.

Hysteroscopy is a valuable diagnostic and therapeutic modality in management of infertility and at present is considered as the gold standard for the evaluation of endometrial cavity in infertile patients.[1]

Still hysteroscopy is not included as a part of basic infertility work-up by the working groups in Human Reproductive Medicine (ESHRE, RCOG).[2]

The five basic steps, which form the cornerstone of infertility evaluation are:[3]

- Semen analysis
- Assessment of ovulation
- Hysterosalpingography (HSG)
- Laparoscopy
- Post-coital test.

The RCOG guidelines for fertility management state "women should not be offered hysteroscopy on its own as a part of initial investigations unless clinically indicated because the effectiveness of surgical treatment of uterine abnormalities on improving pregnancy rates has not been established."

In this chapter we discuss the usefulness of hysteroscopy as a screening method in infertility evaluation as it appears to be the most reliable method for determining the nature of intracavitary abnormalities and is also a very effective treatment modality.

COMPARISON OF HYSTEROSCOPY WITH OTHER DIAGNOSTIC MODALITIES FOR INFERTILITY

Ultrasonography (USG)

USG is a well-accepted procedure because of its minimal invasiveness and fair accuracy. But it is observed that though USG has a sensitivity of 96 percent and specificity of 86 percent in diagnosis of intrauterine abnormalities,[4] the sensitivity and specificity decrease significantly while diagnosing small focal intrauterine pathology, e.g. small polyp, small fibroid, small septum. Furthermore in the diagnosis of intramural extension of submucous myoma which determines the hysteroscopic operability, there was further decrease in sensitivity and specificity to 80 and 69 percent respectively.

Sonohysterography (SHG)

SHG is widely used in the diagnosis of submucous myomas, their size, location and degree of intracavitary growth. It is better and more effective than USG in the diagnosis of intrauterine pathology with a sensitivity of 75 percent in diagnosing the type II submucous fibroids[5] but less effective in diagnosing hyperplastic endometrial pathology, infection and inflammation of endometrium.

Hysterosalpingography (HSG)

HSG is included in basic infertility work-up and for decades it has been used for diagnosis of polyp, myomas, intrauterine adhesions, congenital abnormalities, tubal status in proximal, distal and intrapelvic region. The intrauterine filling defects could also be air bubbles, mucus or asynchronous uterine contractions.

It is well-documented that HSG has a sensitivity of 80.3 percent in revealing intrauterine abnormality and specificity of 70.1 percent, a false-positive rate of 15.6 percent, a false-negative rate of 35.4 percent and with respect to intrauterine adhesions a false-positive rate 54.3 percent when compared with hysteroscopy.[6]

Hysteroscopy should be considered as complimentary to USG and HSG rather than competing with them in the evaluation of infertile patients.[7] It should no longer be considered as second level invasive investigation but with the rapid evolution of hysteroscopic minioptics, office hysteroscopy should be included in basic fertility work-up.[8]

HYSTEROSCOPY BEFORE ART

Embryo transfer is a very important step in success of IVF treatment. All efforts should be made to rule out any intrauterine pathology before enrolling the patient in IVF program, as the presence of intrauterine pathology will definitely impair the implantation rate. The incidence of pathological findings is high (45%) in patients with repeated IVF-ET failures who were enrolled in the program with normal HSG findings.[9]

In addition useful information can be acquired about the direction to follow when transferring embryos so as to check the regularity of the channel and presence of any obstacle to the progression of the catheter. This information is important in order to avoid difficult embryo transfer, which provokes bleeding and uterine contractions.[10]

INSTRUMENTATION

Diagnostic hysteroscopy can be performed in the office, at an outpatient unit or in the operation theater. Pantaleoni initially described hysteroscopy in 1869, but it did not achieve routine gynecologic use due to its poor optic system. However, refinement in optical and fiberoptic instrumentation, along with operative accessories, has dramatically improved visual resolution and operative technique. Today, many hysteroscopic procedures have replaced older, more invasive techniques.

Conventional Diagnostic Hysteroscopy

This procedure is carried out in operation theater under general anesthesia.

A 4 mm 30 degree telescope is the most appropriate to use as it provides a larger and brighter image than the smaller telescopes. Cervical dilatation is done. The telescope along with a 5.5 mm continuous flow sheath is used for diagnostic hysteroscopy. A non-viscous liquid distension medium is used. If a need for intervention arise, the 5.5 mm sheath is replaced by 7-8 mm continuous flow operative sheath with 5-7F semi-rigid instrument, electrosurgical probes or laser fibers.

Office Hysteroscopy

Hysteroscopy in the office is meant for pure diagnostic procedures, without anesthesia and without intervention. It should be performed with a small size hysteroscope. It can be performed by using either flexible or rigid telescopes. The diameter of telescopes ranging from 1.2 to 3.6 mm can be used for office hysteroscopy. During office hysteroscopy, vagal reaction can be prevented with 0.5 mg atropine administered intramuscularly 15 minutes before the procedure. Painful myometrial contractions during the procedure can be prevented by the administration of prostaglandin synthetase inhibitor orally two hours before the procedure.

The Microcolpohysteroscope

It is a complex optical system, which presents the properties of both the telescope and the compound microscope. It can be used at infinity as a telescope or in contact with the epithelium as microscope. The telescope is 4 mm in diameter and 25 cm in length. There are two proximal lenses. The direct lens allows both the observation of conventional panoramic view and view at 60 times magnification if placed in contact with epithelium. The offset lens provides magnification upto 150 times. Microhysteroscopy can be used to determine the histopatology of normal endometrium in proliferative and secretory phase. It can also diagnose abnormal endometrial appearances, e.g. polyp, fibroid, endometritis, endometrial hyperplasia and malignancies.

DIAGNOSTIC HYSTEROSCOPY IN INFERTILITY (FIGURES 16.1 AND 16.2)

Evaluation of Endometrial Cavity

Hysteroscopy gives an assessment of size, shape and regularity of endometrial cavity. It allows direct visualization of proximal tubal ostia. A diagnostic hysteroscopy determines the status of endometrium in terms of presence or absence of intrauterine pathology, endometrial hyperplasia, vascularity and endometritis. The diagnostic accuracy of hysteroscopy when compared with the histological diagnosis showed a sensitivity of 98 percent, specificity of 95 percent, positive predictive value of 96 percent and negative predictive value of 98 percent.[11]

Evaluation of Cervical Canal

Hysteroscopy allows evaluation of cervical mucosal lining and also the channel for embryo transfer.

Diagnosis of Intrauterine Pathology (Fibroids, Polyp)

Hysteroscopy is highly sensitive for diagnosis of even small submucous fibroids or endometrial polyps. In cases of submucous fibroids hysteroscopy helps in diagnosis, nature and extent of pathology.

Depending upon hysteroscopically observed findings, submucous myomas are classified into following types:

ESGE (European Society for Gynaecological Endoscopy) Classification of submucous myoma[12]

Type 0 No intramural extension

Type 1 < 50 percent intramural extension

Type 2 > 50 percent intramural extension.

This classification is a part of preoperative assessment and it plays an important role in determining operative possibility by hysteroscopic myomectomy.

Diagnosis of Endometrial Hyperplasia

The sensitivity of hysteroscopy is poor for diagnosing endometrial hyperplasia (45%) as it has subjective variability. But it offers possibility of visually directed biopsy to study endometrial structure and cyclic development in patients with infertility associated with abnormal uterine bleeding.

Diagnosis of Uterine Malformation

Congenital anomalies of female reproductive tract are seen in 1-2 per 1000 women. In cases of infertility the incidence is 5-10 percent. Uterine anomalies are also associated with recurrent pregnancy losses and failure of IVF treatment. A comprehensive infertility evaluation is necessary prior to concluding anomaly as a cause of infertility.

Uterine anomalies listed by the AFS (American Fertility Society) Classification include aplasia, unicornuate uterus, bicornuate uterus, septate uterus, arcuate uterus and DES-related anomalies. Hysteroscopy alone can diagnose only septate uterus. For diagnosis of the remaining anomalies, a combined hysteroscopic and laparoscopic approach can be used.

In cases of septate uterus, hysteroscopy is essential for determining the extent and thickness of septum.

Intrauterine Adhesions

Diagnosis of intrauterine adhesions can only be made with certainty by hysteroscopy. The AFS classification requires evaluation of extent of cavity, adhesion density and menstrual pattern.

The ESGE classification is based on hysteroscopy and HSG pattern while grade II a and grade IV stages can only be classified by hysteroscopic evaluation.[13]

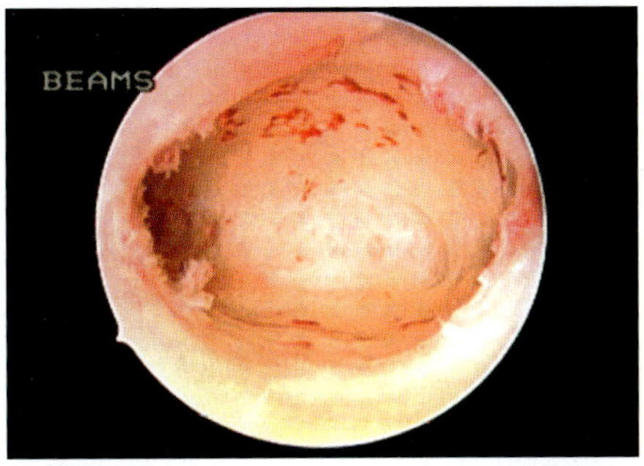

Normal endometrial cavity

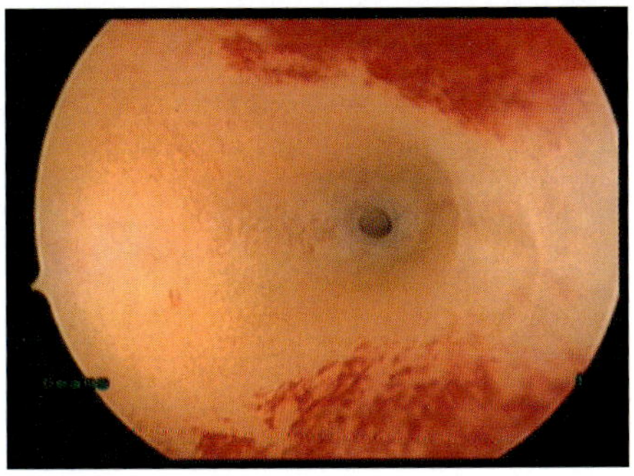
Normal tubal ostium

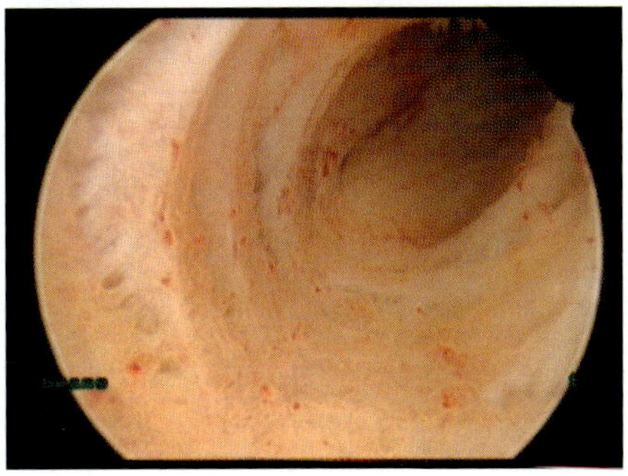
Normal cervical canal

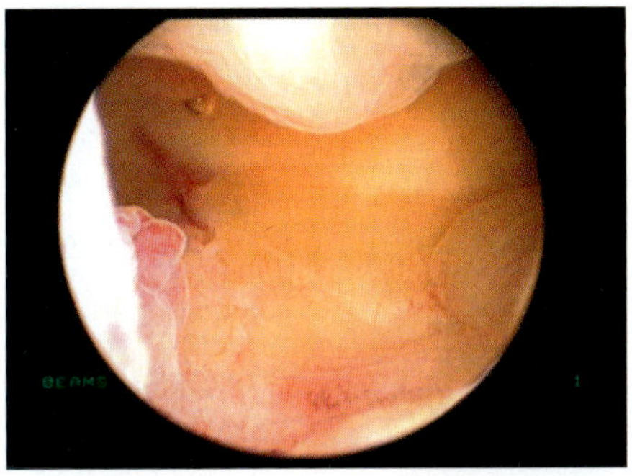
Endometrial hyperplasia

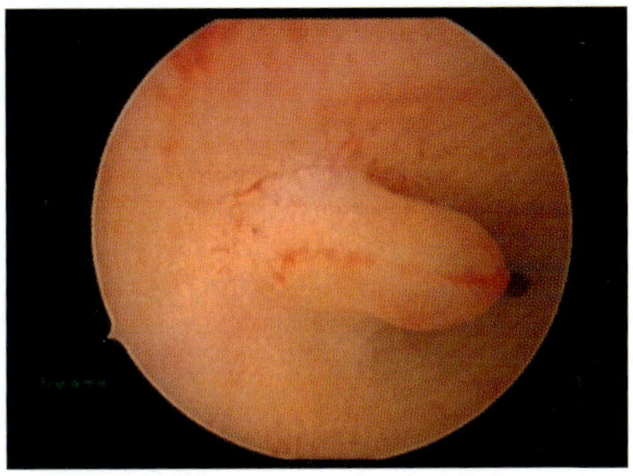
Endometrial polyp

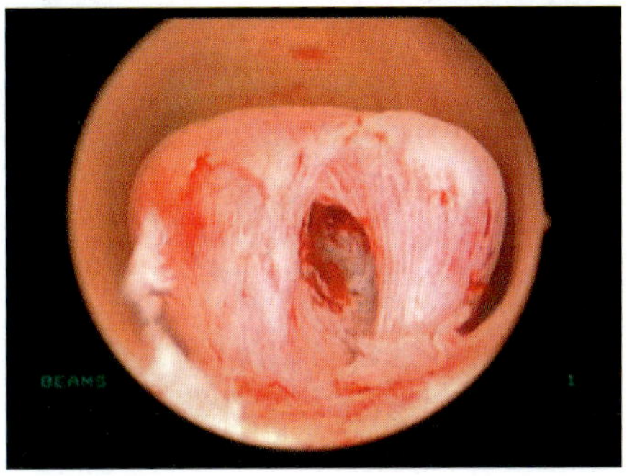
Endometrial polyp

Figure 16.1. Diagnostic hysteroscopy

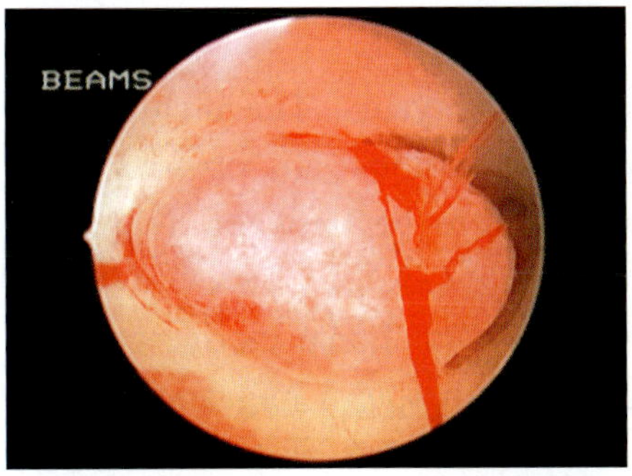

Intracavitary fibroid

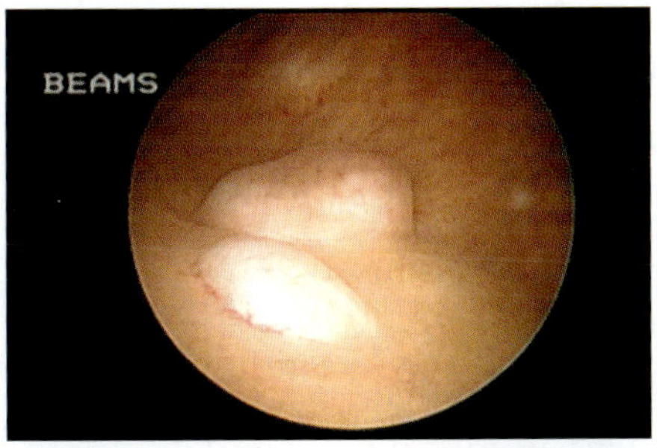

Submucous fibroids on posterior wall

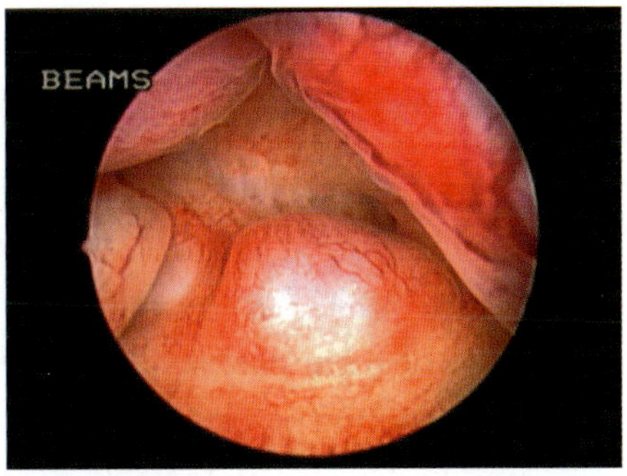

Multiple submucous fibroids

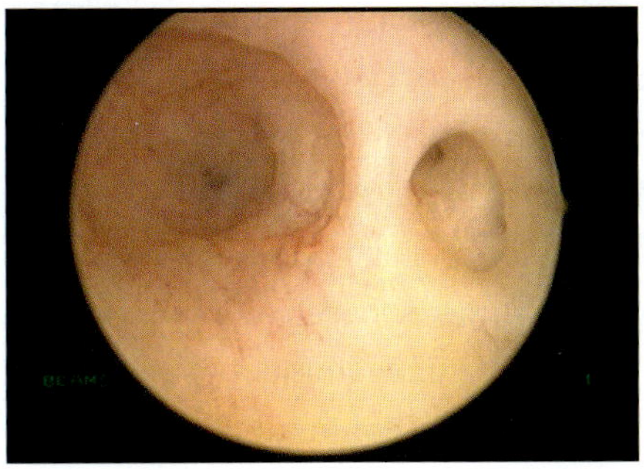
Intrauterine adhesions

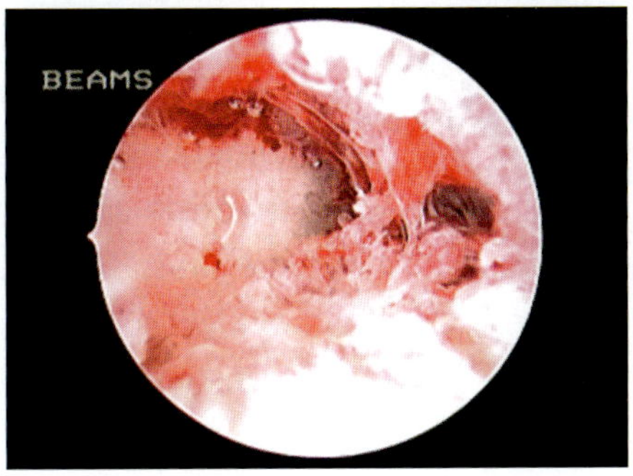

Intrauterine adhesions

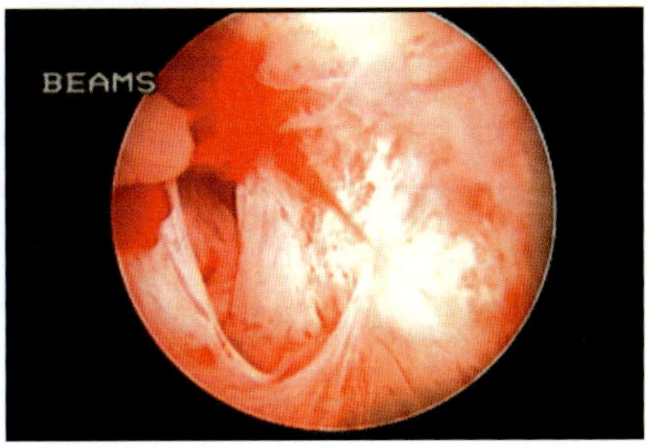

Intrauterine adhesions

Figure 16.2. Diagnostic hysteroscopy

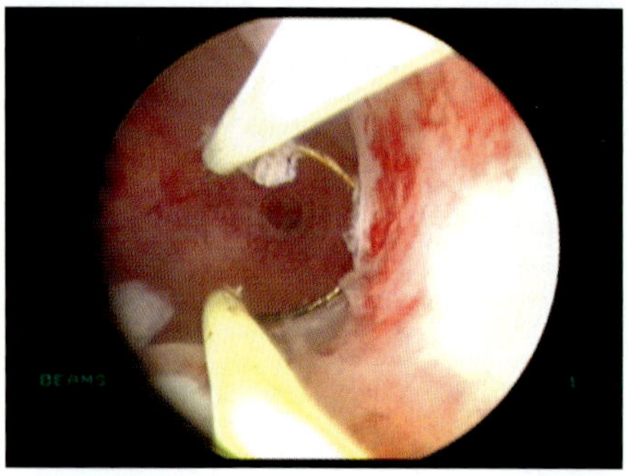

Hysteroscopic biopsy

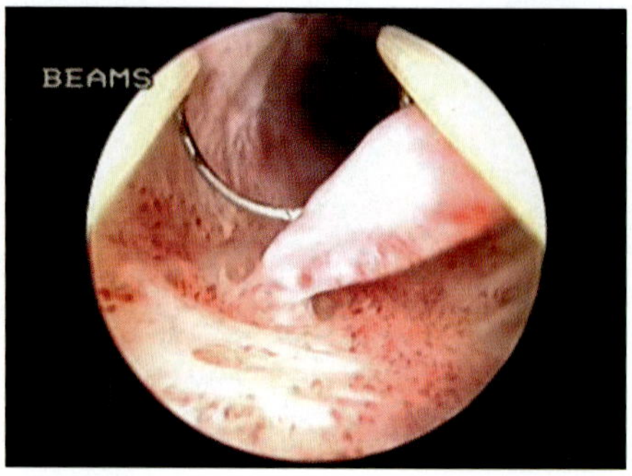

Hysteroscopic polypectomy

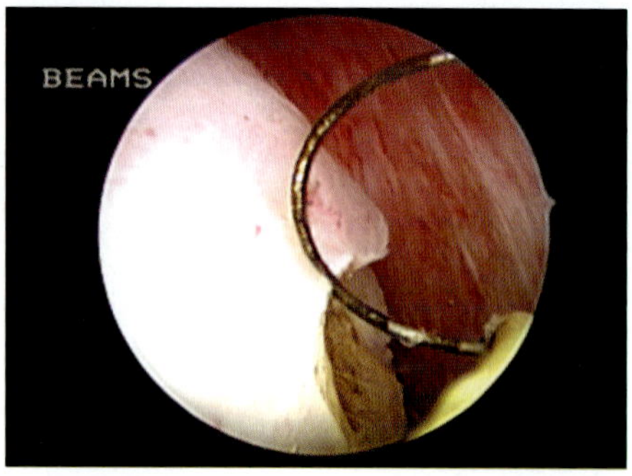

Hysteroscopic myomectomy using resectoscope

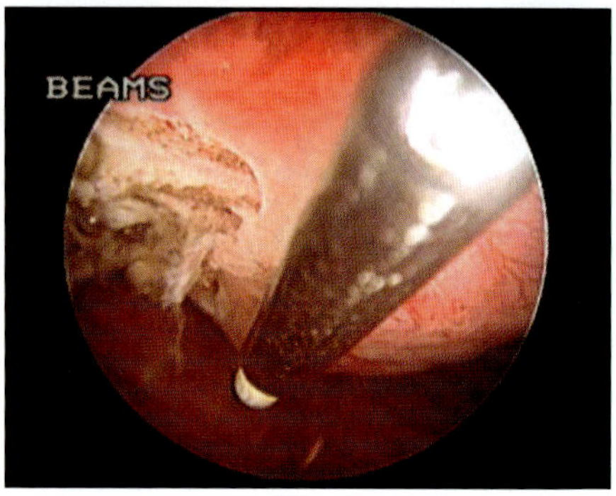

Hysteroscopic myomectomy using bipolar electrode

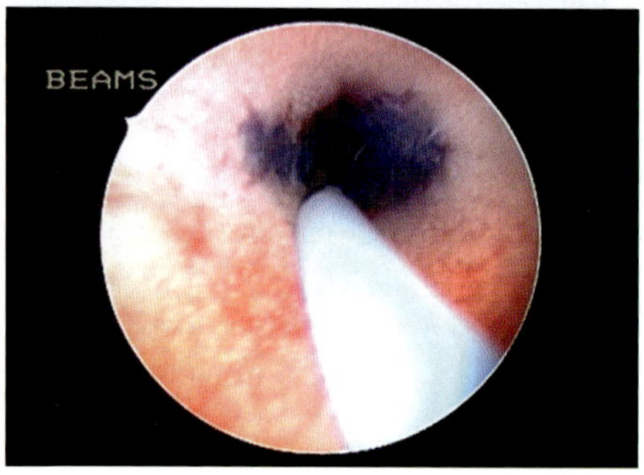

Hysteroscopic tubal cannulation

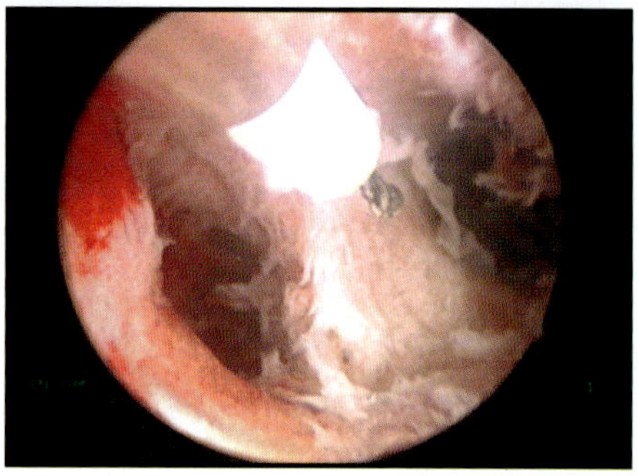
Hysteroscopic adhesiolysis using bipolar electrode

Figure 16.3. Operative hysteroscopy

OPERATIVE HYSTEROSCOPY IN INFERTILITY MANAGEMENT (FIGURE 16.3)

Pantaleoni reported the first hysteroscopic surgery in 1869. Then, in 1925, Rubin added carbon dioxide during evaluation of tubal patency. In the 1970s, hysteroscopy became a common procedure used for office sterilization, and, in the 1980s, distention media was used with hysteroscopy for endometrial ablation. By the mid 1980s, hysteroscopy nearly replaced dilation and curettage (D and C) for diagnosis of intrauterine pathology and now is considered an important therapeutic modality in management of infertility.

HYSTEROSCOPIC MYOMECTOMY

Leiomyoma of the uterus are the most common solid pelvic tumors found in women and are estimated to occur in 20-50 percent of women with increased frequency during the late reproductive years. The incidence of myomas in infertile women without any obvious cause of infertility is estimated to be between 1 and 2.4 percent.[14]

Myomas may cause dysfunctional uterine contractility that may interfere with sperm migration, ovum transport or nidation. Myomas may also be associated with implantation failure or gestation discontinuation due to focal endometrial vascular disturbance, endometrial inflammation, secretion of vasoactive substances or an enhanced endometrial androgen environment. Thus myomas are known to be associated with infertility and the causal relationship in this regard appears to be more evident for submucous myomas. Operative hysteroscopy is the gold standard for treatment of submucous myoma.[15]

A preoperative hysteroscopic evaluation is necessary for the classification of submucous myoma and to determine its operability by hysteroscopic myomectomy.

Neuwirth and Amin were the first to report use of the resectoscope for removal of submucous fibroids. Several different instruments are often used for hysteroscopic myomectomy. They include the resectoscope, bipolar electrodes, scissors, and the laser.

PREOPERATIVE ENDOMETRIAL REDUCTION

The efficacy of preoperative medical treatment with danazol, gonadotrophin releasing-hormone agonists (GnRHa) or progestins in facilitating surgery and improving the long-term results of myomectomy has been proved. Regardless of the type of submucous fibroid, preoperative endometrial reduction allows greater precision during resection and better recognition of low profile fibroids that may be otherwise hidden by the endometrium.[16]

For small fibroids danazol 400-600 mg daily is given preoperatively for 3 weeks. Treatment with biodegradable GnRH agonist implants injected subcutaneously at week 0, 4, 8 help in reducing the fibroid area by an average of 38 percent[17] with a range being reported at 4-95 percent. This treatment is especially helpful in cases with fibroid having largest portion located inside the myometrium that require a two-step surgery.

Pretreatment with GnRH agonists helps by[18]

1. Reducing the vascularity of the fibroid
2. Reducing size of the fibroid
3. Reducing operative time and associated risk of intravasation of distension medium.
4. Reduction of symptoms and anemia.

INSTRUMENTATION

The operative hysteroscope contains the optical system, inflow and outflow channels for the distension medium and the channel for instruments or the laser fibers. The most commonly used telescopes are 4 mm in diameter with a 30° angle.

The irrigation fluids used are low viscosity fluids such as solutions of normal saline, glycine, mannitol or sorbitol. It provides excellent vision and distension of the uterine cavity. Amongst the various distending media that have been tried and tested for operative hysteroscopy the most commonly used media are:

- Normal saline for diagnostic hysteroscopy and operative hysteroscopy using bipolar technology.
- 1.5 percent glycine for operative hysteroscopy using monopolar current.

The complication of media intravasation exists. It is therefore critical to monitor the fluid intake carefully. Continuous flow hysteroscopy is the essence of maintaining a clear view and faster completion of surgery. The continuous irrigation fluid management systems allow efficient monitoring of distension medium intake and output as well as precise control of the intrauterine pressure throughout the procedure.

EQUIPMENT

All the procedures in our center are carried out using a digital Storz camera along with a high intensity Xenon light source to create a high resolution image on a monitor. All procedures are done under general anesthesia and intraoperative monitoring includes strict fluid input and output measurement, pulse oxymetry, electrocardiography with S-T analysis, noninvasive blood pressure, $ETCO_2$, temperature, agent monitoring.

Different surgical modalities can be used for hysteroscopic myomectomy:

1. *Monopolar resectoscope:* It is the most commonly used technique for hysteroscopic myomectomy. The resectoscope with a forward or reverse angled loop depending upon the site of myoma is used. The current used is 90 watts unmodulated monopolar current. Recently bipolar resectoscope has been introduced. The advantages of bipolar over monopolar technology in hysteroscopy is the use of saline solution rather than non-ionic distension media (i.e. glycine, sorbitol, mannitol, etc.), as well as the reduction of energy spread through the tissue during resection.[19]
2. *Bipolar electrodes:* A 5 Fr. bipolar electrical probes can be used to treat endometrial polyps ranging

between 0.5 and 4.5 cm, as well as submucosal and partially intramural myomas between 0.6 and 2.0 cm. The combination of a new generation small diameter hysteroscope and a new bipolar 5 Fr. electrode enables the gynecologist to treat intrauterine pathologies in an office setting without anesthesia.

3. *Laser:* Nd: YAG, KTP, Ho: YAG Lasers have been successfully used for the resection of submucous fibroids. However, Nd: YAG stands out as the laser of choice for myolysis of intramural portion of fibroid because of its ability to penetrate the tissue to a controlled depth upto 7 mm.

The popular CO_2 laser used in gynecological laparoscopy cannot be transmitted through flexible optic fibers and liquid distension media, thereby making its use in operative hysteroscopy impossible.

SURGICAL TECHNIQUE

1. *Intracavitory fibroids:* This type of fibroids is removed using a resectoscope or bipolar electrodes. Pedunculated fibroid is resected keeping the stalk intact. This helps in stabilizing the fibroid while the resection is carried out. The stalk is resected after fibroid is completely resected. Resected bits of fibroid are removed using ovum forceps. In cases of sessile intracavitory fibroids, small fibroids upto 2 cm can be vaporized using a bipolar electrode. Larger fibroids are removed using a resectoscope.
2. *Fibroids with < 50 percent intramural extension:* Literature says that for this type of fibroids preoperative endometrial reduction using GnRH agonists for 6-8 weeks is helpful. This allows vascular transformation and consequent volume reduction, which facilitates the operative procedure and the shrinkage of endometrial cavity after GnRHa treatment makes it relatively easy for the fibroid to be separated from the myometrium.

   At our center we do not give pretreatment with GnRHa to patients as we find these fibroids are easy to resect and with the maintenance of adequate intrauterine pressure the bleeding is observed to be very minimal. Also, cervical dilatation is more difficult in cases of GnRHa pretreatment.
3. *Fibroids with > 50 percent intramural extension:* In literature, a two-step operative hysteroscopy is proposed in cases of submucous fibroids for which the largest portion is not inside the uterine cavity but inside the uterine wall.

   After 8 weeks of pretreatment with GnRHa, partial myomectomy is carried out by resecting the salient portion of myoma protruding in the cavity. The intramural portion is devascularized by introducing laser fiber into the myoma to a depth of 5-10 mm depending upon the depth of remaining intramural portion. The distance between the deepest portion of myoma and the uterine serosa is evaluated by uterine echographic examination done one day prior to the surgery. The end point of laser coagulation is identifiable by the observation of distinct 'craters' with brown borders on all fibroid areas. This technique of inducing an 'iatrogenic necrobiosis' is called transhysteroscopic myolysis.

   After the first operative procedure, the patient is given another 8 weeks of GnRH agonist therapy. At second look hysteroscopy; the hysteroscopic view of the cavity shows a white avascular fibroid remnant protruding in the lumen, as if the shrinkage of uterus induced by the continued GnRHa therapy had virtually expelled the residual necrotic fibroid. This remnant fibroid is resected and the second step of the procedure is completed.

   Again, at our center, we find it fairly easy to do one-step myomectomy hysteroscopically for fibroids with > 50 percent myometrial extension. We do not give GnRHa to these patients. Adequate intrauterine pressure prevents bleeding. The fibroid is completely resected in one step. The end point of resection is the visualization of myometrial fibers.
4. *Multiple submucous myomas:* For cases of multiple submucous fibroids, each myoma is either separated from the surrounding myometrium or totally

coagulated. Intraoperative injection of PGF2α during hysteroscopic myomectomy has been used to induce myometrial contraction thus allowing the myoma to be extruded in the cavity.

Postoperative estrogen therapy is indicated after resection of multiple myomas especially if the myomas are on the opposing wall as there is a risk of formation of adhesion between the two raw surfaces.

PREGNANCY RATES AFTER HYSTEROSCOPIC MYOMECTOMY

Many studies have assessed fertility rates after hysteroscopic myomectomy and have noted pregnancy rates similar to those after abdominal myomectomy, approximately 60 percent. Again, no studies include expectantly managed control groups.

PREGNANCY RATES IN PATIENTS UNDERGOING HYSTEROSCOPIC MYOMECTOMY

Author	*Year*	*Study size*	*Pregnancy rate*
Donnez et al	1990	24	67%
Goldenberg et al	1995	15	47%
Vercellini et al	1999	40	37%
Fernandez et al	2001	59	27%
Bernard et al	2000	31	35%

A significant difference in pregnancy rates between infertile women with and without myomas (11% versus 25%)is found while comparing spontaneous conception in infertile women with and without myomas in whom andrological and tubal infertility factors have been excluded.[20] This shows that infertile women with myomas have better pregnancy rates after myomectomy (42%) than infertile women with untreated myomas (11%).

HYSTEROSCOPIC POLYPECTOMY

The incidence of small endometrial polyps detected hysteroscopically in an infertile eumenorrheic population is 15 percent.[21]

All polyps <0.5 cm can be removed using 5 Fr. mechanical instruments (sharp scissors and/or crocodile forceps). Larger polyps are removed intact, with the bipolar twizzle electrode, only if the internal cervical os size is wide enough for their extraction. Otherwise, they are sliced from the free edge to the base into two/three fragments large enough to be pulled out through the uterine cavity using 5 Fr. grasping forceps with teeth. To remove the entire base of the polyp without going too deep into the myometrium, in some cases the twizzle electrode can be bent by 25-30°, enough to obtain a kind of hook electrode. In cases of infertility, polyps are vaporized using bipolar electrode to prevent thermal damage to endometrium.

HYSTEROSCOPIC SYNECHIOLYSIS

Ashermann syndrome was identified in 1948 as uterine synechiae. These intrauterine adhesions are often associated with amenorrhea or infertility. Hysteroscopy can be used for diagnosis and treatment of these adhesions. The filmy adhesions are often lysed with distension media alone, whereas the dense adhesions often require cutting or excision with blunt, sharp, electrodiathermy, or laser techniques.

Hysteroscopic visualization of the uterine cavity allows for directed lysis. If extensive lysis is indicated, laparoscopy can be used as an aid for decreasing the risk of perforation by visualizing the illuminated cavity intra-abdominally. Overall live delivery rates according to stage of intrauterine adhesions were 33.3 percent, 44.4 percent and 46.7 percent for stages I, II and III respectively. Similar cumulative delivery rates were achieved in patients with no additional infertility factors who attempted to conceive naturally after adhesiolysis using the versapoint (71.7%) or the resectoscope (60%). Hysteroscopic treatment can increase the risk of abnormal placentation (e.g. accreta, percreta, increta, previa).[22]

Follow-up hysterosalpingogram or diagnostic hysteroscopy following withdrawal bleeding has been recommended.

HYSTEROSCOPIC METROPLASTY

Mullerian anomalies usually come to medical attention when they cause recurrent pregnancy losses. Septate uteri have been associated with infertility, recurrent pregnancy loss, and obstetric prematurity, though in many cases a uterine septum may be totally asymptomatic.[23] Most of these complications require surgical correction. The most commonly presenting anomaly is the double uterus which can be the source of recurrent abortion and preterm deliveries. The Strassman, Jones and Tompkins metroplasties have been shown to greatly improve the rate of successful deliveries in these patients. Hysteroscopic metroplasty, using scissors, resectoscope or laser is now the recommended treatment for most septate uteri due to its relative simplicity, low morbidity and excellent reproductive outcome.

- The first method uses the resectoscope, a straight 5 mm loop electrode, and an unmodulated current of 90 watts. The septum is transected until small areas of bleeding are observed, indicating that myometrium has been reached.
- A second method is to use a 5 to 7 mm operative hysteroscope and small scissors to transect the septum until those important small bleeding areas are observed. The intrauterine pressure helps in expanding the septum as it is cut.
- A newer, third, method involves use of a bipolar vaporizing electrode that can be used in isotonic sodium chloride solution. The added benefit is that while the septum is completely removed the thermal damage to the endometrium is less because of less lateral spread of current.

CONCLUSION

Hysteroscopy is a safe and efficient diagnostic and treatment modality. It is one of the most rewarding diagnostic tools in basic reproductive evaluation and we recommend that hysteroscopy should be a part of basic infertility workup. Hysteroscopic surgery is the treatment of choice for submucous myomas, polyps, intrauterine adhesions, and proximal tubal blocks and is known to enhance fertility in these patients. Improved technology now enables us to perform many operative procedures in office setting without anesthesia thus improving efficacy and patient acceptability of the procedure. We believe that hysteroscopy is a minimally invasive surgery in the true sense.

REFERENCES

1. Donnez J, Mathieu PE, Bassil S, Smets M, Nisolle M, Berlière M. Fibroids: Management and treatment: The state of the art. Hum Reprod 1996;11:1837-40.
2. RCOG guidelines, Fertility assessment and treatment of people with fertility problems, 2004.
3. Glatstein IZ, Harlow BL, Hornstein MD. Practice patterns among reproductive endocrinologists: The infertility evaluation. Fertil Steril 1997a;67:443-51.
4. Vercellini P, Cortesi I, Oldani S, et al. The role of transvaginal ultrasonography and outpatient diagnostic hysteroscopy in the evaluation of patients with menorrhagia. Hum Reprod 1997;12:1768-71.
5. Salim R, Lee C. A comparative study of three-dimensional saline infusion sonohysterography and diagnostic hysteroscopy for the classification of submucous fibroids. Hum Reprod 2005;20(1):253-7.
6. Wang CW, Lee CL, Lai YM, et al. Comparison of hysterosalpingography and hysteroscopy in female infertility. J Am Assoc Gynecol Laparosc 1996;3:581-4.
7. Sutton C. Endoscopic Surgery for gynaecologists, Chap 52, Diagnostic Hysteroscopy: Technique and Documentation, page 513.
8. Shushan A, Rojansky N. Should hysteroscopy be a part of basic infertility workup?, Hum Reprod 1999;14(8):1923-4.
9. Oliveira FG, et al. Uterine cavity findings and hysteroscopic interventions in patients undergoing *in vitro* fertilization-embryotransfer who repeatedly cannot conceive. Fertil Steril 2003;80(6):1371-5.
10. Frydman R. Impact of embryotransfer technique on implantation rates. J Gynaecol Obstet Biol Reprod 2004; 33:S36-9.
11. Ceci O, Bettocchi S, et al. Comparison of hysteroscopy and hysterectomy findings for assessing the diagnostic accuracy of office. Hysteroscopy Fertile Steril 2002;78(3): 628-31.
12. Wamstakere, et al. Hysteroscopy Training Centre, Spaarne Hospital, Haarlem, The Netherlands 1993.

13. Sutton C. Endoscopic Surgery for gynaecologists, Chap 52, Diagnostic Hysteroscopy: Technique and documentation, page 514.
14. Donnez J, et al. What are the implications of myomas on fertility? Human Reproduction 2002;17(6):1424-30.
15. Fernandez H, Sefrioui O, Virelizier C, Gervaise A, Gomel V, Frydman R. Hysteroscopic resection of submucosal myomas in patients with infertility. Hum Reprod 2001;16: 1489-2.
16. Parazzini F, Vercellini P, Giorgi O, et al. Efficacy of preoperative medical treatment in facilitating hysteroscopic endometrial resection, myomectomy and metroplasty: Literature review. Hum Reprod 1998;13(9):2592-7.
17. Sutton C. Endoscopic Surgery for gynaecologists, Chap 55: Treatment of dysfunctional uterine bleeding by Nd: YAG Laser: J Donnez et al 1998; Second edition, page 544.
18. Sutton C. Endoscopic Surgery for gynaecologists, Chap 55: Treatment of dysfunctional uterine bleeding by Nd: YAG Laser: 546-7.
19. Bettocchi S, Ceci O. Advanced operative office hysteroscopy without anaesthesia: Analysis of 501 cases treated with a 5 Fr. bipolar electrode, Human Reproduction 2002;17(9):2435-8.
20. Bulletti C, De Ziegler D, Polli V, Diotallevi L, Del Ferro E,. Flamigni C. The role of leiomyomas in infertility. J Am Assoc Gynecol Laparosc, 1999;6:441-5.
21. Shokeir TA, Shalan HM. Significance of endometrial polyps detected hysteroscopically in eumenorrheic infertile women. J Obstet Gynaecol Res 2004;30(2):84-9.
22. Zikopoulos KA,Kolibianakis EM. Live delivery rates in subfertile women with Asherman's syndrome after hysteroscopic adhesiolysis using the resectoscope or the Versapoint system. Reprod Biomed Online 2004;8(6):720-5.
23. Pellicer A. Shall we operate on Müllerian defects? An introduction to the debate. Hum Reprod 1997;12:1371-2.

Section Three

TUBES

17 Laparoscopic Surgery for Distal Tubal Occlusion

Pravin Patel, Manish Banker, Tejas Dave, Manish Shah

INTRODUCTION

Even though last quarter of the previous century witnessed considerable advances in management of distal tubal occlusion, the pregnancy outcome after repair of post infections distal tubal disease are not surpassing that if IVF/ARTS. In 1970s several team worldwide laid down principals for microsurgery and later on laparoscopy started to get a place in DTOS. With advancing field of Laparoscopy, laparoscopic microsurgery (Dr. Koh) soon became the reality. In this chapter the laparoscopic surgical treatment for distal tubal infertility is discussed.

SURGICAL ANATOMY

From a surgical viewpoint the tube lateral to ampullary-isthmic junction is considered the distal tube. It is 5-8 cm, elastic and sinous, ending in the funnel shape infundibulum (2-3 cm). The infundibulum opens in the peritoneal cavity via abdominal ostium which is covered by 12-15 fimbriae. The relaxed abdominal ostium is 2-3 mm but can be stretched. The stretched luminal diameter of ampulla is about 1cm. The mesosalpinx ends short of infundibulum, allowing the terminal end of tube to move freely over ovary.

The ampullary mucosa is having primary longitudinal folds with many secondary and tertiary folds on primary ridges. The folds are supported on subepithelial lamina propria. Ciliary cells are move on apices and folds and in the interfold spaces are nonciliated cells.

Muscularis is thin with outer longitudinal and inner circular layer.

PATHOLOGY (TABLE 17.1)

Distal tubal occlusions are mostly following pelvic inflammatory diseases, other cause includes tuberculosis, endometriosis, previous pelvic abdominal or tubal surgeries, rarely schistosomiasis, congenital anomalies.

Table 17.1. Etiology of distal tubal occlusion

A.	Pelvic inflammatory disease
B.	Endometriosis and primary peritoneal neoplasia
C.	Pelvic and abdominal surgery
D.	Tubal surgery-tubal pregnancy, fimbriectomy, and tuboplasty
E.	Parovarian and ovarian cysts
F.	Pelvic hemoperitoneum

There are two types of occlusions:

- Partial stenosis with some degree of permeability
- Complete occlusion with hydrosalpinx

The morphological sequeal of the damaged distal tube can be out lined as follow:

- Intraluminal and fimbrial adhesions
- Infundibular constriction ring or tubal phimosis
- Fimbrial encapsulation by ampullary or other peritoneum

- Complete occlusion of the terminal tubal opening with accumulation of tubal fluid, and formation of hydrosalpinx
- Fibrosis of tubal wall (thick wall hydrosalpinx)
- Pelvic adhesions
- Complete fusion of pelvic organs

CLASSIFICATION OF DTOs

Universally accepted classification for distal tubal occlusion does not exist but still the classification is required for planning and execution of therapeutic approach. The morphological classification by tubal surgeons takes in account fimbrial status and abdominal ostium.

a. Preserved fimbria
   - Fimbrial agglutination
   - Fimbrial encapsulation
   - Mild tubal phimosis
b. Absent fimbria
   - Severe tubal phimosis
   - Thin walled hydrosalpinx
   - Thick walled hydrosalpinx

The individual fimbrial lappets are fused in fimbrial agglutination or conglutination. The fimbria may be sequestered by the rolled over ampullary peritoneum or peritubal adhesions or the distal tubal end may adhere to one of the pelvic organs in fimbrial encapsulation.

In mild tubal phimosis the peritoneal constriction rings reduces the size of ostium. On laparoscopy, the ampullary distension with infundibular stenosis and normal fimbria can be seen.

In severe phimosis the ring totally occludes the ostium and sparse fimbria may be noticed on examinations, which neither have connection to the ampullary tubal folds nor have any functional significance.

When this process totally occludes the ostium (with complete loss of fimbria) the hydrosalpinx formation starts; 3-5 ml of the tubal fluid escapes through uterine (intramural) ostium into the uterus. Subsequently edema of the intramural endosalpinx prevents this escape resulting in hydrosalpinx.

There are different anatomical categories of hydrosalpinx:

HYDROSALPINX SIMPLEX

Moderately dilated ampulla with clear yellow fluid. The tubal wall is thinned with atrophy of mucosa but no adhesions between mucosal folds.

HYDROSALPINX FOLLICULARIS

The lumen is divided by adhesions forming septa and folds may be agglutinated or adhered together.

HYDROSALPINX WITH PACHYSALPINX

Here the progression has replaced the muscularis with fibrous tissues. This produces thickened tubal wall with local tubal sclerosis.

This distinction between thin wall and thick wall is important from prognostic viewpoint; later giving less pregnancy rates following surgery.

Depending upon the diameter of tube, four different categories are diagnosed on laparoscopy:

a. Patent tubes with conglutination or phimosis of fimbria.
b. Complete distal occlusion but the diameter of the tube remains normal.
c. Complete distal occlusion with ampullary diameter less than 25 mm.
d. Complete distal occlusion with ampulla more than 25 mm.

Preoperative Evaluation

The complete clinical evaluation and psychological assessment of the couple are essential. This includes following:

Couple Fertility

All male-female factors for infertility should be investigated. These include spermogram, ovulation documentation, hormonal assays and testing for infections especially for *N. gonorrhea* and *Chlamydia trachomatis*.

Basal body temperature and post-coital test are mentioned for the sake of exclusion. All invasive procedure can be carried out later during same sitting prior to surgery.

Hysterosalpingography (HSG)

The role of HSG is very vital before undertaking surgery. It gives information about tubal health by following parameters. Length of ampulla, size of ampulla, passage of dye from ampulla towards ostium and most importantly presence or absence of mucosal folds. In one study the presence of mucosal fold was found to be single most preoperative indicator for successful pregnancy. The pregnancy rate was 60.7% amongst patients with mucosal pattern in HSG compared to 7.3% for tube without mucosal patterns. In one study of 300 patients only women with normal mucosal pattern on HSG conceived.

In addition HSG gives clue for uterine and proximal tubal disease like salpingitis isthmica nodosa (SIN).

Hysteroscopy

This is a complementary procedure for intrauterine conditions like submucosal myoma, intrauterine polyps, synechiae and congenital anomalies.

Salpingoscopy

Salpingoscopy should be performed at the time of Laparoscopy. The small endoscope (2.0 m or 2.9 mm) is inserted through an abdominal ostium. Tube is distended with normal saline or glycine.

Following five patterns are identified:

1. Normal mucosal fold
2. Major-minor folds are preserved but there is slight flattening of variable degree.
3. Major or minor folds are preserved but there are focal lesions like adhesions or agglutination.
4. Extensive lesion of major or minor folds like adhesions, stricture of lumen and formation of pseudospaces.
5. Fold pattern totally lost, lumen is dilated with rigid walls.

Treatment Options

Depending upon the result of the investigations various scoring systems have been devised. Out of them French tubal scoring system (Table 17.2) and Boer-Meisel classification are commonly used.

Table 17.2. French tubal scoring system

Tube premeability	*Ampullary mucosa*	*Wall of ampulla*
Phimosis 2 Hydrosalpinx 5	Folds remaining 0 Folds reduced 5 No folds 10	Normal 0 Thin 5 Thick or sclerotic 10
Stage: 1: 2-5 2: 6-10	Surgery	
Stage: 3: 11-15 4: >15	IVF (Arts)	

Boer-Meisel Classification

Only ampullary mucosa considered

Group 1: Normal mucosa with regular folds

Group 2: Moderate alteration; here normal ampullary mucosa intersperse with areas where folds are non-existent

Group 3: Mucosa considerably damaged. Here folds are absent and/or replaced by intratubal synechia.

This classification does not take in account the size of ampulla and as such seems to be the simplest one.

The result according to both the system as compared by Dubuisson (in 1994) are as under (Table 17.3).

Operative Techniques

The three important surgical techniques are usually performed in DTO (a) Adhesiolysis (b) fimbrioplasty (c) salpingostomy

Adhesiolysis

The first part is to inspect the pelvic cavity and abdominal cavity for any inflammatory lesions, tuberculosis, adhesions and endometriosis. Liver bed must be evaluated for presence of adhesions (Fitz-Hugh-Curtis syndrome) suggesting chronic infective process.

Table 17.3. Dubuisson's comparison of results

Results according to the French tubal scoring system

		Intrauterine Pregnancy		Ectopic Pregnancy	
Tube Score	*Number*	*(N)*	*(%)*	*(N)*	*(%)*
1	15	9	60.0	0	0.0
2	29	15	51.7	2	6.9
1 + 2	44	24	54.5	2	4.5
3	16	2	12.5	1	6.2
4	21	0	0.0	1	4.7
3 + 4	37	2	5.4	2	5.4

Results according to Boer-Meisel classification

		Intrauterine Pregnancy		Ectopic Pregnancy	
Tube Score	*Number*	*(N)*	*(%)*	*(N)*	*(%)*
Group 1	32	17	53.1	0	0.0
Group 2	27	9	33.3	4	14.8
Group 1 + 2	59	26	44.0	4	6.7
Group 3	22	0	0.0	0	0

Whether fimbrioplasty or salpingostomy is required, they are usually associated with adhesiolysis. Certain general principles of adhesiolysis should be kept in mind.

- Adhesions should be placed under tension before lysis.
- Proceed from midline to laterally (towards adnexa)
- Lysis should be done layer wise cutting superficial adhesions first.
- Simple adhesions should be freed first.
- Round ligament insertion is an important anatomical landmark in case of difficult adhesiolysis.
- Avoid injury to peritoneum as far as possible.
- The aim of adhesiolysis is to restore pelvic anatomy to normal and to have free fallopian tube and ovary maintaining their relationship.

Hemostasis is vital and frequent irrigation with suction is essential. One can use monopolar or bipolar electrical currents or use LASER depending upon individual choice and availability.

Fimbrioplasty

The principle of fimbrioplasty is to restore the original anatomy of infundibulum by treating phimosis and agglutination.

a. Where the fimbria are encapsulated and hidden by fibrotic bands, the antimesentric border is incised to remove fibrotic bands and expose the fimbria.
b. In case of agglutination where the folds are stuck together a small incision is put at the center of agglutination. Now dilate the opening by introducing atraumatic forceps in closed position and opening it in different directions. Any small fibrotic bands can be lysed as mentioned earlier.
c. In tubal phimosis-an atraumatic forceps is introduced inside the infundibulum. By opening the jaws, the adhesion bands in the infundibulum can be seen. They are incised with mono/bi-polar or CO_2 laser.

At the end of operation hemostasis is to be confirmed. Any small oozers are controlled by submersing the infundibular portion of tube in warm (37°C) normal saline for few minutes. Any residual oozers are controlled by bipolar fine coagulation. Care is taken to avoid damage to the mucosa. Severe phimosis is treated by salpingostomy.

Laparoscopic Salpingostomy

There are two types of salpingostomy:

a. Cuff salpingostomy for thin wall hydrosalpinx
b. Flap salpingostomy for thick wall hydrosalpinx

Latter procedure is usually not done as the results are not convincing as compared to ARTs for thick walled hydrosalpinx.

Cuff Salpingostomy

This operation is usually subdivided into three parts:
a. Opening (incising) the tube
b. Eversion of mucosa
c. Stabilizing the eversion

Opening the Tube (Figures 17.1 and 17.2)

Initially the methylene blue dye is injected to see the end of tube. The central whitish fibrotic area is now exposed. This point is now incised with monopolar current or laser. Once the lumen is opened the dye comes out and soils the field. Operative field is made clear and incision is extended in a cruciate manner. If possible incision should be placed in between mucosal folds to avoid bleeding and if bleeding occurs it has to be controlled with minimum fine bipolar coagulation.

Everting the Mucosa (Figure 17.3)

After opening the tube infundibulum is assessed for presence of adhesions. If present they are lysed as mentioned earlier.

Now through the ipsilateral port, the tubal serosa is catch hold of and with contralateral port, babcock's grasping forceps is introduced in the lumen of tube. By gradually exerting pressure in opposing direction with each graspers, the mucosa of infundibulum is everted making lumen fairly prominent in the center.

If incision put is too small eversion will be difficult producing more damage to mucosa and if incision is too large-eversion will not be maintained properly.

Stabilizing the Eversion

There are different techniques:
a. Coagulation of serosa with bipolar forceps, lowest power setting should be used to coagulate only serosa and prevent damage to everted mucosa.

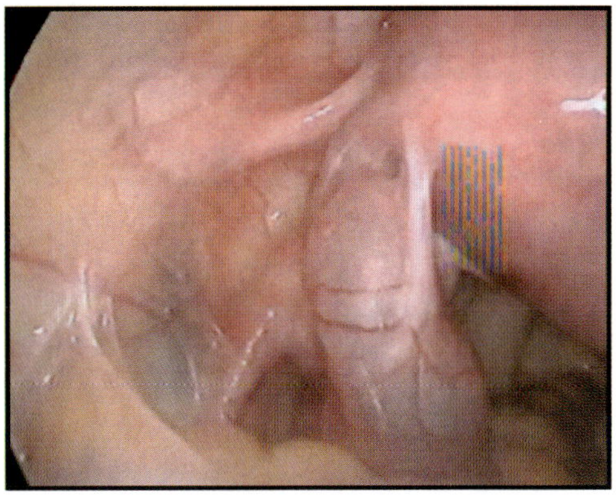

Figure 17.1. Hydrosalpinx

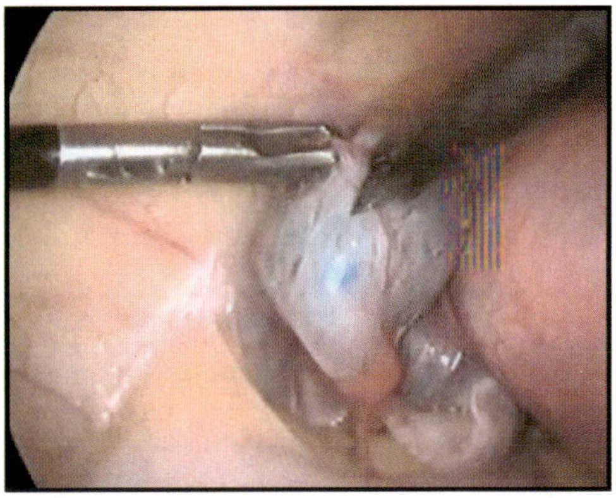

Figure 17.2. Incising the tube

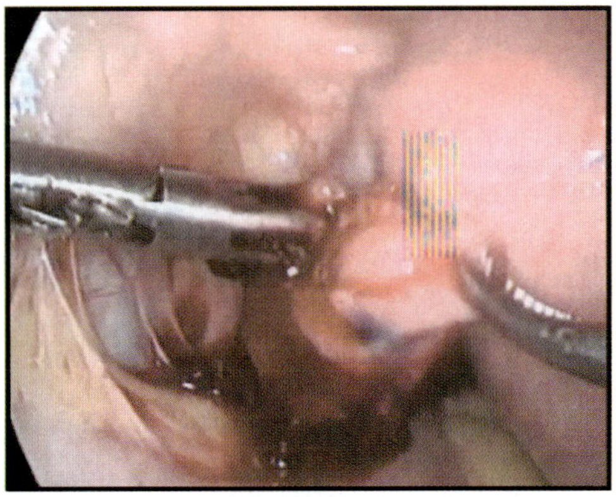

Figure 17.3. Eversion of mucosa

b. Vaporisation of the tubal serosa with focused shot from laser beam.
c. Suturing with 3 to 4 interrupted sutures with 6/0 non-absorbable material. The results are mostly equal, but suturing is usually preferred in our setup to avoid any lateral thermal damage to mucosa.

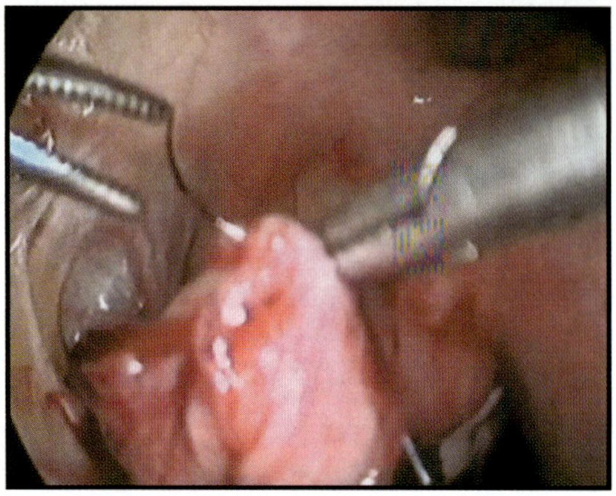

Figure 17.4. Suturing the everted

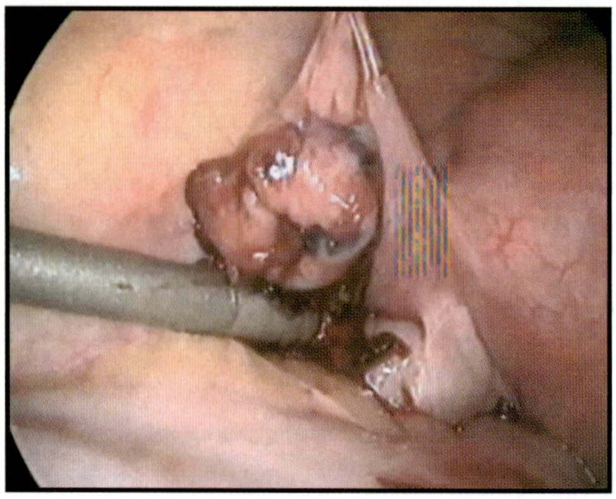

Figure 17.5. End result

Salpingectomy

In the patients who are to undergo IVFs for thick walled hydrosalpinx or any other reasons, salpingectomy is advisable for improving embryo implantation and reducing the chances of ectopic pregnancy. The mesosalpinx is cauterized very close to tube to avoid damage to ovaries.

Results

Fertility results postlaparoscopic tubal surgery are shown in Table 17.4.

Table 17.4. Laparoscopic adhesiolysis: Fertility results

Authors	*Year*	*Number*	*Intrauterine Pregnancies (N)*	*(N)*	*Ectopic Pregnancies*	
Mettler et al	1979	44	13	29	-	-
Palmer	1979	144	34	23.6	11	7.6
Mintz et al	1979	65	34	52.3	-	-
Gomel	1983	92	54	58.7	5	5.4
Audebert	1983	50	15	30	0	0
Fayez	1983	50	30	60	2	4
Bruhat et al	1983	93	48	52	7	7.5
Feste	1985	17	6	35.3	-	-
Diamond et al	1986	9	0	0.0	-	-
Reich	1987	27	21	78	1	4
Serour et al	1989	25	3	12.0	-	-
Fimbrioplasty by Laparoscopy: Fertility Results						
Gomel	1983	40	20	50	2	5
Dubuisson et al.	1990	31	5	25.8	4	12.9
Total		**71**	**28**	**39.4**	**6**	**8.5**

contd...

Table contd.

Salpingostomy by Laparoscopy: Fertility Results

Authors	*Year*	*Number*	*Pregnancies*	*Intrauterine pregnancies* (%)	*Ectopic pregnancies* (%) (%)
Gomel	1977	9		44.4	0
Metter et al	1979	38	26	-	-
Fayez	1983	19	10	-	10
Daniell and Herbert	1984	21	24	19	5
Audibert et al	1991	55	20	-	15
Canis et al	1991	87		33.3	6.9
McComb and Paleologou	1991	22	22.7	-	?
Nezhat et al	1992	42	35.7	-	15.4
Dubuisson et al	1994	81	37	32.1	4.9

Most pregnancies are achieved within 1st year or surgery

CONCLUSION

The development of laparoscopic surgery and assisted reproductive techniques have given new hope for patients of distal tubal infertility.

The fertility prognosis is directly correlated with condition of the distal tube. Laparoscopic surgery is the choice for periadnexal and pelvic adhesiolysis and distal tubal plasties. IVF should be strongly considered from the outset in patient with badly deteriorated fallopian tube.

SUGGESTED READING

1. Andersion AN, et al. Low implantation rate after IVF in patient with hydrosalpinges diagnosed by USG: 1994. (Human Reproduction 1935-1938).
2. Boer Meisel ME. Predicting the pregnancy outcome in patients treated for hydrosalpinx prospective study. Fertility and Sterility 45:23-9.
3. Bruhat MA, et al. Laparoscopic procedure to promote fertility: salpingolysis 93 cases. Acta Europaea Fertilitatis 14:13-5.
4. Brosens Ivo. Tubal infertility 1989;11:24-2.
5. Canis M, Mage G. Laparoscopic distal tuboplasty: 87 cases 4 yrs experience. Fertility Sterility 56:616-21.
6. Chapron C, Dubaisson JB. Treatment and causes of female infertility. Lancet 1994a;344:333-4.
7. Daniell JF. Laparoscopic salpingostomy utilising CO_2 laser. Fertility Sterility 1984;41:558-63.
8. Dubuisson JB. Terminal tuboplasties by Laparoscopy 65 consecutive cases. Fertility Sterility 1990;54:401-3.
9. Dubuission JB. Laparoscopic salpingostomy: Fertility results according to tubal mucosal appearance. Human Reproduction 1994;9:334-9.
10. Fleming C. Impaired implantation after IVF treatment associated with hydrosalpinx. British Journal of Obs and Gyne 1996;103:265-7.
11. Gomel V. Salpingostomy by laparoscopy. Journal of Reproductive Medicine 1977;18:265-7.
12. Henry Suchet J. Prognostic value of tuboscopy vs Hysterosalpingography before tuboplasty. Journal of Reproductive Medicine 1984;29:602-12.
13. Mage G, et al. A preoperative classification to predict the intrauterine and ectopic pregnancy rates after distal tubal microsurgery. Fertility Sterility 1986;46:807-10.
14. Mc comb PF. The intussusception salpingostomy techniques for therapy of distal oviductal occlusion at Laparoscopy. Obstetric and Gynecology 1991;78:443-7.
15. Reich H. Laparoscopic treatment of extended pelvic adhesions including hydrosalpinx. Journal of Reproductive Medicine 1987;32:736-42.
16. Rock JA. Factors influencing the success of salpingostomy techniques for distal fimbrial occlusion. Obstetrics and Gynecology 1978;52:591-9.

18 Current Trends in the Management of Ectopic Pregnancy

B Ramesh

INTRODUCTION

Ectopic pregnancy is a pregnancy implanted at a site other than the endometrial cavity. Although extrauterine pregnancy can be affixed to cervix, ovary, bowel or other structures the most common location is the fallopian tube, more than 95 percent of ectopics occurs in the oviduct.

DIAGNOSIS

The triad of abdominal pain, Vaginal bleeding and adnexal mass was the corner stone in the diagnosis for decades but is present in less than half of these women. In fact, the so called classic triad may represent mostly advanced cases. Early diagnosis is critical to lessen serious morbidity.

Frequencies of implantation sites for ectopic pregnancies are (Figure 18.1): Ampulla – 78 percent, Isthmus – 12 percent, Fimbriae – 5 percent, cornual, interstitial or Intramural Area – 2 percent and Abdominal, Cervical or Ovarian – 3 percent.[1]

How is an early diagnosis made? The two tests which help in early diagnosis are serum human chorionic gonadotropin (hCG) levels and transvaginal ultrasound.

Beta hCG is a very sensitive blood test, which can detect the presence of pregnancy as early as 1 week after implantation. Measured serially, a rise of less than 66 percent over a 48 hours interval is highly suggestive of either an abnormal intrauterine pregnancy or ectopic pregnancy.[2,3]

Vaginal ultrasound (TVS) can detect an intrauterine pregnancy when the serum hCG level has reached 1500 mIU/ml. When an IUP was not seen on ultrasound (TVS) and hCG levels exceeded the so called discriminatory zone, ectopic pregnancy was present 86 percent of the cases.[4]

When beta hCG and ultrasound (TVS) are inconclusive diagnostic laparoscopy comes to the rescue of clinician in the diagnosis. Even in laparoscopy the presence of ectopic pregnancy (EP) could be undetected in 3-4 percent of women.[5] Salpingoscopy may confirm the presence of tubal pregnancy when it is too small to detect laparoscopically.[6]

TREATMENT

In the past, salpingectomy was the standard management for ectopic pregnancy. But recently, technical advances with earlier diagnosis and treatment allow definitive management of unruptured ectopic pregnancy, there by preserving the tube and increasing the chance of subsequent intrauterine pregnancy.

Selecting the best therapy for a patient depends on her desire for future pregnancy, her surgical history, previous pregnancy outcome, general medical and gynecological history and the skill of the gynecologist.

MANAGEMENT OPTION INCLUDE

- Expectant management

- Chemotherapy
- Surgical management
  - Laparotomy
  - Laparoscopy
  - Conservative
  - Radical

Expectant Management

Management by observation and monitoring may be chosen in selected women.[7] A substantial number of EP's die and resorb without treatment. Spontaneous resolution is most likely in women with declining and low levels of hCG – less than 1000 mIU/ml.[8]

Inclusion Criteria

1. Asymptomatic patients
2. Initial beta-hCG level < 1500 mIU/ml
3. No evidence of pregnancy by TVS
4. Serial beta-hCG estimation show falling levels.

Exclusion Criteria

1. Sonographic evidence of adnexal mass with transverse diameter > 4 cm.
2. Extrauterine fetal heart beat on TVS.
3. Documentation of free fluid on USG > 100 ml.
4. Hemodynamic instability
5. Abdominal pain.

Method

Patients are monitored with serial sonographic examinations and hCG determinations twice per week for the first 2 weeks and then once a week until the level has fallen < 4 mIU/ml. Intervention is required if peritoneal signs or hemodynamic instability was noted.

Success

In properly selected patients the chance of spontaneous resolution is 70-80 percent.

CHEMOTHERAPY

Methotrexate a competitive inhibitor of folinic acid is effective in the management of ectopic pregnancy in selected patients.[9]

Inclusion Criteria for Chemotherapy

a. Desire for future fertility
b. Sac size < 3 cm
c. Peak hCG values < 15,000 mIU/ml
d. No active bleeding, unruptured ectopic
e. No cardiac activity on USG
f. Selected cases of cervical or cornual pregnancy.

Contraindications

- Poor patient compliance
- Active hepatic or renal disease
- Active peptic ulcer disease
- Blood leukocyte < 3000/cumm
  Or
- Platelet < 1,00000/cumm.

Success Rate

The success rate of single dose regime is 85 percent:

The success rate of variable dose regimen is 93 percent.

The chance of subsequent intrauterine pregnancy is 60 percent.

The chance of subsequent ectopic pregnancy is 7-8 percent.

Direct Injection

Cytotoxic drugs can be injected in to the ectopic sac by laparoscopy or by TVS guided injection.

Drugs used

- Prostaglandin F2 – 85 percent success rate.[10]
- Methotrexate
- Potassium chloride.

Method	*Follow-up*
Single dose regimen Methotrexate 50 mg/M2, 1M	• Beta-hCG on day 4 and 7 • If difference is > 15 percent repeat beta-hCG until < 15 mIU/ml • If difference is < 15 percent repeat the dose of MTX • Surgical treatment – if Beta-hCG does not decrease
Variable dose regimen	*Follow-up*
Methotrexate 1mg/kg IM on days 1, 3, 5, 7 Leucovorin 0.1mg/kg IM on days 2, 4, 6, 8	Continue alternate day injections till Beta-hCG levels decrease > 15 percent in 48 hours Repeat beta-hCG levels weekly until < 5 mIU/ml

SURGICAL MANAGEMENT

Laparotomy or Laparoscopy

Now it is established that laparoscopy is the gold standard in the surgical management of ectopic pregnancy. With adequate practice and surgical experience in operative laparoscopy, ectopics can be treated successfully by laparoscopy regardless of the gestation's size or location or tubal rupture.[11]

The advantages of laparoscopic surgery over laparotomy are:

- Improved fertility due to decrease adhesion formation
- Shorter recovery period
- Less postoperative pain and all the benefits of minimally invasive surgery.

Laparoscopic surgery is contraindicated in the following situations, where laparotomy is a preferred approach.

- Hemodynamically unstable patient
- Massive hemoperitoneum
- Gynecologists not trained in laparoscopic surgery.

LAPAROSCOPIC APPROACH

At laparoscopy the location, the size and the nature of the tubal pregnancy are ascertained. Ruptured tubal pregnancies can be treated laparoscopically if the bleeding has stopped or can be arrested adequately (Figure 18.2). Once the bleeding is controlled the products of conception and blood clots are removed.

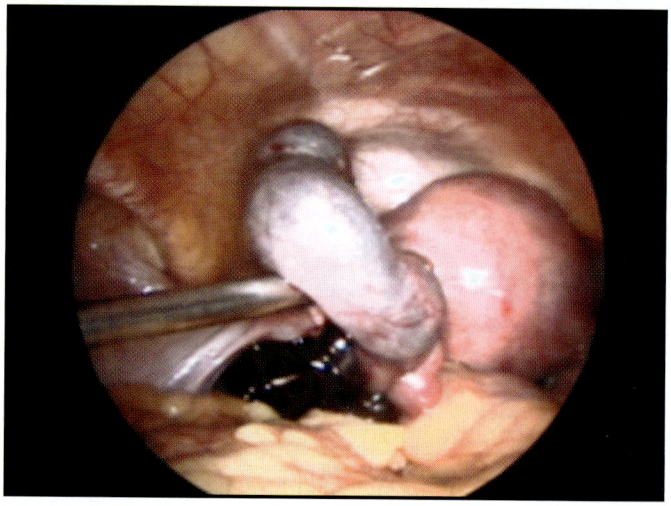

Figure 18.1. Left ampullary ectopic pregnancy

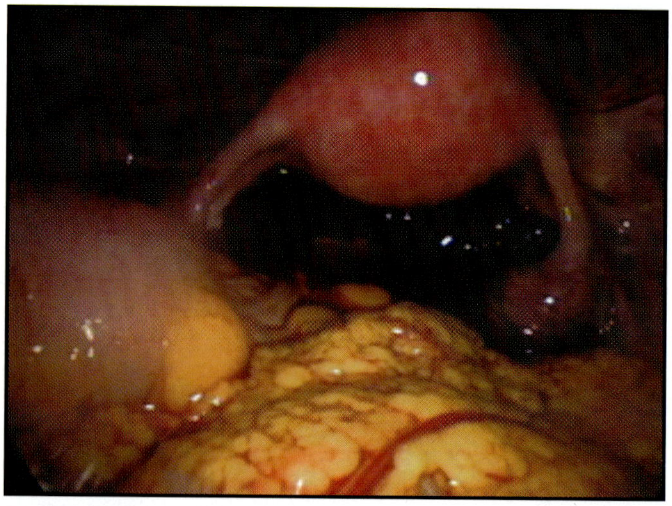

Figure 18.2. A laparoscopic view of ruptured ectopic pregnancy

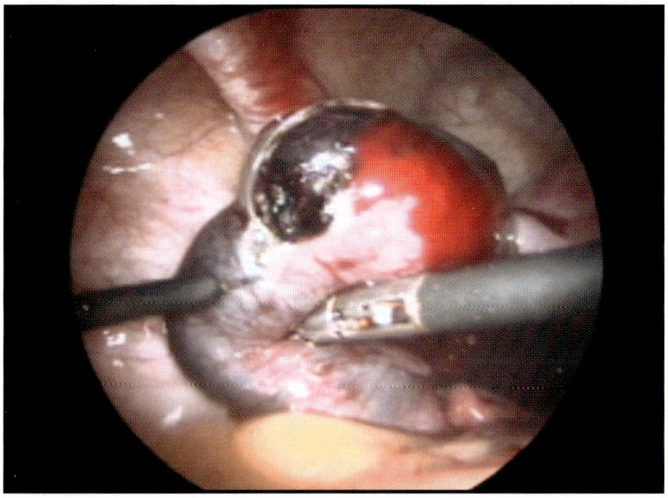

Figure 18.3. Salpingostomy for ampullary ectopic

SALPINGOSTOMY (FIGURE 18.3)

For unruptured tubal pregnancies the tube is indentified and mobilized. To minimize bleeding 5-10 ml of diluted Pitressin is injected in the mesosalpinx just below the ectopic pregnancy. Using monopolar microelectrode a linear incision is made on the antimesenteric surface. The pregnancy usually protrudes through the incision, it may be teased gently out using hydrodissection or with atraumatic grasper. As pregnancy extrudes from the tube some of the products of conception can adhere to the implantation site, using bipolar forceps the structure should be coagulated before removing the tissue. Oozing from the tube is common but usually stops spontaneously or with pressure. The incision is left unsutured to heal by secondary intention. The risk of subsequent ectopic pregnancy is slightly higher than the methotrexate group, around 10 percent. The chance of subsequent intrauterine pregnancy is 60 percent.

SEGMENTAL RESECTION

Segmental resection is done for ruptured tube or isthmic pregnancy, because the lumen of the isthmus is relatively small and gestational tissue is often completely or partially extraluminal.[12]

SALPINGECTOMY

Salpingectomy can be done if the patient has completed the family, ruptured ectopic, ectopic in badly damaged tube or when the contralateral tube is healthy.

Laparoscopic salpingectomy is a simple technique which is done by progressively coagulating and cutting the mesosalpinx beginning with proximal isthmic portion progressing to the fimbrial end of the tube.

REPRODUCTIVE OUTCOMES

In patients treated with methotrexate 82 percent of the patients revealed patency in the involved tube and those attempting pregnancy, 79.6 percent conceived with 87 percent intrauterine and 13 percent repeat ectopics.[13] Following linear salpingostomy by laparoscopy 62 percent conceived with 16 percent repeat ectopics.[14]

CONCLUSION

Ectopic pregnancy is a persistent and challenging problem. Methods of treatment continue to evolve, as of now chemotherapy and laparoscopy are the first line of treatment with preservation of fertility where ever applicable.

REFERENCES

1. Leach Residence, Ory SJ. Modern management of ectopic pregnancy. J Reprod Med 1989;34:324.
2. Kadar N, Devore G , Remoero R. Discriminatory hCG Zone: Its use in the sonographic evaluation for ectopic pregnancy. Obstet Gynaecol 1981;58:156.
3. Kadar N, Caldwell BV, Romero R. A method of screening for ectopic pregnancy and its indications. Obstet Gynaecol 1981;58:162.
4. Romero R, et al. diagnosis of ectopic pregnancy: Value of discriminatory hCG zone. Obstet Gynecol 1985;66:357.
5. Samuelson S, Sjovall A. A laparoscopy in suspected ectopic pregnancy. Acta Obstet Gynecol Scand 1972;51:31.
6. Gurgan T, Yarali H, Urman B. Diagnosis of early tubal pregnancy by salpingoscopy. J Am Assoc Gynaecol Laparososc 1995;2:217.
7. Leach Residence, Ory SJ. Modern management of ectopic pregnancy. J Reprod Med 1989;34:324.

8. Gomel V. For tubal preg, surgical treatment is usually best. Clin Obstet Gynaecol 1995;38:353.
9. Schafer D, et al. Trophoblast tissue culture of human intrauterine and ectopic pregnancies and treatment with methotrexate. Human Reprod 1992;7:311.
10. Paulsson G, et al. Laparoscopic Prostaglandin injection in ectopic pregnancy. Fertile Steril 1995;63:473.
11. Nezhat C, Nezhat F. Conservative management of Ectopic gestation. Fertil Steril 1990;53:382.
12. Senterman M , Jibldh R, Tulandi T. Histopathologic Study of Ampullary and Isthmic tubal ectopic pregnancy. Am J Obstet Gynaecol 1988;159:939.
13. Stovall TG, Ling FW. Single dose methotrexate and expanded clinical trial. Am J obstet Gynecol 1993;168: 1759.
14. Decherney AH, Diamond MP. Laparoscopic Salpingostomy for Ectopic Pregnancy. Obstet Gynecol 1987;70:948.

19 Hysteroscopic Cannulation for Proximal Tubal Block

Sulbha Arora, Gautam N Allahbadia

INTRODUCTION

Tubal disease accounts for 25-35 percent of infertility in women, and salpingitis is believed to account for >50 percent of these cases.[1] Proximal blockage of the fallopian tube occurs in 10-25 percent of women with tubal disease and is mainly due to salpingitis isthmica nodosa (SIN), chronic salpingitis, intratubal endometriosis, amorphous material (e.g. mucus plugs), or spasm.

In 1954, Rubin discussed the difference between tubal obstruction and occlusion. Obstruction is a time-limited process that may be reversible, such as tubal spasm or plugging by amorphous material, and occlusion is organic pathology that is permanent, such as SIN.[2]

HISTORICAL REVIEW

Obstruction of the proximal tube has been a well-recognized entity in gynecology since the early 1800s. WT Smith reported the first transcervical tubal cannulation in 1849.

By means of a hollow silver tube... the point of the instrument was conveyed to the corner of the uterus and made to pass into the tube.

— W Tyler Smith, 1848

The procedure was done blindly, using a whalebone bougie to open a proximally occluded fallopian tube.[3] It relied on tactile feedback as the bougie was advanced through the cervix and uterus. The procedure was described as 'a new uterine operation' and, ironically, is an early, rudimentary form of selective salpingography and transcervical cannulation.[4] He does not say whether the patient became pregnant. Though not widely used, its importance was in the concept of mechanical dilatation of proximally obstructed tubes. In 1896, Watkins performed the first tubal implantation in a patient with a myoma blocking the uterotubal junction. After the procedure, a pregnancy was reported, but resulted in a miscarriage.[5] In 1921, a case report described a uterotubal implantation that resulted in the first living child after this procedure.[6] However, success after surgical repair remained uniformly poor, prompting investigations to bypass the tube entirely. With this in mind, Estes described a procedure for direct approximation of the ovary into a uterine window (Estes' operation). It was abandoned because of poor outcomes. A similar procedure involved placement of the ovary into the uterine cavity (Tuffier's procedure) and had similar poor results.[7]

Despite poor outcomes and pregnancy rates ranging from 0 to 30 percent, the lack of alternative therapies prompted a continued interest in tubal implantation procedures through the 1940s.[8] Mohri et al attempted transcervical passage of a fiberoptic endoscope, called a 'tubaloscope', hoping to view the ovum in the fallopian tube. Insertion into the tubal ostium was 'not easy', and intratubal mucosal bleeding was described.[9] Interest in the transcervical approach to access the tube continued, primarily for developing a transcervical sterilization technique.[10] In 1961, van Ikle described an isthmic implantation into a small cornual aperture.[11] In 1965, Ehrler found that in proximal tubal obstruction the intramural segment is rarely affected and usually patent.[12,13] These findings, along with the concept that as much tube as possible should be preserved, led to the suggestion that tubocornual anastomosis was the optimal procedure.

Advances in microsurgery led to the abandonment of implantation procedures in favor of the less invasive anastomosis. Microsurgical tubocornual anastomosis is technically difficult, but in experienced hands it gives a pregnancy rate of 57 percent and 11 percent ectopic pregnancy rate.[14] But these surgical procedures involve laparotomy resulting in significant patient discomfort and convalescent period. IVF is another alternative for tubal factor infertility, but it is inconvenient to the patient, time consuming and results in 20-25 percent pregnancy rate per attempt. Additional procedures are required for subsequent pregnancies.

The first reported attempt at correcting proximal obstruction by selective salpingography (SS) was performed in 1977 at Hôpital Saint-Antoine in Paris.[15] In 1985, Platia and Krudy reported the first transcervical catheterization (TC) of a proximal tube under fluoroscopic guidance.[16] Transcervical balloon tuboplasty (TBT) was described next by Confino et al in 1986, using a prototype catheter (Cook Co., Bloomington, IN) in a manner similar to balloon angioplasty.[17] Daniel and Miller reported the first term birth after hysteroscopic correction of cornual occlusion in 1987.[18] The patient had bilateral SIN on hysterosalpingography (HSG), and she conceived inspite of perforation at the right cornu. In the same month, Sulak et al[19] published a report of two patients who were treated by hysteroscopic cannulation. Both patients had bilateral proximal blockage documented by HSG and laparoscopy. One became pregnant two months after operation and was delivered at term; the other was lost to follow-up. After the initial case report, larger series began to appear, with six reports[20-25] independently published in 1990 alone.

Transcervical fallopian tube cannulation and selective salpingography for diagnosis and treatment of proximal tubal disease have become well-established tools. Successful cannulations have since been performed with assorted instruments under fluoroscopic, hysteroscopic, falloposcopic, and sonographic guidance. The procedures are clinically effective, minimally invasive, and cost-effective. Furthermore, continued improvements in equipments and methodology improve technique and outcomes. Assisted reproductive technologies have led to the abandonment of microsurgical procedures for PTO after failed canalization or recurrent obstruction. If obstruction persists after a canalization, IVF is the next step.

THE NORMAL FALLOPIAN TUBE

Normal Gross and Histologic Anatomy

The fallopian tubes or oviducts are musculomembranous canals that range from 7 to 14 cm in length.[26] The tubal wall consists of three layers: The internal mucosa (endosalpinx), the intermediate muscular layer (myosalpinx), and the outer serosa, which is continuous with the peritoneum of the broad ligament and uterus, the upper margin of which is the mesosalpinx. The intramural segment ranges from 1.5 to 2.5 cm, with an average luminal diameter of 100 μm. Sweeney described the course of the intramural tube in 100 hysterectomy specimens and found it to be quite variable.[27] A tortuous route to the fundus was seen in 69 percent, a simple straight route in 23 percent, and a curved path in 8 percent. The isthmic segment begins at the uterotubal junction and extends for 2-3 cm, with an average luminal diameter of approximately 500 μm.

Vasen[28] suggested that the intramural tube promotes the passage of fertilized ova toward the uterus, while it also inhibits the uterine contents from entering the abdominal cavity. He described a loop of muscle and vascular rings around the distal intramural tube, which exert a constricting effect on the larger part of the tube. Peristaltic waves are always preceded by a dilation of the tubal lumen, facilitating the passage of gametes through the narrow intramural tube. The thick muscular wall and convoluted intramural course, in addition to the physiologic constrictor mechanism, make the uterotubal junction (UTJ) a likely site for blockage by uterine debris.[29]

Normal Tubal Physiology

Much of tubal physiology is inferred from work done in animals, particularly rabbits.[30-32] Estrogen, progesterone and prostaglandins also are known to modulate tubal function.[33] Estrogen activates α-adrenergic receptors, reducing transisthmic flow in the animal model; hence, stimulation of the outer layers of the UTJ during the phase of estrogen dominance can cause spasm. Paucity of cilia and a narrow lumen at the interstitial segment, as well as this adrenergic contractile mechanism, may predispose to stasis of refluxed material at this site.

PATHOPHYSIOLOGY

Most of the proximal tubal obstructions are thought to be caused by inflammatory processes or endometriosis which leads to local fibrosis. The histology of obstruction is unique in that in 40-60 percent of patients with clinical PTO, the tubal lumen is patent when studied histologically.[34] The presence of a discrete plug of amorphous material resulting in PTO is as high as 75 percent.[35,36] The debris is of unknown etiology and often appears as casts. Such plugs may have no clearly established clinical origin and may be treated by selective salpingography or cannulation. There is also the phenomenon of tubal spasm or pseudo-obstruction. Sulak et al identified amorphous material as causing obstructions in 3 of 6 resected fallopian tube segments. Based on these figures, De Cherney extrapolated guardedly that nonfilling may be due to obstruction in half of all patients and to tubal occlusion in the other half.[37] In another study, in 7 out of 18 cases, the surgically resected segment of the occluded tube showed an organic pathology. In the rest of the cases the tubes appeared normal or with moderate fibrosis or inflammation. So a surgical correction is not warranted in majority of proximal tubal blocks since there is no true block. This is the basis for tubal cannulation.

CLINICAL CORRELATES

PTO is a silent process with no overt clinical manifestations. The abnormalities come to clinical attention only in the evaluation for infertility. Two classification systems of PTO have been proposed, both intended to assist the clinician and the patient in deciding upon the appropriate therapy (cannulation or IVF). The first is based on the appearance of the tubal isthmus and isthmic-cornual junction. This system is based on results of falloposcopy and laparoscopy and classifies PTO into three categories. Category 1 is non-nodular or complete fibrotic occlusion resulting from an inflammatory process; category 2 is nodular obstruction such as that which results from salpingitis isthmica nodosa or endometriosis; and category 3 is tubal obstruction resulting from polyps or amorphous debris within the tubal lumen. These classifications enable the categorization of proximal tubal obstruction into entities that are best managed by tubal cannulation or IVF (category 1); are amenable to medical management using GnRH analogs (category 2); or tubal cannulation and catheterization (category 3).

The second system is based on the anatomic site of obstruction, whether intraluminal, intramural, or extramural. Intraluminal obstruction is secondary to debris, polyps, amorphous plugs, or parasitic infections. Intramural obstruction includes abnormalities in the mucosa, muscularis, and serosa, such as muscular spasm, fibrosis, salpingitis isthmica nodosa, endometriosis, and congenital atresia. Extramural abnormalities include leiomyomas, intrauterine synechiae, and osteal polyps that block the opening of the proximal tube into the uterus. This classification system also provides a means of differentiating those patients who would benefit from cannulation or IVF. Neither system has been evaluated regarding its predictive power nor been formally adopted. Entities such as mucosal agglutination, amorphous debris, or muscle spasm are most likely to respond to cannulation. Chronic salpingitis, SIN, and endometriosis are less likely to respond. Luminal fibrosis, leiomyomas, or any occlusion secondary infectious processes rarely responds to cannulation techniques.

Bipolar obstruction involves blockage at both proximal and distal tubal segments. In such cases, referral for IVF should be made. Combination of tubal catheterization for proximal obstruction and microsurgery for distal obstruction has poor results.

DIAGNOSIS OF PROXIMAL TUBAL BLOCKAGE

The most common method of diagnosis of PTO is HSG. Proximal tubal blockage, suggested by failure of contrast medium to enter the intramural or isthmic portion of either tube, is diagnosed in 10-20 percent of HSGs performed for infertility.[38,39] One shortcoming of HSG is that it does not reliably differentiate potential spasm from obstruction or occlusion. Excessive injection pressure may lead to the occurrence of iatrogenically introduced corneal spasm, and to a false positive. The false positive rate for PTO on HSG is as high as 25 percent. Characteristic findings are seen only in SIN, where a stippled or honeycomb appearance on HSG indicates retained contrast medium in small diverticular projections. Confirmation of proximal tubal blockage requires a second HSG, selective salpingography or chromopertubation by laparoscopy. Repeated examination with prostaglandin antagonists such as aspirin and β_2 agonists such as isoxsuprine and terbutaline in addition to spasmolytic agents such as diazepam, glucagon, amylnitrate and morphine has been suggested,[40,41] but their efficacy has not been established.[42]

TUBAL CANNULATION

A variety of terms have been used for techniques of probing the proximal tubal segment, including cannulation, recannulation, catheterization, and cannulization. These terms are similar in their clinical implications and imply the passage of a catheter, guide wire, or balloon apparatus into the proximal segment under fluoroscopic, ultrasound, or hysteroscopic control to diagnose PTO and establish proximal patency.

Tubal recanalization by hysteroscopic control offers a number of advantages over other techniques. First the guidance of the tubal catheter into the tubal ostia is simple because it is done under direct vision. Second, since it is done along with a laparoscopy the presence of distal tubal disease can be diagnosed and treated simultaneously. So it offers a one-step evaluation and treatment in infertile patients with proximal obstruction.

HYSTEROSCOPIC CANNULATION

Hysteroscopic cannulation is a relatively simple technique. Different custom made catheter systems are available. Essentially it consists of a flexible guide wire to negotiate the intramural portion of the tube and a cannula to direct it towards the tubal ostia. A flexible or rigid hysteroscope can be used. Hysteroscopic cannulation is done under GA if a simultaneous laparoscopy is performed.

TECHNIQUE

The technique of cannulation of the proximal tubal segment with a variety of wires, catheters, and balloons is effective therapy for PTO.[43-50] The largest series involved fluoroscopically guided tubal cannulation, but several series describe hysteroscopic and ultrasound guidance.[51] There are no data to suggest that the use of a balloon is more advantageous than a wire.[52,53]

We use a 21 Fr rigid hysteroscope with a 7 Fr operating channel. Guide wire is Terumo guide wire (Radifocus guide wire M diameter 0.89 mm) and cannula is a 7Fr outflow catheter. Hysteroscopy is performed and the ostia identified. The 7 Fr outflow catheter is now introduced through the operating channel and aligned towards the ostia (Figures 19.1 and 19.2). Terumo guide wire is then introduced through the outflow catheter.

The hysteroscope and outflow catheter are positioned in such a way that, if the guide wire is pushed it should enter the ostia (Figure 19.3). The flexibility of the guide wire is altered by varying the length of the guide wire protruding from the outer catheter.

The guide wire is now pushed into the ostia for 2-3 cm, always keeping the outflow catheters almost in a straight line for easy sliding. If difficulty is encountered, laparoscopic control may be used. It is not necessary to cannulate the ampullary portion of tube because it can damage the delicate mucosa. The procedure is repeated on the other side. The hysteroscope is withdrawn and

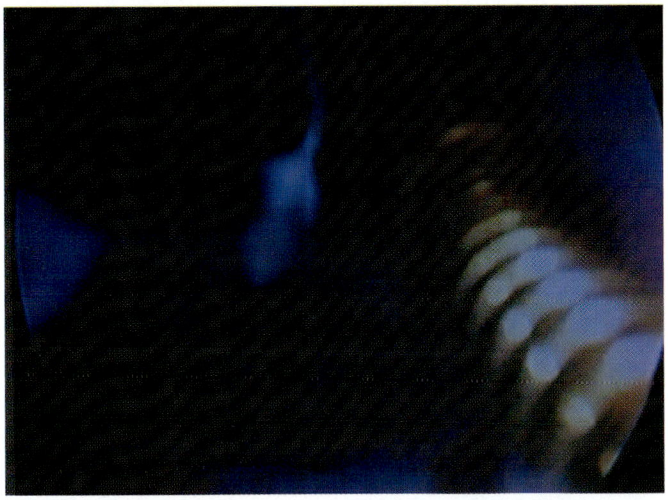

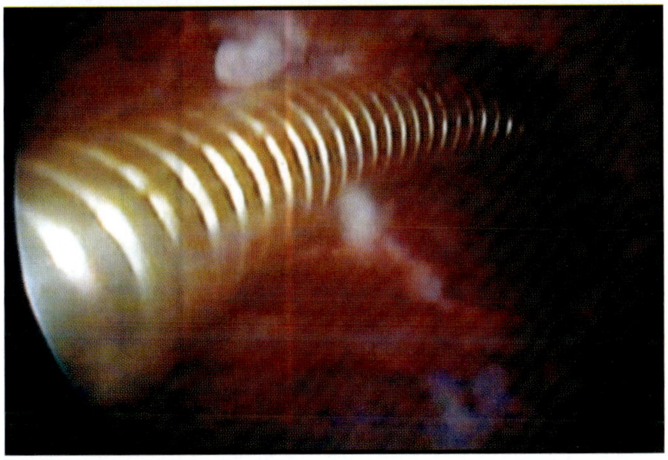

Figures 19.1 and 19.2. Hysteroscopic view of the flexible guide cannula being moved towards the internal tubal ostium. Note the bulbous atraumatic head of the cannula

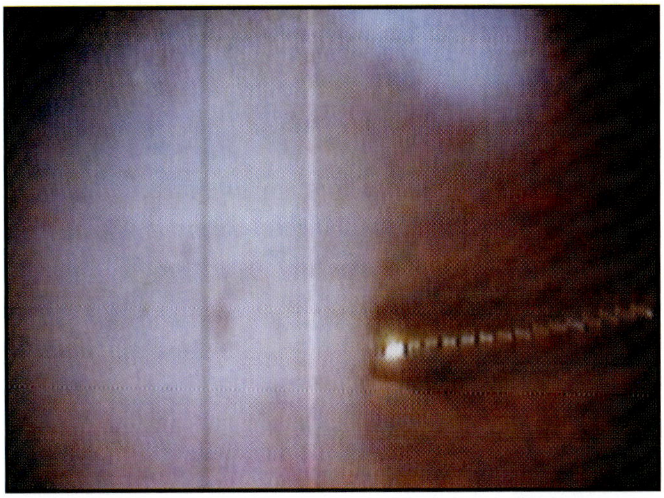

Figure 19.3. Hysteroscopic view of the flexible guide cannula lodged securely into the internal tubal ostium

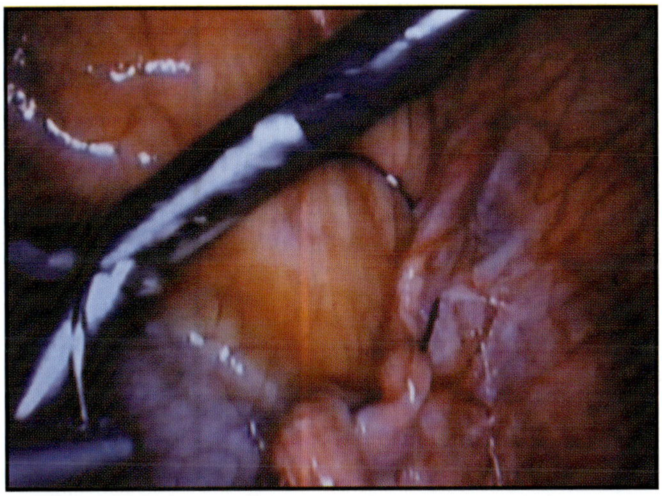

Figure 19.4. Laparoscopic view of the exit of the 0.018 inch hydrophilic guide wire through the fimbrial end of the fallopian tube

chromopertubation done and observed through the laparoscope to confirm the result of cannulation (Figure 19.4).

Another catheter system available is Novy set which includes an external catheter with a memory, a 3 Fr catheter to cannulate the orifice and a guide wire to catheterize the fallopian tube. Angioplasty catheter can also be used for cannulation. The balloon can be distended to give a long lasting mechanical dilatation.

We had reported our initial experience of hysteroscopic cannulation in 17 cases (34 tubes) of proximal tubal obstruction.[54] Cannulation could be attempted in 30 tubal ostia and was successfully accomplished in 15 cases. The instances in which we could not cannulate the tubal ostia (2 patients) were not failures of cannulation but failures to visualize the internal tubal ostia because of thick endometrium. Four of our patients conceived following this procedure and delivered at term.

COMPLICATIONS AND CONTRAINDICATIONS

Complications occur in 6 percent of cases.[55] Perforation is the most frequent and requires no intervention. Use of appropriate flexible catheter may decrease the risk of perforation. When perforation occurs, it is left to heal spontaneously. Febrile morbidity and gram-negative sepsis have been described, but are rare. Cannulation should not be performed in the presence of known pelvic infection. All patients should be given prophylactic antibiotics (100 mg Doxycycline twice a day) on the day before, on the day of, and the day after the procedure. The procedure should not be attempted in patients with known distal tubal disease as it increases the chances of developing an ectopic pregnancy.

CONCLUSION

Proximal tubal block is a common infertility problem and needs confirmation by a repeat HSG or laparoscopy. The diagnosis and management of PTO has undergone considerable change in the recent years. Considering the simplicity of the procedure, hysteroscopic cannulation should be tried as the first procedure for proximal tubal block. If the procedure is not successful, or a pregnancy is not achieved, IVF is recommended. Laparotomy and microsurgical anastomosis is indicated in few cases where other simpler methods fail, where IVF is not an acceptable option on religious grounds; and technical expertise is available.

REFERENCES

1. Musich J, Behrman S. Surgical management of tubal obstruction at the uterotubal junction. Fertil Steril 1983;40:423-40.
2. Honore GM, Holden AE, Schenken RS. Pathophysiology and management of proximal tubal blockage. Fertil Steril 1999;72:950-1.
3. Smith TW. New method of treating sterility by the removal of obstructions of the fallopian tube. Lancet 1849;1:603.
4. Letterie GS. Proximal tubal obstruction. In: Taylor and Francis, Surgery, Assisted Reproductive Technology and Infertility, 2005;351-73.
5. Greenhill JP. Evaluation of salpingostomy and tubal implantation for treatment of sterility. Am J Obstet Gynecol 1937;2:39-51.
6. Shaw R. Uterotubal implantation. Bull Johns Hopkins Hospital1921;32:305-7.
7. Sovak FW. Operations for the correction of sterility. In: Davis CH, (Ed): Gynecology and obstetrics. Hagarstown, MD: WF Prior, 1946.
8. Kistner RW, Patton GW. Surgery of the oviduct. In: An Atlas of Infertility Surgery. Boston: Little, Brown, 1975;145.
9. Mohri T, Mohri C, Yamadori F. Tubaloscope: Flexible glassfiber endoscope for intratubal observation. Endoscopy 1970;4:226-30.
10. Flood JT, Grow DR. Transcervical tubal cannulation: A review. Obstet Gynecol Surv 1993;48:768-76.
11. Ikle FA. Pregnancy after implantation of the ovary into the uterus. Gynaecologia 1961;151:95-9.
12. Ehrler P. Anastomose intramurale de la trumpe. Bol Federal Soc Gynaecol Br Empr 1965;17:866-72.
13. Green-Armitage VB. Tubo-utero implantation. J Obstet Gynaecol Br Empr1957;64:47-50.
14. Dubuisson JB, Chapron C, Ansquer Y. Proximal tubal occlusion: Is there an alternative to microsurgery? Human Reprod 1997;12:692-8.
15. Rouanet JP, Chalut J. An application of selective catheterization: Salpingography. Preliminary note [letter]. Nouv Prés Med 1977;6:2785.
16. Platia MP, Krudy AG. Transvaginal fluoroscopic recanalization of a proximally occluded oviduct. Fertil Steril 1985;44:704-6.
17. Confino E, Friberg J, Gleicher N. Transcervical balloon tuboplasty. Fertil Steril 1986;46:963-6.
18. Daniell J, Miller W. Hysteroscopic correction of cornual occlusion with resultant term pregnancy. Fertil Steril 1987;48:490-2.
19. Sulak PJ, Letterie GS, Hayslip CC, Coddington CC, Klein TA. Hysteroscopic cannulation and lavage in the treatment of proximal tubal occlusion. Fertil Steril 1987;48:493-4.
20. Confino E, Tur-Kaspa I, DeCherney A, Corfman R, Coulam C, Robinson E, et al. Transcervical balloon tuboplasty. A multicenter study. J Am Med Assoc. 1990;264:2079-82.
21. Kumpe DA, Zwerdlinger SC, Rothbarth LJ, Durham JD, Albrecht BH. Proximal fallopian tube occlusion: Diagnosis and treatment with transcervical fallopian tube catheterization. Radiology 1990;177:183-7.
22. LaBerge JN, Ponec DJ, Gordon RL. Fallopian tube catheterization: Modified fluoroscopic technique. Radiology 1990;176:283-4.
23. Thurmond AS, Rosch J. Nonsurgical fallopian tube recanalization for treatment of infertility. Radiology 1990;174:371-4.
24. Lang EK, Dunaway HEJ, Roniger WE. Selective ostial salpingography and transvaginal catheter dilatation in

the diagnosis and treatment of fallopian tube obstruction. Am J Roentgenol 1990;154:735-40.

25. Segars J, Herbert CM, Moore DE, Hill GA, Wentz AC, Winfield AC. Selective fallopian tube cannulation: Initial experience in an infertile population. Fertil Steril 1990;53:357-9.
26. Chiari H. Zur pathologischen anatomie des eileitercatarrhs. Z Heilkunde 1887;8:457-73.
27. Sweeney W. The interstitial portion of the uterine tube—its gross anatomy, course, and length. Obstet Gynecol 1962;19:3-8.
28. Vasen L. The intramural part of the fallopian tube. Int J Fertil 1959;4:309-14.
29. Herschlag A, Diamond MP, DeCherney AH. Tubal physiology: An appraisal. Gynecol Surg 1989;5:3-25.
30. Strom C, Edin R, Dahlstrom A, Ahlman H. *In vivo* studies of the motility of the isthmic segment in the perfused rabbit oviduct. Acta Physiol Scand 1981;113:491-8.
31. Strom C, Dahlstrom A, Lindblom B, Ahlman H. Adrenoceptor modulated flow through the rabbit ampulloisthmic region studied *in vivo* and *in vitro*. J Neural Transm 1986;66:209-19.
32. Spilman G, Harper M. Comparison of the effects of adrenergic drugs and prostaglandins on rabbit oviduct motility. Biol Reprod 1974;10:549-54.
33. Elder M, Myatt L, Chandhun G. The role of prostaglandins in the spontaneous motility of the fallopian tube. Fertil Steril 1977;28:86-90.
34. Sulak PJ, Letterie GS, Coddington CC, et al. Histology of proximal tubal obstruction. Fertil Steril 1987;48:437-40.
35. Capitanio GL, Ferraiolo A, Croce S, et al. Transcervical selective salpingography: A diagnostic and therapeutic approach to cases of proximal tubal injection failure. Fertil Steril 1991;55:1045-50.
36. Tur-Kaspa I. Pathophysiology of the fallopian tube. In: Gleicher N (Ed). Tubal catheterization. New York: Wiley-Liss, 1992.
37. DeCherney AH. Anything you can do I can do better—or differently! Fertil Steril 1987;48:374-6.
38. Winfield AC, Pittaway D, Maxson W, Daniell J, Wentz AC. Apparent corneal occlusion in hysterosalpingography: reversal by glucagon. Am J Roentgenol 1982;139:525-7.
39. Haney AF, Hammond MG. Infertility in women exposed to diethylstilbestrol *in utero*. J Reprod Med 1983;28:851-6.
40. World Health Organization. A new hysterographic approach to the evaluation of tubal spasm and spasmolytic agents. Fertil Steril 1983;39:105-7.
41. Thurmond AS, Novy M, Rosch J. Terbutaline in diagnosis of interstitial fallopian tube obstruction. Invest Radiol 1988;23:209-10.
42. Cooper JM, Rigberg HS, Houck R, Aiken M. Incidence, significance, and remission of tubal spasm during attempted hysteroscopic tubal sterilization. J Reprod Med 1985;30:39-42.
43. Lang EK, Dunaway HE Jr, Roniger WE. Selective osteal salpingography and transvaginal catheter dilatation in the diagnosis and treatment of fallopian tube obstruction. Am J Roentgenol 1990;154:735-40.
44. Rosch J, Thurmond AS, Uchida BT, Sovak M. Selective transcervical fallopian tube catheterization: Technique update. Radiology 1988;168:1-5.
45. Ataya K, Thomas M. New technique for selective transcervical osteal salpingography and catheterization in the diagnosis and treatment of proximal tubal obstruction. Fertil Steril 1991;56:980-3.
46. Hurd WW, Randolph JF Jr, Smith YR, et al. Transcervical tubal cannulation: A comparison of two techniques. Fertil Steril 1992;58:1068-70.
47. Hovsepian DM, Bonn J, Eschelman DJ, et al. Fallopian tube recanalization in an unrestricted population. Radiology 1994;190:137-40.
48. Nakamura K, Ishiguchi T, Maekoshi H, et al. Selective fallopian tube catheterization in female infertility: Clinical results and absorbed radiation dose. Eur Radiol1996;6:465-9.
49. Hepp H, Korell M, Strowitzki T. Proximal tubal obstruction– is there a best way to treat it? Hum Reprod 1996;11:1828-31.
50. Hayashi M, Hoshimoto K, Ohkura T. Successful conception following fallopian tube recanalization in infertile patients with a unilateral proximally occluded tube and a contralateral patent tube. Hum Reprod 2003;18:96-9.
51. Bloechle M, Schreiner T, Gouma E, Lisse K. Comparison between hysterosalpingo-contrast sonography and sonographically controlled selective tubal catheterization. Hum Reprod 1996;11:1423-6.
52. Gleicher N, Redding L, Parrilli M, et al. Wire guide cannulation alone is no treatment of proximal tubal occlusion. Hum Reprod 1994;9:1109-11.
53. Gazzera C, Gallo T, Faissola B, Zanon E. Tubal catheterization and selective salpingography. Rays 1998;23:735-41.
54. Allahbadia GN, Mangeshikar P, Pai Dhungat PB, Desai SK, Gudi AA, Arya A. Hysteroscopic fallopian tube recanalization using a flexible guide cannula and hydrophilic guide wire. Gynaecological Endoscopy 2000;9:31-5.
55. Lang EK, Dunaway HH. Recanalization of obstructed fallopian tube by selective salpingography and transvaginal bougie dilatation: Outcome and cost analysis. Fertil Steril 1996;66:205-9.

20 Falloposcopy and Salpingoscopy in Tubal Evaluation for Infertility

Sunita R Tandulwadkar

INTRODUCTION

The importance of tubal obstruction as a major cause of infertility was recognized by Burns in 1809.[1] Since that time a number of methods of demonstrating tubal blockage have been described,[2] like transcervical insufflation with gas, hysterosalpingography, hydrotubation with dye controlled by laparoscopy, etc. In the investigation of tubal infertility, the goal must be to test the function of the fallopian tubes rather than to demonstrate their patency as patency of the distal tube does not necessarily equate with normality of the mucosa. Conventional methods used in tubal assessment provide only indirect information about tubal patency and do not evaluate tubal mucosal status and there may be discrepancies between the findings at hysterosalpingography, laparoscopy and intra-luminal endoscopy in the presence of peritubal adhesions or endometriosis.[3] Pathological lesions may be missed if more accurate methods of tubal assessment are not employed.

Though hysterosalpingography should be the initial test of tubal function in the investigation of infertility, if investigation is limited to hysterosalpingography alone, proximal tubal obstruction may be over diagnosed and consequently over treated.[4,5]

Tubal endoscopy enables a more specific assessment of the tubal mucosa, further refining the prediction of successful tubal function.[6-8]

The first attempts at transvaginal endoscopic examination of the fallopian tube were made by Mohri in Japan in 1970.[9] Technical limitations and the thickness of the endoscope (2.4 mm) prevented cannulation beyond 3 cm in most of his cases.

Falloposcopy using the coaxial technique was first described by Kerin et al.[10] Subsequently, Bauer et al[11] developed a falloposcopic method that uses the linear eversion technique.

INDICATIONS FOR TUBAL ENDOSCOPY

Proximal Tubal Disease

Falloposcopy may be used in the investigation of the status of the proximal tubal segment. It is usually performed as an out-patient procedure avoiding the need for anesthesia. In patients in whom hysterosalpingography suggests the presence of obstructive or non-obstructive proximal tubal disease falloposcopy may accurately define the site and nature of the lesion.

In addition to its value in assessing the proximal tubal segment it also has a potential for effecting recanalization and tuboplasty in cases of proximal tubal obstruction.

In untreated proximal tubal obstruction, trans-abdominal salpingoscopy is the only technique which allows examination of the distal tubal segment prior to reconstructive tubal surgery. Lesions of the ampullary mucosa have been seen in 50 percent of cases of proximal tubal obstruction and restoration of patency in these cases results in a 60 percent pregnancy rate.[12]

Pelvic Inflammatory Disease (PID) Affecting the Distal Tubal Segments

In cases of suspected PID the mucosa of the distal segments may also be assessed by falloposcopy but salpingoscopy allows better visualization and also allows assessment of the peritubal structures.

Pelvic inflammatory disease is frequently associated with lesions in the ampullary tubal mucosa. Peritubal and periovarian adhesive disease cause distal tubal blockage. The damage to the tubal mucosa may be a secondary feature.[13] While the presence of peritubal adhesive disease may suggest intratubal damage, the correlation between the external and internal appearances of the tube is poor. Mild adhesive disease may be associated with severe mucosal damage and there may be marked differences between the degree of involvement of the two tubes.[14] The degree of damage to the tubal mucosa may be used to predict the possibility of intrauterine or ectopic pregnancy. It is therefore essential to examine the full length of both tubes to ascertain the degree of mucosal damage.

Endometriosis

Endometriosis may be associated with adhesive disease and the tube is frequently involved in severe endometriosis. The tubal obstruction is more often caused by compression or stricture than by mucosal adhesions. Salpingoscopy in endometriosis usually reveals a normal mucosal architecture.

Ectopic Pregnancy

The prevalence of recurrence of ectopic pregnancy after conservative surgery depends on the underlying disease rather than the operative technique. Tubal endoscopy is recommended in the investigation of patients with a history of a previous ectopic pregnancy.

Unexplained Infertility

Tubal mucosal lesions may be detected in patients whose fallopian tubes appear normal and patent at laparoscopy or hysterosalpingography.

Prior to Assisted Fertilization

Tubal endoscopy may be used to confirm tubal normality in cases where intrauterine insemination, gamete or early embryo transfer to the tube are being considered.

Techniques of Intraluminal Tubal Endoscopy

Intraluminal tubal endoscopy may be performed by transvaginal (falloposcopy) or transabdominal (salpingoscopy) approach.

FALLOPOSCOPY

Falloposcopy using the coaxial technique was first described by Kerin et al.[10] Subsequently, Bauer et al[11] developed a falloposcopic method that uses the linear eversion technique.

Patient Preparation

The optimal time for performing falloposcopy is during immediate post-menstrual phase of the menstrual cycle because the ostium can be visualized most easily in the absence of blood and a thick endometrial lining.[10] While previously antibiotic prophylaxis was given, the majority of recent studies report not using antibiotics and not encountering infection after falloposcopy.[15,16] Various kinds of anesthesia for falloposcopy have been described in the literature. Initially, general anesthesia was used when suspected abnormal tubes were examined by falloposcopy, especially if concurrent laparoscopy was performed.[16,17] Office falloposcopy, however, is gaining greater acceptance like office hysteroscopy, though adequate explanation and counseling to patient before office falloposcopy is needed.

Falloposcope

Modern technological advances have enabled the development by Kerin in 1989-1990 of endoscopes with greatly improved optical properties and yet outer diameters of as little as 0.5 mm.[10,18]

The falloposcope is a flexible high resolution micro-endoscope of 0.5 mm diameter and 1.73 m length that contains a bundle of 2000 optical fibers and eight to twelve illuminating fibers. The falloposcope is capable of magnifying up to fifty times.

The Coaxial Technique

The coaxial technique of falloposcopy described by Kerin[10,18] required hysteroscopically directed tubal cannulation with a flexible guidewire (of diameter 0.3-0.8 mm) followed by serial passage of a Teflon cannula (of diameter up to 1.3 mm) over the guidewire. The guidewire is then removed and the falloposcope passed down the lumen of the Teflon cannula. Irrigation with Ringer's Lactate solution facilitates movement of the endoscope within the cannula and lifted the tubal mucosa of the lens allowing better vision. The best way to view the tubal lumen is during withdrawal of the endoscope and cannula.

When Kerin et al performed falloposcopy using the coaxial system on 75 patients (112 tubes), there were no intraoperative or postoperative complications related to the falloposcopic procedure.[17] When direct balloon tuboplasty procedure was attempted, there were five instances of partial and one instance of complete tubal perforation. The perforations were all small and without external bleeding, and had only minor endotubal bleeding that resolved spontaneously.[17]

The Linear Everting Catheter System Technique (Figures 20.1A to C)

The linear everting catheter (LEC) system is an alternative to the coaxial system and is gaining greater acceptance. Use of the linear everting catheter system with sedation is now usually regarded as an office procedure that does not need laparoscopy or hysteroscopy. The linear everting catheter consists of inner and outer catheter bodies (of diameters 0.8 mm and 2.8 mm, respectively) that are joined circumferentially at their distal tips by a distensible polyethylene membrane. The pressure within the enclosed space (the balloon space) is controlled by a fluid-filled syringe. The falloposcope is advanced within the inner catheter and the membrane and introduced into the uterus.

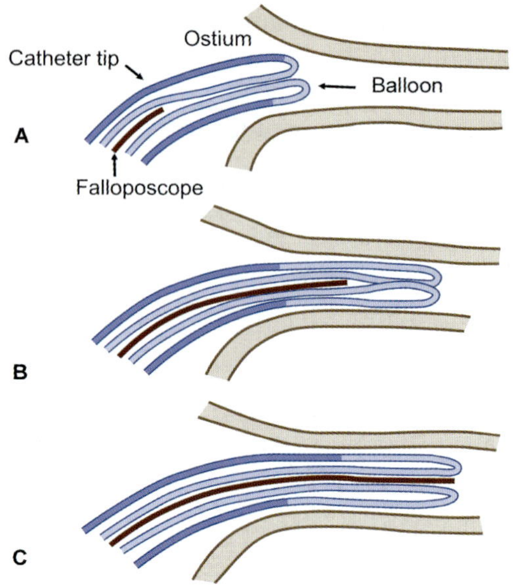

Figures 20.1A to C. Mechanism of eversion with the linear everting catheter system. A. balloon is pressurized; B. inner body is advanced carries falloposcope forward; C. complete eversion: falloposcope reaches tip of balloon

Once the ostium is identified, the outer catheter is held in position and pressure is applied to the membrane by using the fluid-filled syringe; the inner catheter pushed forward, resulting in the linear eversion of the balloon into the fallopian tube.

As the balloon has a double layered wall the endoscope moves forward at twice the speed of the balloon tip. It is crucial to keep the endoscope tip behind the balloon during eversion. Hence, it is important to move forward in a coordinated series of 1-2 cm steps with the endoscope being withdrawn 1-2 cm each time it reaches the balloon tip. This requires a good understanding of the mechanism of hydraulic pressure in the balloon. The pressure in the balloon needs to be raised in order to advance the balloon tip. This "grips" the endoscope preventing movement independent of the balloon and the pressure within the balloon needs to be reduced each time the endoscope is withdrawn. Flushing the lumen with a crystalloid solution assists in the advancement of the endoscope by providing lubrication.

If there is difficulty in everting and advancing the balloon, the balloon tip should be identified visually with the endoscope which is then withdrawn a little and used to support the pressurized balloon thus aiding its advancement. Attempting to force the advancement of the balloon and endoscope may damage the balloon, the endoscope or the wall of the fallopian tube. If performed properly, the technique allows cannulation to a distance of 10 cm. Tubal damage is unlikely because the balloon exerts no shear force on the tubal wall unless the endoscope is allowed to project beyond the balloon during eversion.

Imaging of the endotubal surface is performed in a retrograde manner from fimbrial end to proximal end using the lens-fluid interface.[19,20] As the balloon and endoscope are withdrawn along the tube, the tip of the endoscope is kept approximated to the tip of the balloon. Less pressure is needed within the balloon during withdrawal and so by flushing with a saline solution simultaneously, it is possible to constantly wind forward the endoscope during withdrawal at a rate which keeps the tips of the balloon and endoscope approximated to one another. The flush also lifts the tubal mucosa off the endoscope lens allowing better vision. Imaging can be carried out in this way until the endoscope and balloon re-enter the catheter within the uterine cornu.

The linear everting catheter system confers a few advantages over the coaxial system. Firstly, the eversion balloon is unrolled into the fallopian tube without exerting any shearing force between the balloon and the tubal epithelium. The everting balloon will seek the path of least resistance and negotiate any tubal tortuosity. This process greatly minimizes the risk of tubal injury, which is associated with guide wire cannulation in the coaxial system. Secondly, the falloposcope advances automatically during balloon eversion and can be moved independently to optimize visualization. Thirdly, there is no need for any hysteroscopy or cervical dilatation, and falloposcopy using the linear everting catheter system can be accomplished as an out patient procedure that requires only local anesthesia. Finally, the falloposcope is well protected inside the balloon and is kept coaxially aligned along the tubal lumen.

RESULTS FROM FALLOPOSCOPY

In the classification system, each of the four segments of the fallopian tube (intramural, isthmic, ampulla, and fimbria) are assessed according to the following five parameters: patency (patent, stenosed, or obstructed); epithelium (normal, atrophic, or flat and featureless); vascularity (normal or pale); adhesion (none, thin, or thick); and dilatation (none, minimal, or hydrosalpinx). The scores 1, 2, or 3 assigned to the three options for each parameter reflecting normal findings, mild to moderate abnormalities, and severe abnormalities, respectively. The total scores of each tube are then added; a total score of 20 reflects normality, 21 to 30 means mild to moderate disease, and a total score of >30 signifies severe disease. This score correlates inversely with subsequent pregnancy rate. This method of scoring the tubal status is based on methods of assessment which are considered as having prognostic significance in the treatment of distal tubal disease by a number of authors (Table 20.1).[8,10,21,22]

Kerin et al[17] examined 112 'diseased' tubes in 75 patients. Falloposcopy showed 52 (46%) tubes to be normal, 33 (29%) tubes to have mild to moderate disease, and 27 (24%) tubes to have severe to obstructive disease. Follow-up showed that within one year of the procedure, six (21%) of the 28 women in whom at least one tube was normal had conceived and two (9%) of the 22 who had mild to moderate disease had conceived, while none of the 16 patients with severe endotubal disease had no conception (Table 20.2). Thus, severe tubal disease, as identified by falloposcopy, carries a poor prognosis for pregnancy.[17]

Table 20.1. Falloposcopic classification and localization of tubal lumen disease

	Right tube				Left tube			
Site of disease	Intramural	Isthmic	Ampullary	Fimbrial	Intramural	Isthmic	Ampullary	Fimbrial
PATENCY Patency....1 Stenosis...2 Fibrotic....3 Obstruction								
EPITHELIUM Normal....1 Pale,atropic..2 Flat, featureless..3								
VASCULARITY Normal.........1 Intermediate..2 Poor pallor....3								
ADHESIONS None...........1 Thin, weblike..2 Thick............3								
DILATATION None.............1 Minimal..........2 Hydrosalpinx..3								
OTHER.......2-3								
Cumulative score								
Total score	Right tube:		(Normal=20)		Left tube:		(Normal=20)	

Cumulative score for each tube

20 = Normal tubal lumen

> 20 but < 30-Moderate endotubal disease

> 30 = Severe endotubal disease

Mucus plugs or tubal debris, endotubal polyps, endometriosis, salpingitis isthmica nodosa, inflammatory, infective, neoplastic conditions and absent tubal segments are each assigned a score of 2 to 3 depending on the significance of the lesion

Table 20.2. Relationship of tubal score and subsequent pregnancy rates

Falloposcopy score and 12 months pregnancy rate		
Healthy tube	Score = 20	6/28 (21%)
Mild/moderate disease	Score = 21-30	2/22 (9%)
Severe disease	Score > 30	0/16 (0%)

Pitfalls of Scoring System

Despite its popularity, the classification system has its shortcomings. Firstly, a score cannot be given if the tube cannot be cannulated along its full length. If a patient has a history of tubal surgery and reanastomosis, then part of the tube may be missing and a score cannot be given. Secondly, the transition from one segment of the tube to another can be difficult to distinguish, especially if tubal damage is present. Thus, an individual description of all four segments may not give reproducible findings and scores.

Management of Fallopian Tubal Luminal Disease

If pseudo proximal tubal occlusion by a mucous plug or debris is confirmed, the occlusion can usually be dislodged by passage of the falloposcope or by aqua dissection.

A mild to moderate adhesion or a stenosis may be divided by balloon dilatation techniques.[23]

In the case of dense fibrotic obstruction, either *in vitro* fertilization or tubal resection followed by microsurgical anastomosis should be considered. Tubal surgery is warranted only in patients with mild to moderate tubal disease. Previously, the endosalpinx status could be assessed only during operation. Using falloposcopy, however, a more accurate assessment of the tubal status can be made before subjecting the patient to tubal surgery.

Falloposcopic findings can lead to a change in patient management in more than 60 percent of cases.[15,24,25]

Potential Therapeutic Applications of Falloposcopy

The direct visualization and identification of each segment of the fallopian tube allows the non-incisional transfer of gametes or embryos into the ampulla during assisted reproductive procedures.[26] In selected patients who have tubal occlusion, pregnancies have been achieved after tubal recanalization using falloposcopic tuboplasty.[27] In addition, direct instillation of methotrexate or an alternative medication in tubal pregnancy can be performed.

Complications of Falloposcopy

The duration of falloposcopy depends on the experience and skill of the operator. Six instances of minor tubal perforation among the 122 'diseased tubes' in 75 patients (i.e. a perforation frequency of 4.9% per tube and 8% per patient) have been detected by the coaxial system using guide wire cannulation.[18] No other major complications have been reported. Thus, falloposcopy can be considered a safe and atraumatic procedure, particularly when the linear everting catheter system is used.

SALPINGOSCOPY

Detailed examination of the mucosa of the distal segment of the fallopian tube has an important role in the investigation of infertility. The intact fold structure of the mucosa with its secretary and ciliated cells is essential for normal gamete transport and fertilization. Pathological lesions in the distal tube are associated with infertility and ectopic pregnancy. The mucosa may show changes such as flattening of the folds, deciliation, fine or dense adhesions, fibrosis and occlusion of the lumen. Flattening of the folds and deciliation occurring in thin walled hydrosalpinx may be reversible when tubal patency has been restored. Pregnancy can occur after the flattened mucosal folds and stretched myosalpinx have recovered.

Instruments

In salpingoscopy the rigid salpingoscope is introduced through the operating channel of the laparoscope.[28,29]

The component parts of the salpingoscopy are:

1. A 11 mm operating laparoscope.
2. The salpingoscope sheath which is 5 mm in diameter and has a Luer connector at the proximal end for a saline infusion. The sheath fits into the operating channel of the laparoscope and protrudes 8 cm from the distal end.
3. An obturator with a conical distal end which facilitates introduction of the sheath into the tubal ostium.
4. The salpingoscope which is a 2.8 mm diameter telescope, is 5 cm longer than the sheath and has a 0° distal lens. The salpingoscope may have a variable proximal lens similar to the Hamou microcolpohysteroscope which allows the tubal mucosa to be examined under 60x magnification. The telescope moves freely within its sheath. This allows it to be advanced 5 cm beyond the tip of the sheath to visualize the full length of the ampulla.
5. A 500 ml bag of normal saline and connecting tubing with which to instill fluid through the sheath and distend the tube.
6. Atraumatic tube-holding forceps which are used to align the tube with the salpingoscope and to grasp it over the salpingoscope to form a water-tight seal.

7. The normal accessory equipments for laparoscopy including light source, fibroptic cables and camera , CO_2 insufflator, electrosurgical generator.

Technique

1. Standard diagnostic laparoscopy is performed which should include a full, systematic examination of the upper and lower abdomen and the pelvic organs.5 mm secondary trocar and cannula is inserted to carry ancillary forceps.
2. If there is pelvic adhesive disease, the adhesions should be divided and the adnexa fully mobilized. Salpingoscopy can be easily performed if the distal tube is patent.
3. The instruments are assembled. The salpingoscope sheath with its obturator is inserted into the operating channel of laparoscopic and the saline bag connected. Fluid is run through the system to prime it.
4. The right tube is manipulated until it is aligned with the laparoscope. The fimbrial opening may be found by following the fimbriae ovaricae from the ovary towards the tube. The ostium is close to the anti-mesenteric border. The tip of the laparoscope is now brought close to the tube and the salpingoscope sheath slowly advanced out of the operating channel towards the fimbriae.
5. When the tip of the sheath is seen to enter the fimbrial opening, the atraumatic tube holding forceps are used to gently draw the tube over the sheath. When the sheath is secured in the tube the forceps are closed over the full circumference of the tube and sheath to form a water tight seal. The position of the sheath within the tube can be confirmed by allowing saline to flow into the tube which may be seen to distend. The saline should be stopped again before the next step.
6. The obturator should be withdrawn and the salpingoscope inserted into the sheath. The light cable and camera are transferred from the laparoscope to the salpingoscope and the saline infusion commenced. An image of the distal end of the sheath and the tubal mucosa should appear on the screen.
7. Under direct visual control the salpingoscope is advanced out of its sheath into the tubal infundibulum and along the ampulla. The ampulla normally has one or two bends in its lumen but with care these can be negotiated and the full length of the segment examined as far as the isthmo-ampullary junction.
8. Proximal tubal patency can be confirmed by chromopertubation with dilute methylene blue dye. The dye can be seen to pass along the tube and stain the mucosa.
9. By similar technique left tube is examined. It is usually easier to examine the right tube because the left adnexa are often hidden behind the sigmoid colon.
10. In case of fimbrial block, fimbrioplasty should be performed before proceeding for salpingoscopy.

Findings

Normal Structure

The infundibulum has a concentric structure of folds. In the normal tube the folds are well formed and move freely in the distending fluid. In the ampulla there are 4-6 major folds each about 4 mm in height. Accessory folds arise from their sides giving a complex appearance. On high power examination the accessory folds are seen to be well vascularized but neither the cellular pattern nor the cilia can be visualized. Several minor folds each about 1mm in height lie between the major folds. When the junction of ampulla and isthmus is reached the major folds give way to three or four rounded folds each about 0.2-0.4 mm in height which continue into the isthmic segment.

Tortous Tubes

Occasionally a convoluted or tortuous tube may be seen. The folds are flattened and the tubal wall appears very thin. This abnormality is probably due to herniation of the tubal mucosa through areas where the myosalpinx is deficient. The abnormality may involve part of or the whole ampulla. It may be erroneously interpreted as hydrosalpinx at hysterosalpingography. It is not believed to be a cause of infertility as it is found in parous women.

Accessory Ostia

Occasionally an accessory ostium is seen on the anti-mesenteric border of the tube. Very rarely the accessory ostium is not patent in which case an oocyte could be trapped in it and unable to reach the tubal lumen.

Vascular Abnormalities

Vascular abnormalities of the small vessels in the folds have been described but their significance is uncertain.[30] Marked vascularization with hemorrhagic spots are suggestive of chronic inflammation.

Adhesions and Fibrosis

The most significant abnormal findings are adhesions and fibrosis of the tubal walls. Filmy adhesions may be found between otherwise normal folds. They are avascular and may be focal or diffuse. Thick fibrous vascularized adhesions may produce distortion of the fold structure. They are usually extensive and involve the whole ampulla. Fibrosis is the end result of a chronic severe infectious process and results in a rigid tubal wall with complete loss of the normal fold pattern.

These changes have been classified as follows:[29]

- Grade 1 Normal fold pattern
- Grade 2 Separation and flattening of major folds
- Grade 3 Peripheral filmy and focal adhesions
- Grade 4 Fibrous adhesions across more than 50 percent of the lumen
- Grade 5 Fibrosis of the tubal walls with loss of the fold system.

DISCUSSION

Conventional methods that use hysterosalpingography or laparoscopy to assess tubal infertility are inadequate due to their high rate of both false positive and false negative results.

Tubal endoscopy has a role to play in the fine assessment of tubal disease and should be part of the protocol for investigating patients with proximal tubal obstruction, pelvic inflammatory disease, ectopic pregnancy, unexplained infertility and prior to tubal surgery and some forms of assisted conception, thus avoiding unnecessary surgery in these cases.

Falloposcopy allows the direct visualization of the endosalpinx and can diagnose and correct tubal occlusion; the method can also detect non-obstructive tubal disease. The increased accuracy of the tubal assessment helps in the allocation of patients to the most appropriate treatment . The development of the linear everting catheter system has enabled falloposcopy to be performed as an office procedure under local anesthesia. The technique is safe and atraumatic, but is still in its infancy. By giving operators the appropriate training, the use of falloposcopy can be increased; pregnancy rates could thereby be improved and the cost and time spent on unnecessary surgical intervention or assisted reproductive procedures could be reduced.

Salpingoscopy enables a more specific assessment of the distal tubal mucosa, further refining the prediction of successful tubal function.[6,8,29]

REFERENCES

1. R Burns CL. Principles of Midwifery. Longman, Hurst, Rees and Orme, London 1809;131-2.
2. Maguiness SD, Djahanbakhch O, Grudzinskas JG. Assessment of the fallopian tube. Progress in Obstet Gynaec 1993;10.
3. Donnez J, Langerock S, Lecart CI, Thomas K. Incidence of pathological factors not revealed by hysterosalpingography but disclosed by laparoscopy. Euro J Obstet Gynaec Reprod Biology 1982;13:369-75.
4. Sulak PJ, Letterie GS, Coddington CC, Hayslip CC, Woodward JE, Kein TA. Histology of proximal tubal occlusion. Fert Ster 1987;48:437-40.
5. Marana R, Muzii L, Paielli FV, Lucci FM, Dell'Acqua S, Mancuso S. Proximal tubal obstruction: Are we overdiagnosing and overtreating? Gynae Endo 1993;1:99-101.

6. Henry-Suchet J, Loffredo V, Tesquier L, Pez J, et al. Endoscopy of the tube (=tuboscopy): Its prognostic value for tuboplasties. Acta Europ Fert 1985;16:139-45.
7. Brosens I, Boeckx W, Delattin Ph, Puttemans P, Vasquez G. Salpingoscopy: A new pre-operative diagnostic tool in tubal infertility. British Journal of Obstetrics and Gynaecology, 1987;94:768-73.
8. Shapiro BS, Diamond MP, DeCherney AH. Salpingoscopy: An adjunctive technique for evaluation of the fallopian tube. Fertil Steril 1988;49:1076-9.
9. Mohri T, Mohri K, Yamadori F. Tubaloscope. Flexible glassfiber endoscope for intratubal observation. Endoscopy 1970;4:226-30.
10. Kerin J, Daykhovsky L, Segalowitz J, et al. Falloposcopy: A microendoscopic technique for visual exploration of the human fallopian tube from the uterotubal ostium to the fimbria using a transvaginal approach. Fertil Steril 1990;54:390-400.
11. Bauer O, Diedrich K, Bacich S, et al. Transcervical access and intra-luminal imaging of the fallopian tube in the non-anaesthetized patient; preliminary results using a new technique for fallopian access. Hum Reprod 1992;7(Suppl 1):7S-11S.
12. Dubuisson JB, Chapron C, Morice P, Aubriot FX, Foulot H, de Joliniere JB. Laparoscopic salpingostomy: Fertility results according to the tubal mucosal appearance. Human Reprod 1994;9:334-9.
13. Woodruff JD, Pauerstein CJ. The fallopian tube: Structure, function, pathology and management. Baltimore, The Williams and Wilkins Company, 1969.
14. Brosens IA. Salpingoscopy. In: Gordon AG, Lewis BV, DeCherney AH (Eds): Atlas of Gynecologic Endoscopy, 2nd Edition. London, Mosby-Wolfe, 1995;21-6.
15. Venezia R, Zangara C, Knight C, Cittadini E. Initial experience of a new linear everting falloposcopy system in comparison with hysterosalpingography. Fertil Steril 1993;60:771-5.
16. Grow DR, Coddington CC, Flood JT. Proximal tubal occlusion by hysterosalpingogram: A role for falloposcopy. Fertil Steril 1993,60:171-4.
17. Kerin JF, Williams DB, San Roman GA, Pearlstone AC, Grundfest WS, Surrey ES. Falloposcopic classification and treatment of fallopian tube lumen disease. Fertil Steril 1992;57:731-41.
18. Kerin J, Surrey E, Daykhovsky L, Grundfest WS. Development and application of a falloposcope for transvaginal endoscopy of the fallopian tube. J of Laparoendoscopy 1990;1:47-56.
19. Scudamore IW, Dunphy BC, Cooke ID. Outpatient falloposcopy intra-luminal imaging of the fallopian tube by trans-uterine fibreoptic endoscopy as an outpatient procedure. Br J Obstet Gynaecol 1992;99:829-35.
20. Pearlstone AC, Surrey ES, Kerin JF. The linear everting catheter: A nonhysteroscopic, transvaginal technique for access and microendoscopy of the fallopian tube. Fertil Steril 1992;58:854-7.
21. DeBruyne F, Puttemans P, Boeckx W, Brosens I. The clinical value of salpingoscopy in tubal infertiltiy. Fertil Steril 1989;51:339-40.
22. The American Fertility Society. The American classifications of adnexal adhesions, distal tubal occlusion secondary to tubal ligation, tubal pregnancies, mullerian abnormalities and intrauterine lesions. Fertil Steril 1988; 49:944.
23. Kovacs G, Kerin J, Scudamore I, Wood C. Falloposcopy—a non-invasive method of salpingostomy. Gynaecol Endosc 1992;1:159-60.
24. Dunphy B, Pattinson HA. Office falloposcopy; a tertiary level assessment for planning the management of infertile women. Aust NZ J Obstet Gynaecol 1994;34:189-90.
25. Surrey ES, Adamson GD, Nagel TC, et al. Multicenter feasibility study of a new coaxial falloposcopy system. J Am Assoc Gynecol Laparosc 1997;4:473-8.
26. Bauer O, Diedrich K, Al Hasani S. Non-surgical tubal transfer techniques In: Sueoka K, Asada H, Tsuchiya S, Kobayashi N, Kuroshima M (Eds): Ann Prog Reprod Med 1993;10:95-106.
27. Yoshimura Y. Falloposcopic tuboplasty for bilateral tubal occlusion. A novel infertility treatment as an alternative for *in vitro* fertilization? Hum Reprod 1998;13:71-4. 1996:72-86.
28. Cornier E. L'ampulloscopie per coelioscopie. Journal de Gynecologie, Obstetrique et Biologie de la Reproduction. 1985;14:459-66.
29. Brosens I, Boeckx W, Delattin Ph, Puttemans P, Vasquez G. Salpingoscopy: A new preoperative diagnostic tool in tubal infertility. British Journal of Obstetrics and Gynaecology 1987;94:768-73.
30. Maguinness SD, Djahanbaksh O. Salpingoscopic findings in women undergoing sterilisation. Human Reprod 1992;7:269-73.

21 Role of Laparoscopic Tubal Recanalization in Modern Era of ART

Sanjay Patel, Yogendra Jhala

INTRODUCTION

Laparoscopic microsurgery is a new discipline that synergizes the potential of classical microsurgery and laparoscopy. It can overcome the deficiencies in each of the techniques. Advent of microsurgical technique began by Swolin in 1967. First microsurgical reversal of the sterilization was done by Gomel and Winston in 1977.

Around 25-30 percent of the subfertile females have tubal damage and quite a few of them seek tubal micro-reconstruction for fertility enhancement, also those with tubal sterilization procedure seeking reversal for further child bearing are better candidates. This can now be achieved with principles of laparoscopic microsurgery.

ADVANTAGES OF LAPAROSCOPIC TUBAL ANASTOMOSIS

- All microsurgical principles are well maintained like magnification, tissue handling, hemostasis and lavage
- Avoids laparotomy and tissue trauma associated with packing and retractors
- Minimal tissue handling and trauma
- Adhesions are minimal
- Cosmetically far better
- Faster recovery
- Single step procedure as compared to IVF where multiple sittings may be required.

PREOPERATIVE WORK UP

- Semen Analysis: to rule out male factor.
- Day 3 Serum FSH level to know the ovarian reserve.
- HSG to know the length and condition of the proximal tube.
- Saline infusion sonography and hysterosalpingography may be helpful.

INDICATIONS

- Reversal of tubal sterilization procedure
- Mid-tubal block secondary to various pathology
- Tubal occlusion secondary to ectopic pregnancy treatment
- Salpingitis isthmica nodosa
- Failed tubal cannulation for proximal tubal block
- Failed previous macrosurgical sterilization reversal.

CONTRAINDICATIONS

Absolute Contraindications

- Aged 40 years or older
- Decreased ovarian reserve or ovarian failure
- Tubal infertility not amenable to tubal reconstruction
- Extensive tubal damage
- Hydrosalpinx with a diameter of more than 3 cm
- Inadequate proximal or distal tubal segment for reanastomosis.

- Projected tubal length of less than 3 cm after the reconstruction procedure
- Extensive pelvic/peritubal adhesions
- Abnormal uterine cavity
- Any contraindication to pregnancy or surgery
- Severe male factor infertility or male sterility.

EQUIPMENTS AND INSTRUMENTS

Magnification, Resolution and Digital Enhancement

- **25-40X** magnification is essential to identify healthy mucosa of the fallopian tube. **10-15X** magnification is adequate for micro suturing.
- Use of endoscope, digital three chip camera with monitor has a ***'Multiplier Effect'*** and the magnification can be achieved up to **20-25X.**

Micro-Instrumentation

- It is collectively known as ***'Koh ultramicro series'*** (Figure 21.1).
- Terminal serration of the jaw is specially treated so that micro suture material does not get crushed.
- Handle design should be such that least friction and max transmission of hand movement occur to the instrument tip. 130° angle between handle and shaft of the instruments provides better movements.

Sutures, Needles and Energy

- More rigid needles are better for micro-endosuturing.

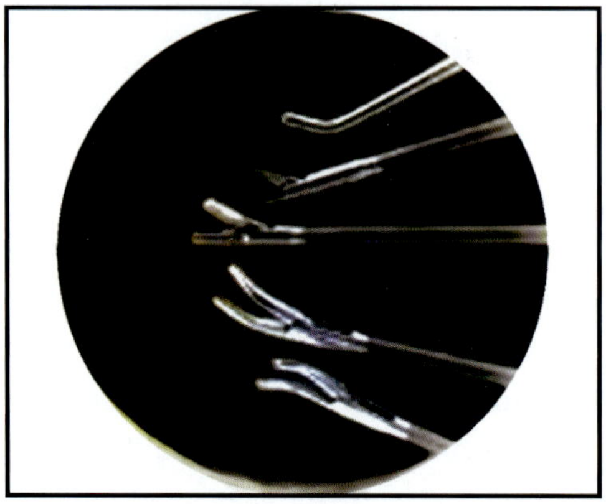

Figure 21.1. Koh ultramicro series

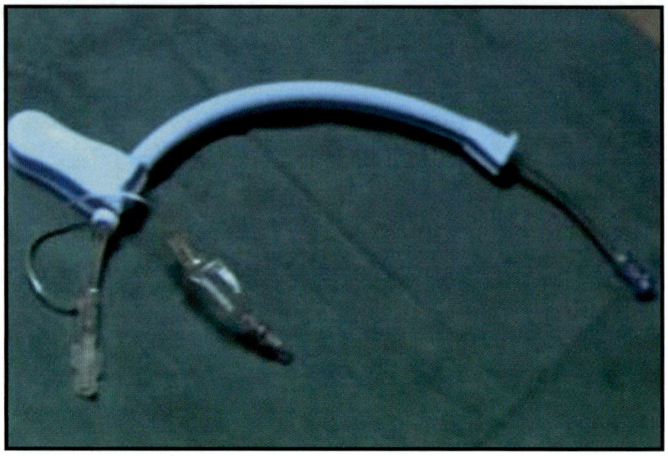

Figure 21.2. Handlin's uterine manipulator

- The suture material should be 6-0 to 8-0 polypropylene, depending upon the surgeon's experience of material handling and preference.
- Electrosurgery: 15-20 W for cutting and 15 W for fulguration, use minimum cautery to preserve subtubal vasculature (Figure 21.12).
- ***Handlin's uterine manipulator*** is a fine disposable instrument (Figure 21.2), which allows administration of the dye and manipulation of the uterus without causing any significant trauma.

SELECTION OF CASES

Length of Tubal Damage in Various Methods of Ligation

Type of TL	*Length*	*Case type*
Monopolar diathermy	50 mm	Unfavorable
Falope Ring TL (Figure 21.5)	40 mm	Unfavorable
Pomeroy's method	30 mm	Intermediate
Bipolar diathermy (Figure 21.4)	30 mm	Intermediate
Hulka clip	7 mm	Favorable
Filshie's clip (Figure 21.3)	4 mm	Most favorable

Other non-suitable cases are pathological tubes with PID, Salpingitis isthmica nodosa and Failed tubal cannulation.

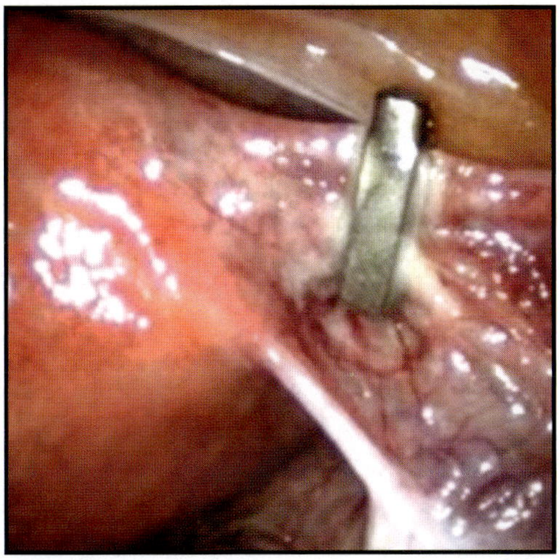

Figure 21.3. Filshie's clip TL

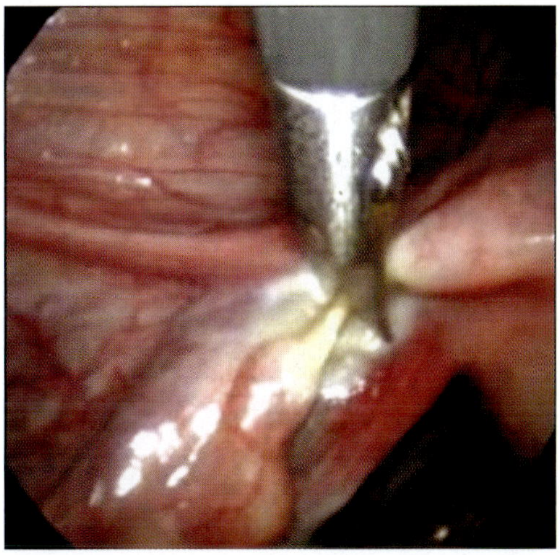

Figure 21.4. Tubal ligation with bipolar

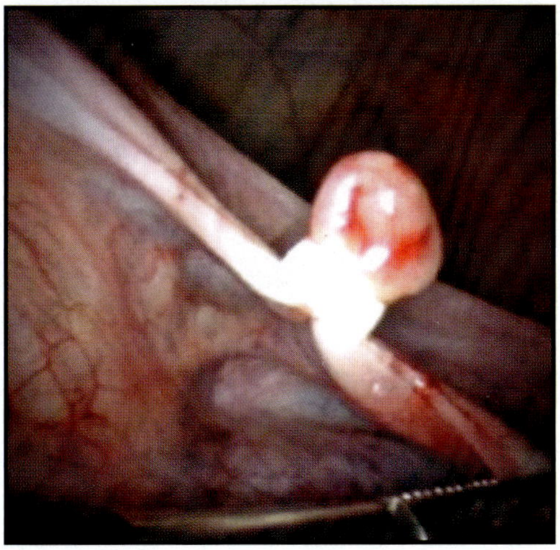

Figure 21.5. Falope ring tubal ligation

INTRAOPERATIVE EVALUATION

Before proceeding for the tubal reconstruction one must evaluate the inside of the tube, so as to be confirmed that the anastomosis is going to be fruitful or not at all worthwhile. This involves *Salpingoscopy and Falloposcopy.*

- Salpingoscopy allows direct inspection of tubal mucosa in the ampullary part.
- The degree of tubal mucosal damage is probably the major factor in establishing the prognosis for tubal surgery.
- *Brosen's classification* is useful for evaluation according to degree of mucosal atrophy and mucosal adhesions.

Salpingoscopy Grade 1 (Figure 21.6)

Normal intraluminal findings with healthy. Major (Primary) and Minor (Secondary) folds.

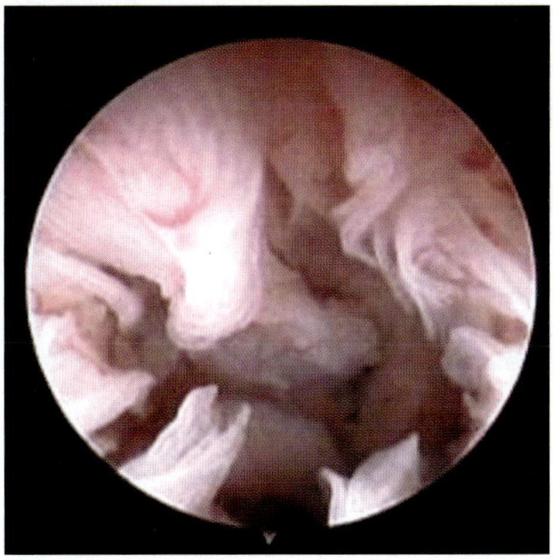

Figure 21.6. Salpingoscopy grade I (normal)

Salpingoscopy Grade 2 (Figure 21.7)

Mucosal nuclear staining with Methylene blue dye.

Salpingoscopy Grade 3 (Figure 21.8)

Minimal flattening and minimal adhesion of endosalpinx.

Salpingoscopy Grade 4 (Figure 21.9)

Moderate flattening of endosalpinx with intraluminal adhesion.

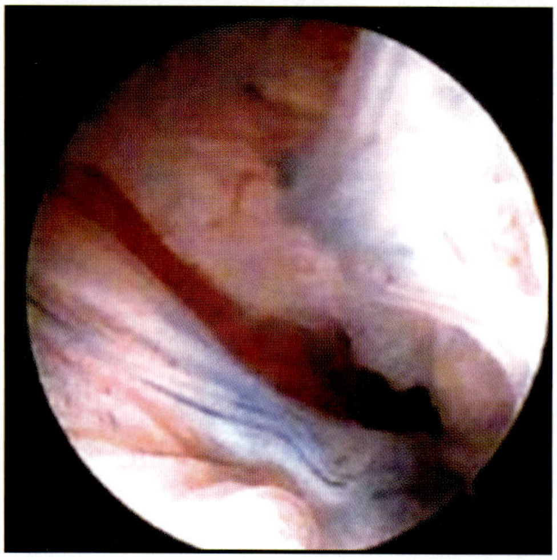

Figure 21.7. Salpingoscopy grade 2 (staining)

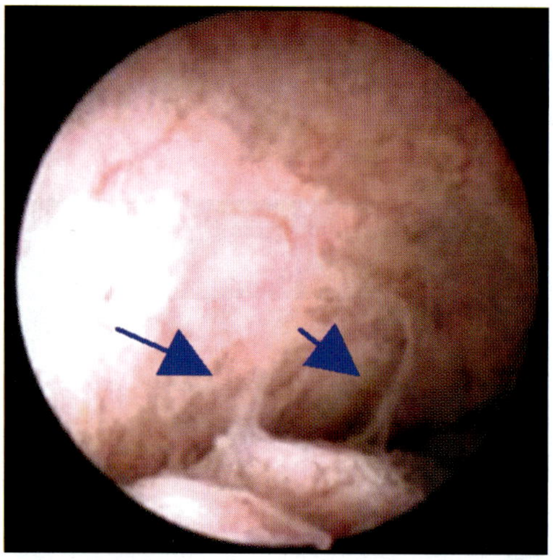

Figure 21.8. Salpingoscopy grade 3 (focal adhesion)

Salpingoscopy Grade 5 (Figure 21.10)

Severe flattening of mucosa with severe interluminal adhesions.

Surgical Technique (Figure 21.11)

Total 5 ports are used

- 10 mm laparoscope through the primary umbilical port.
- Four ancillary ports, two 5 mm and two 3 mm.
- The lower pelvic port of 5 mm is placed 4 cm medial and above the anterior superior iliac spine, i.e. Ipsilateral Port.

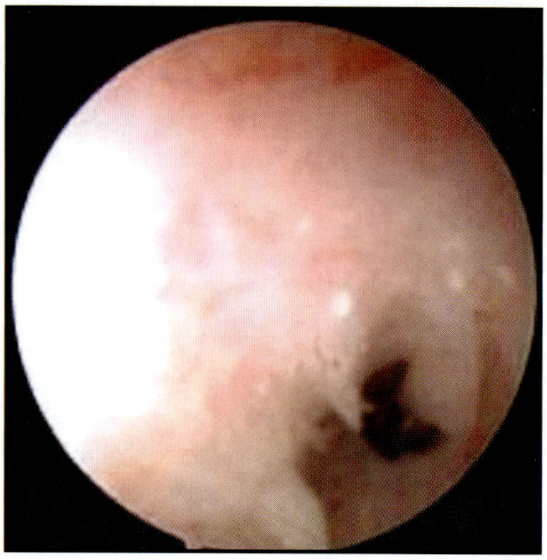

Figure 21.9. Salpingoscopy grade 4

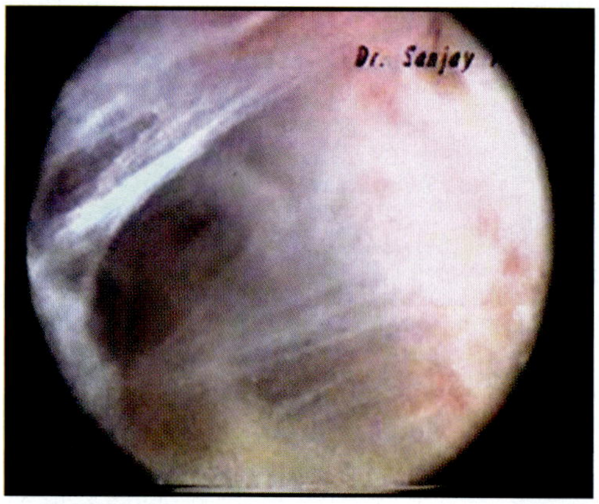

Figure 21.10. Salpingoscopy grade 5

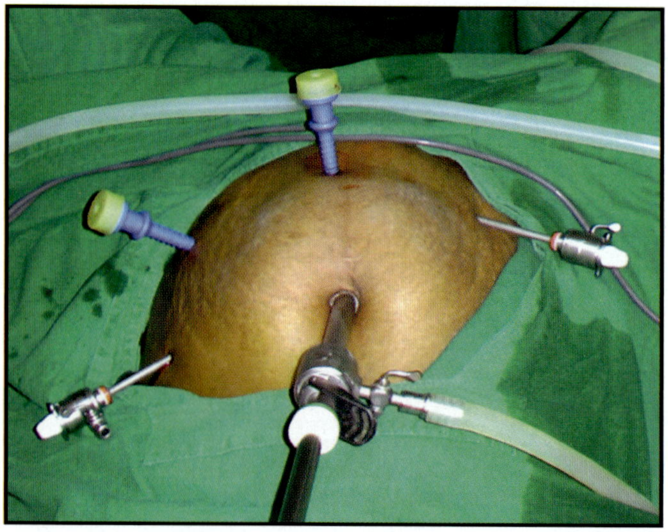

Figure 21.11. Port positioning

- Contralateral port of 3 mm size placed exactly opposite to ipsilateral port.
- Another ipsilateral port of 3 mm is paraumbilical and laterally in the anterior axillary line.
- One 5 mm central port, 2-3 cm above the pubic symphysis.

'The position of the ports is critical in enabling fluent two handed operating as well as suturing. The so-called 'fulcrum effect' is virtually eliminated by adopting specific port positions.'

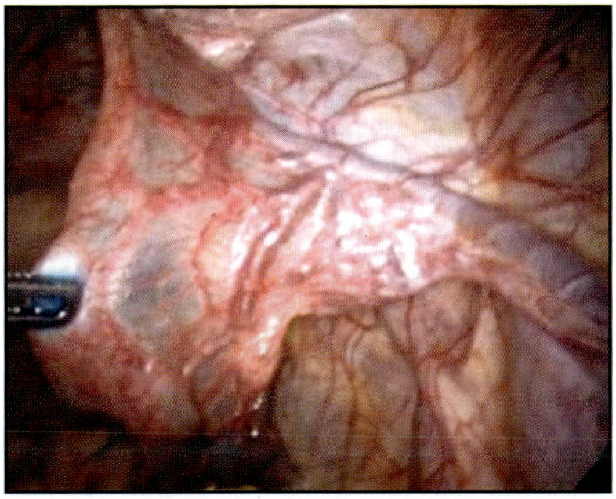

Figure 21.12. Sub-tubal vessels

IMPORTANT SURGICAL STEPS

- Distention of the proximal segment of the tube by transcervical chromo perturbation to know the exact site of the block.
- Excision of pathological segment of the tube (Figure 21.13).
- Make sure that the incision does not extend beyond the mesosalpinx.
- Ensure the right angled cut of the tubal ends for better alignment and approximation (Figure 21.14).
- Free spillage of the dye (Figures 21.15 and 21.16).
- Mesosalpinx is sutured first, using 6-0 polypropylene (Figure 21.17).

Most difficult and important step - end to end anastomosis in two layers.

First layer, the mucosal-muscularis layer.

- Most important is 6 O'clock position stitch (Figure 21.18).
- To keep the knot outside the lumen, stitches are taken from outer to inner side on proximal end and vice versa on distal end (Figure 21.19).
- Rests of the stitches are taken at 12, 3, and 9 O' clock position in the similar manner.

Second layer, the sero-muscularis layer; sutured with 6-0 polypropylene (Figures 21.20 and 21.21).

- Thorough peritoneal irrigation with Ringer's lactate solution throughout the operation.

TYPES OF ANASTOMOSIS

Isthmo- Isthmic Anastomosis

- Lumen size is 500 µm-1mm
- Equal lumen size and thick muscularis allows technically easier and better anastomosis.

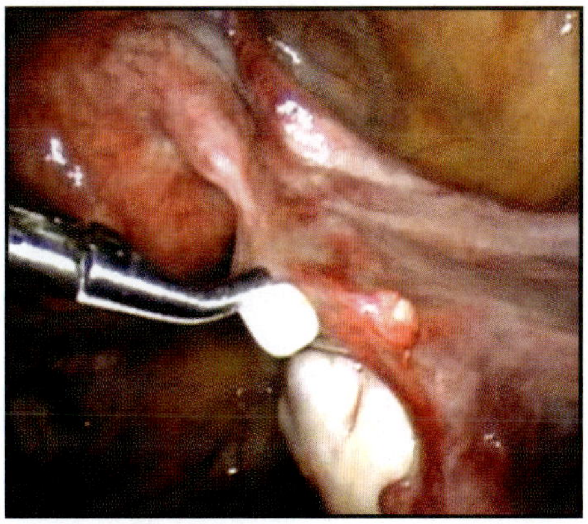

Figure 21.13. Falope ring excision

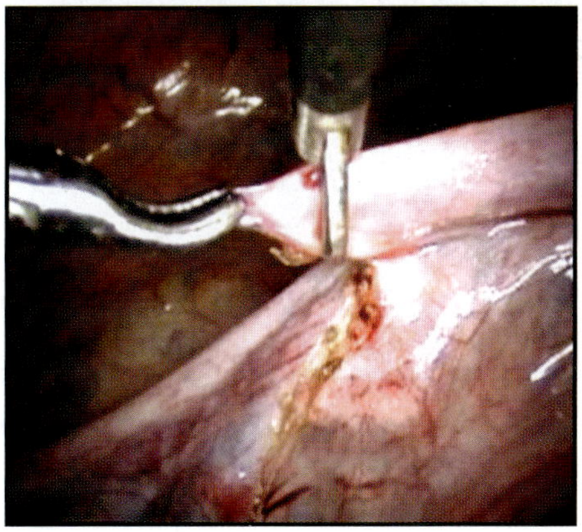

Figure 21.14. Refreshening of edges

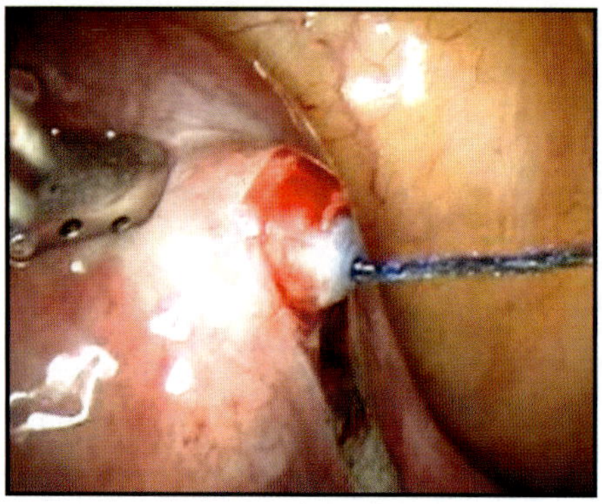

Figure 21.15. Free dye flow

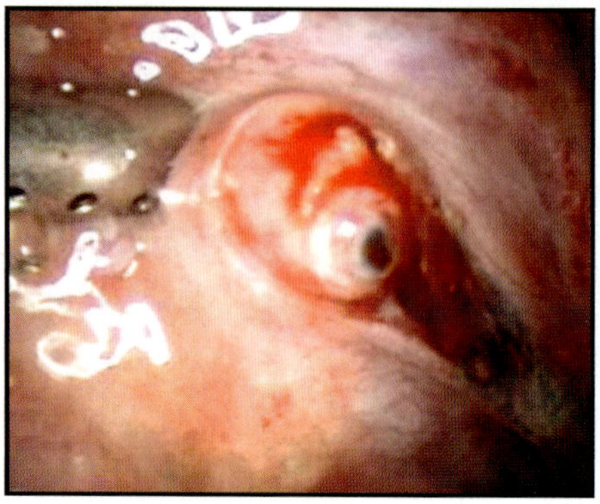

Figure 21.16. Magnified view

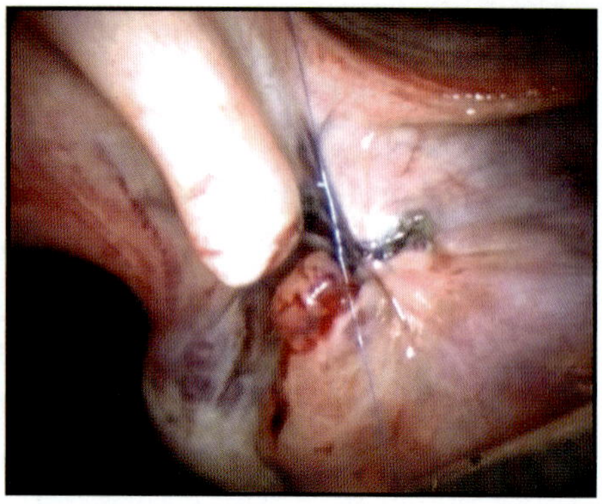

Figure 21.17. Mesosalpinx stitch

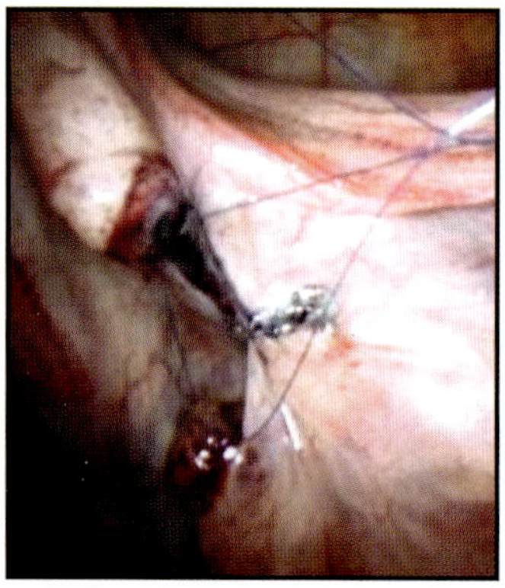

Figure 21.18. 6 O'clock stitch

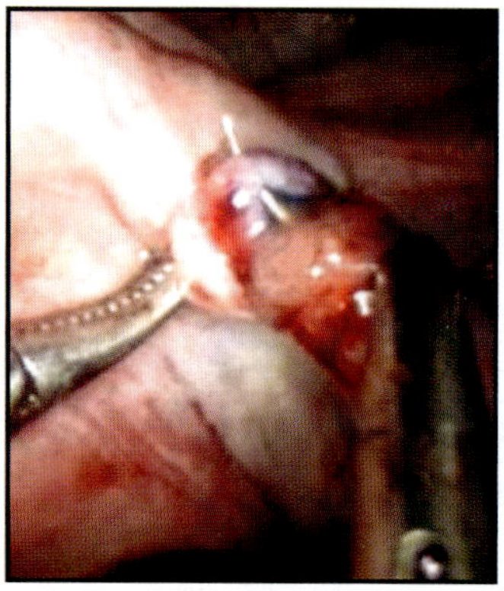

Figure 21.19. 12 O'clock stitch

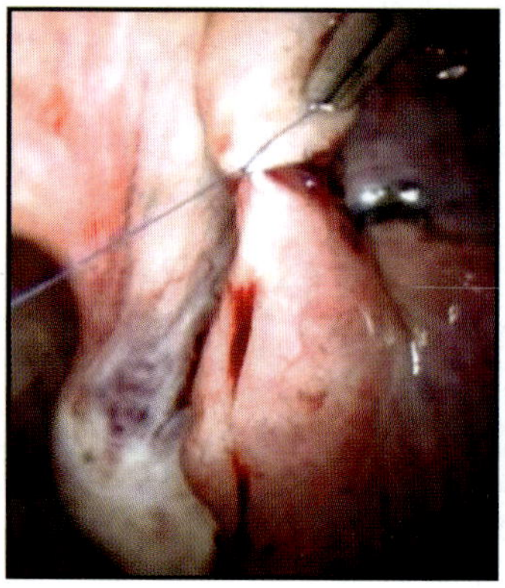

Figure 21.20. Second layer

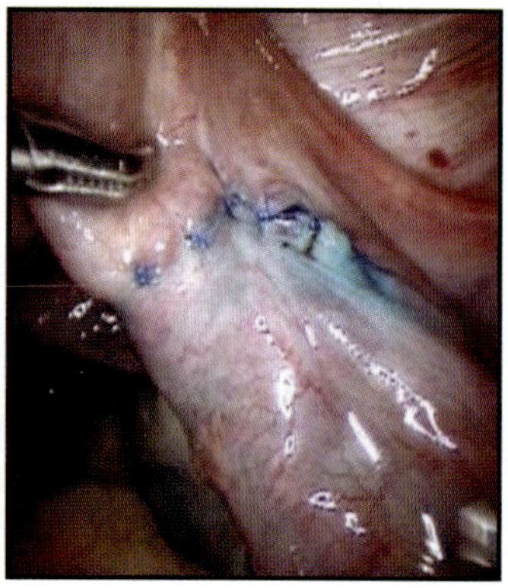

Figure 21.21. End result

Isthmo-Ampullary Anastomosis (Figures 21.22 to 21.25)

- Luminal disparity is the potential problem which can be adjusted by cutting the isthmic end.

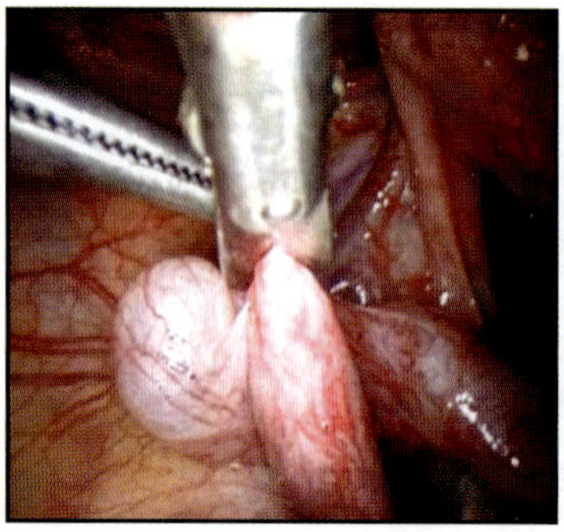

Figure 21.22. Refreshening ends

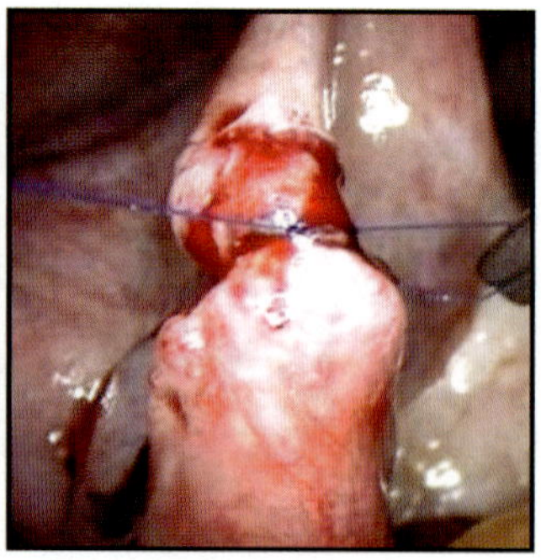

Figure 21.23. First layer

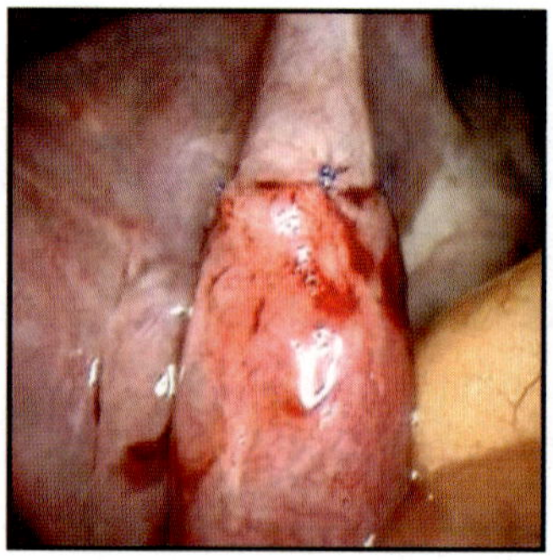

Figure 21.24. Second layer

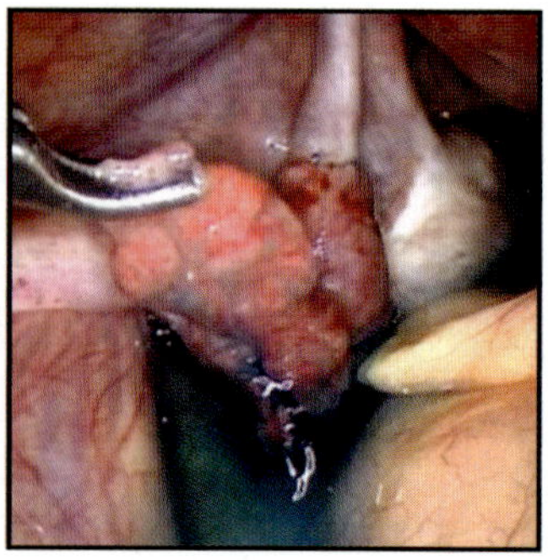

Figure 21.25. Free spill

Ampullo-Ampullary Anastomosis (Figures 21.26 to 21.28)

- Technically difficult anastomosis due to thin muscularis and tendency for mucosal folds prolapse.

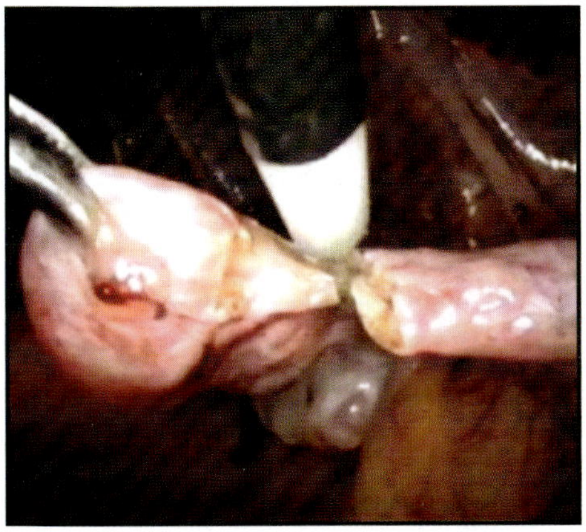

Figure 21.26. Refreshening ends

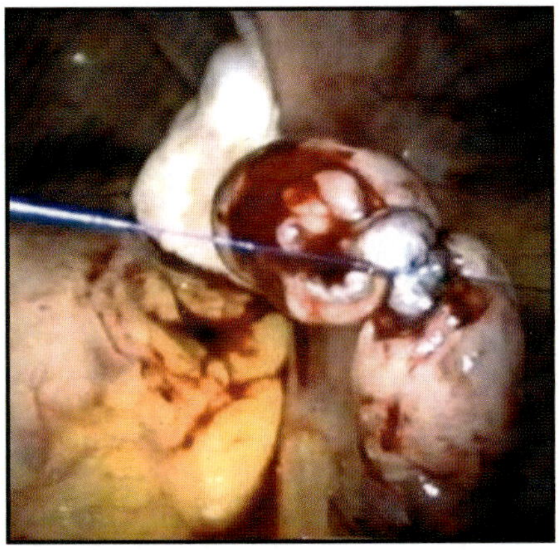

Figure 21.27. First layer

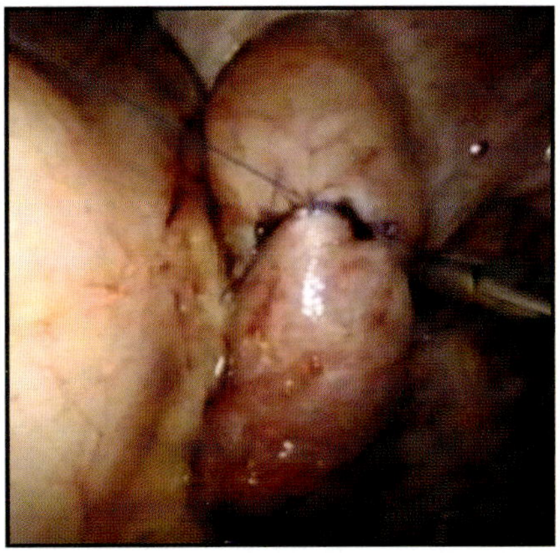

Figure 21.28. Second layer

Tubo-Cornual Anastomosis (Figures 21.29 to 21.35)

- Wedge excision in the cornual end mobilizes good length of interstitial tube.

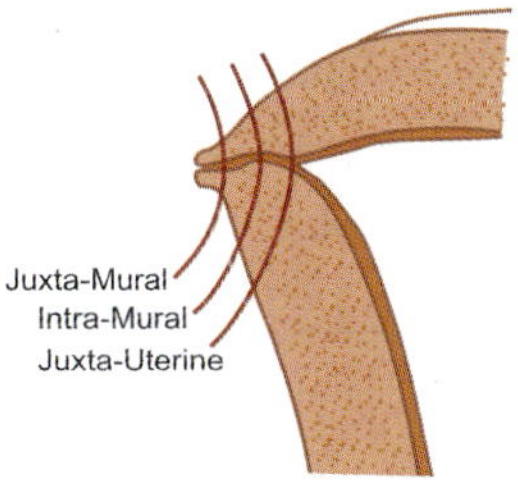

Figure 21.29. Interstitial portion of tube

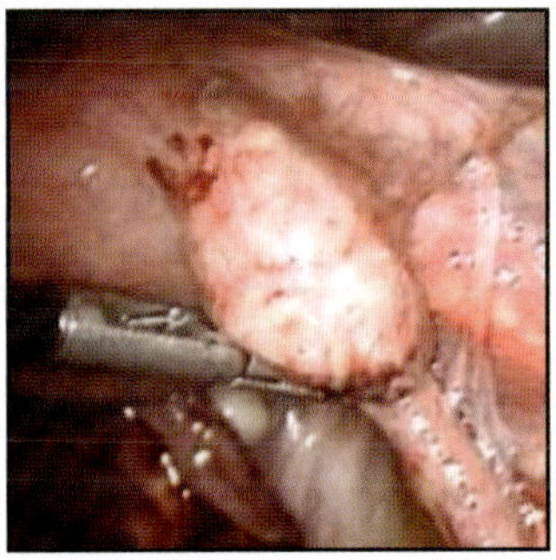

Figure 21.30. Cornual pathology

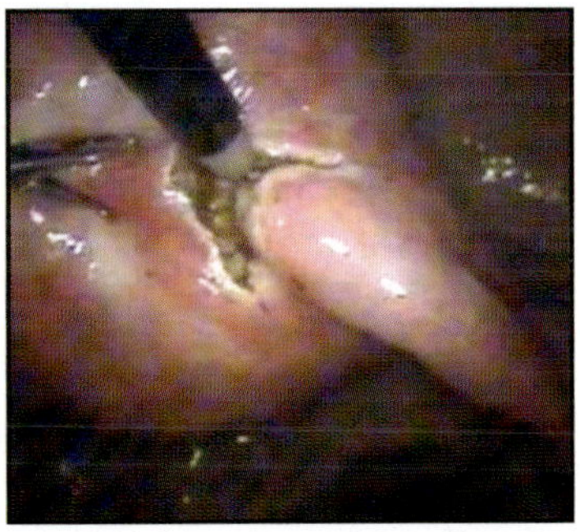

Figure 21.31. Wedge incision

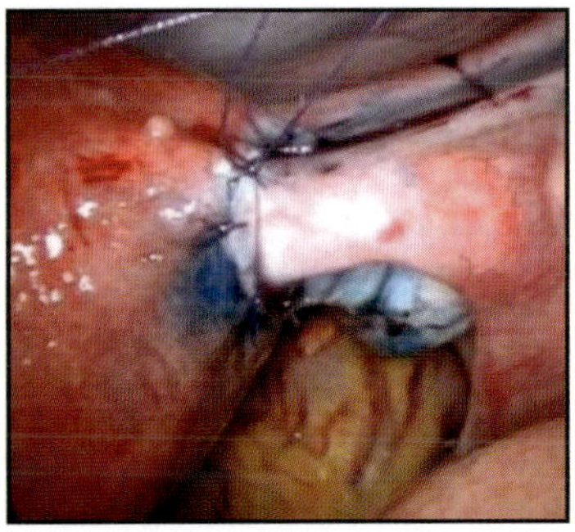

Figure 21.32. Interstitial anastomosis

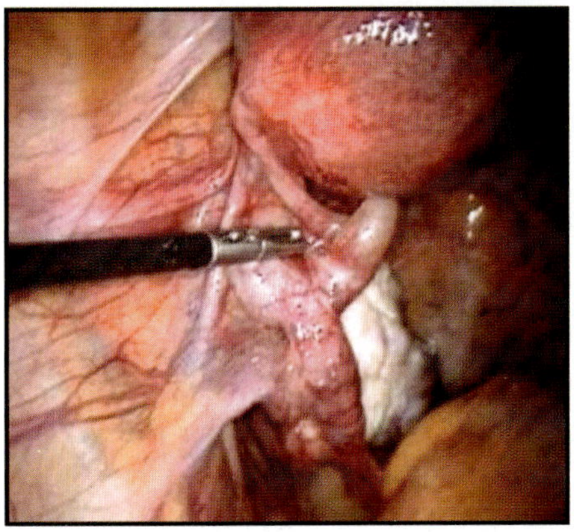

Figure 21.33. Mild hydrosalpinx

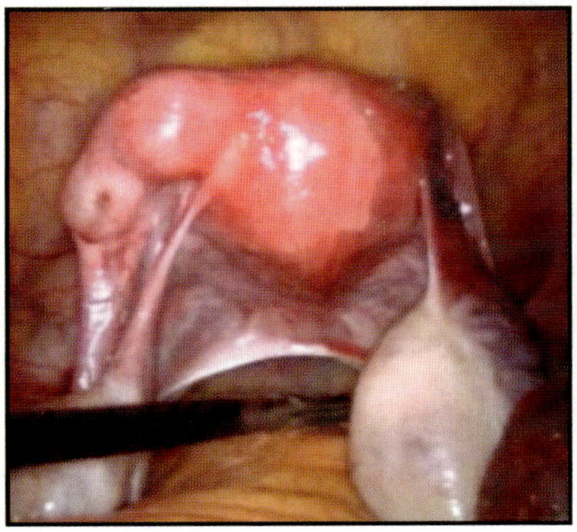

Figure 21.34. Cornual pathology

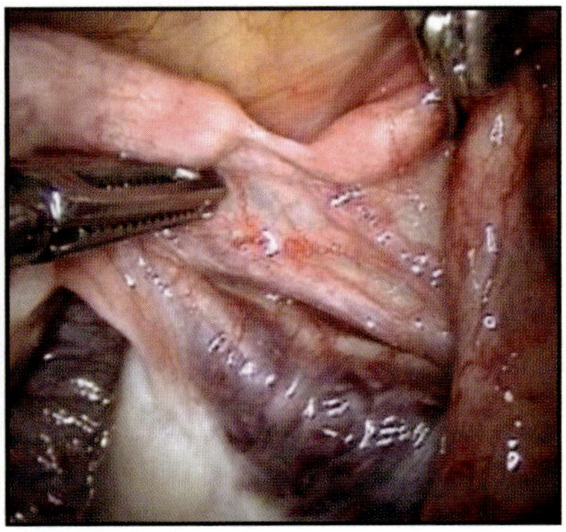

Figure 21.35. Proximal tubal block

PATHOLOGICAL TUBES

Salpingoscopy plays a key role in decision making for reconstructive surgery of such tubes

OUR EXPERIENCE

Study Between 1996 to 2005

TL Reversal	*Tubal block due to PID*	*Tubal block secondary to ectopic pregnancy*	*Failed tubal cannulation for proximal block*	***Total***
126 (68.5%)	38 (20.6%)	7 (3.8%)	13 (7.1%)	**184 cases**

Types of Anastomosis

Bilateral	*Unilateral*	*Incomplete (due to multiple blocks)*	***Total***
137 (74.4%)	39 (21.1%)	08 (4.3%)	**184 cases**

Types of Anastomosis and Its Result

Types of anastomosis	*Isthmo-isthmic*	*Isthmo-ampullary*	*Ampullo-ampullary*	*Juxtamural-isthmic*	*Juxtauterine-isthmic*	*Intramural-isthmic*	***Total***
Total No.	102 (55.6%)	39 (21.1%)	24 (13.1%)	09 (4.7%)	03 (1.6%)	07 (3.8%)	**184**
Cases conceived	93 (91.1%)	34 (87.1%)	12 (50%)	04 (44%)	- -	2 (28.5%)	**145 (78.8%)**

Case Type Vs Result

Out of the 184 successful surgeries, 145 (78.8%) conceived, including 6 cases of ectopic pregnancy (4.2%).

Type of Cases	*TL Reversal (N=126)*	*Pathological Tubes (N=58)*	***Total (N=184)***
Cases conceived	116 (92%)	29 (48%)	**145 (78.8%)**

CONCLUSION

- Pregnancy rates were comparable with open tubal re-canalization.
- Salpingoscopy is very helpful in presence of pathological block.
- In cases of ectopic pregnancies segmental excision is best option as compared to salpingostomy or total salpingectomy, if the ectopic sac is < 2 cm of size.
- There is no place of tubal implantation rather interstitial tubal anastomosis is preferable and more fruitful.
- The average surgical duration was 2 hours and 30 minutes.
- The average hospital stay was 36 hours.
- More cost-effective than IVF in the long run.
- Single step treatment as compare with IVF which requires multiple steps in each cycle.

- Author's results are among the best in the world and exceed pregnancy rates from *in vitro* fertilization.

SUGGESTED READING

1. American College of Obstetricians and Gynecologists: ACOG technical bulletin. Sterilization. Number 222—April 1996 (replaces no. 113, February 1998). Int J Gynaecol Obstet 1996;53(3):281-8.
2. Bateman BG, Nunley WC Jr, Kitchin JD. Fertil Steril 1987;48:523-42.
3. Cetin MT, Demir SC, Toksoz L, Kadayifci O. The effect of laparoscopic reversal of tubal sterilization on pregnancy rate. European Journal of Contraception and Reproduction Health Care 2002;7(3):162-6.
4. Dubuisson JB, Chaperon C, Nos C, et al. Sterilization reversal: Fertility results. Hum Reprod 1995;10(5):1145-51.
5. Gomel V. Microsurgical reversal of female sterilization: A reappraisal. Fertil Steril 1980;33(6):587-97.
6. Mage G, Pouly JL, Bouquet de Jolinière J, Chabrand S, Riouallan A, Bruhat MA. Fertil Steril 1986;46:807-10.
7. Reich H, McGlynn f, Parente C, et al. Laparoscopic tubal anastomosis. J Am Assoc Gynecol Laparosc 1993;(1):16-9.
8. Sauer MV. In: Mishell DR, Davajan V, Lobo RA (Eds): Infertility, Contraception and Reproductive Endocrinology (3rd ed), Blackwell Scientific Publications, Boston 1991;682-707.
9. Swolin K. [50 fertility operations. I. Literature and methods]. Acta Obstet Gynecol Scand 1967;46(2):234-50.
10. Van Voorhis, Bradley J. Comparison of tubal ligation reversal procedures. Clinical Obstetrics and Gynecology 2000;43(3):641-9.
11. Williams TJ. Obstet Gynecol. Clin North Am 1987; 14:1037-48.
12. Yoon TK, Sung HR, Kang HG, et al. Laparoscopic tubal anastomosis: Fertility outcome in 202 cases. Fertilisation 1999;72:1121-6.

Section Four

OVARIES

22 Laparoscopic Electrocauterization of Ovarian Surface

Shyam V Desai, Nikhil S Jani

INTRODUCTION

In 1935, Stein and Levinthal[1] described a symptom complex associated with Oligomenorrhea, Anovulation, Hirsutism, Infertility and Polycystic ovaries. This was named the Stein-Levinthal syndrome. As these symptoms can occur from a host of pathologies like a virilizing tumor of the ovary or an adrenal neoplasm, these symptoms are not pathognomonic of a polycystic ovarian disease.

Polycystic ovarian disease is a heterogeneous group of disorders that may present with a wide variety of clinical syndromes. At one end of the spectrum is a single finding of polycystic ovarian morphology detected by pelvic ultrasound and at the other end is the presentation with symptoms such as obesity, hyperandrogenism, menstrual cycle abnormalities and infertility.

Thus polycystic ovarian disease is diagnosed once neoplasm and enzymatic defects are excluded.

INCIDENCE

The incidence amounts to as much as 20 percent of "normal" adult women (Polson et al 1988).[2] Using ultrasound criteria, PCOD has been shown to account for 60 percent of women with anovulation and upto 92 percent women with hirsutism (Adams et al).[3]

ETIOPATHOLOGY

Classically, elevated levels of pituitary derived serum luteinizing hormone and ovarian derived hyperandrogeniemia characterize PCOD. These set up a self perpetuating vicious cycle of relative luteinizing hormone hypersecretion, leading to ovarian stromal hyperactivity, atresia of antral follicles and disordered ovarian steroidogenesis. High levels of serum testosterone are associated with increased risk of infertility, hirsutism and cycle disturbance. Carey et al (1993)[4] suggested a familial condition possibly autosomal dominant, however, the polycystic gene has not been identified.

Several hypothesis have been suggested for the over secretion of luteinizing hormone. These include:

- Increase pulse frequency of GnRH secretion from the hypothalamus.
- Increased pituitary sensitivity to to GnRH.
- Hyperinsulinemic stimulation of the pituitary.
- Disturbance of the ovarian steroid pituitary feedback mechanism.

None of these theories however, completely explain the luteinizing hormone hypersecretion.

Insulin receptor dysfunction leading to insulin resistance has been shown to be a common association with PCOD, and evidence suggests that this is a primary defect and not a result of hyperandrogenism or obesity. The compensatory hyperinsulinemia, is thought to act by augmenting the LH dependent androgen production by the thecal and stromal tissues. It is possible that it may also be directly associated with the disordered secretion of LH, SHBG and DHEAS. Metabolic and hormonal disturbances such as elevated levels of LH, Testosterone, Insulin, and Prolactin are commonly found in PCOD and these might be associated with long-term sequelae such as diabetes mellitus, hypertension, hyperlipidemia, and endometrial carcinoma.

CLINICAL FINDINGS

In a large series by Balen et al (1995)[5] 1700 women with at least one symptom of PCOS were investigated. He found that:

1. Approx. 38 percent were overweight (BMI >25), these patients were at increased risk of hirsutism and menstrual cycle disturbance.
2. Twenty-six percent of cases had primary infertility and 14 percent had secondary infertility.
3. Only 30 percent had regular menses, where as 50 percent had oligomenorrhea, and 20 percent had amenorrhea.

INVESTIGATIONS

Ruling out ovarian and adrenal neoplasm and enzymic defects may be required for the diagnosis of PCOS.

- FSH and LH – Ratio of 3:1 of LH: FSH is diagnostic.
- Testosterone levels are not increased to more than twice the upper limit of normal range (20-80 ng/ml), any level > 200 ng/ml is s/o adrenal pathology.
- DHEA level is raised but is not more than 700 ng/dl which is also s/o adrenal pathology.
- SHBG levels are increased.
- LDL and triglyceride levels are also increased.
- OGTT levels are altered.
- USG: High resolution USG remains the most important means of diagnosis of PCOS.

Ovarian morphology with the criteria described by Adams (1985) appears to be the most sensitive marker for PCO, (10 or more cysts that are greater than 2 to 8 mm in diameter, arranged in echo dense stroma. Increase in the ovarian size, with a cross-sectional area of >10 cm is also a sign of PCOD. This when combined with features of oligo /amenorrhea, obesity and / or other symptoms of hyperandrogenism are diagnostic of PCOS.

The study by Fox (1991)[6] suggested that transabdominal ultrasonography failed to detect 30 percent of PCO as compared to transvaginal sonography which could detect almost 100 percent cases.

Bridges (1993)[7] showed that PCO was seen in 24 percent of population between 3 and 18 years of age and rate of detection is higher in older girls.

- Doppler ultrasonography—might be effective in predicting the risk of OHSS in patients on gonadotropin therapy.
- Magnetic resonance imaging—useful in obese patients.
- Diagnostic laparoscopy.

TREATMENT

PCOS being a heterogeneous group of disorder appropriate therapy demands those potential etiologies be excluded. Apart from treatment of infertility resulting from PCO, the aim of therapy in women with PCO are to control hirsutism and endometrial hyperplasia. In women with PCO who do not desire pregnancy—intermittent progesterone therapy or oral contraceptives are used to reduce the risk of endometrial hyperplasia and for cycle regulation.

For patients with hirsutism, treatment remains the physical adjuncts like bleaching, electrolysis, etc. Cyclic oral contraceptive pills or continuous suppression with Medroxyprogesterone acetate is recommended.

In women with PCO desirious of pregnancy, weight reduction and treatment of hyperglycemia are very important. Clomiphene citrate is the first choice of therapy to induce ovulation. Due to its simplicity, and high success rate (ovulation rate 75% and pregnancy rate of 35-40%). Reported ovulation and conception rate was 50-60 percent.

Recently some attempts have been made on clomiphene resistant patients to intervene on what has been considered to be the main pathogenic mechanism, Insulin resistance. Analouge of somatostatin, Octreotide which brings about a reduction in the insulin secretion and improvement in the ovarian response to HMG. Similar results have been also shown by the use of

Metformin an agent that increases the peripheral sensitivity to insulin (Malkawi et al[8]). Vandermolen et al[9] reported an ovulation rate of 79.7 percent in their series. Kocak[10] reported that combination of Metformin with CC improved the ovulation rate. Parsanezhad et al[11] reported that treatment with Bromocriptine had on effect on ovulation. Dexamethasone pretreatment improves the ovulation rate in selected patients.

Other potential methods of ovulation induction include use of human chorionic gonadotropin with human menopausal gonadotropin, human purified FSH and hCG, or pulsatile GnRH. No other modality of treatment is more effective than Clomiphene citrate, though rescent data suggests that unresponsive women may ovulate if first supperessed with a GnRH analogue.

Medical methods of ovulation with inducing agents, however, fail in approximately 25 percent of patients, the main reasons being lack of adequate response or exaggerated response, leading to development of OHSS. Multiple pregnancy remains a problem when these agents carry out ovarian stimulation.

SURGICAL MANAGEMENT

- The response to operative laparoscopy has been significantly more compared to CC induction, and the conception rates reported for laparoscopy are comparable to that of gonadotropins (Rajan),[12] surgical therapy has become an important therapeutic approach to PCOD treatment. Surgical management of PCOD begins:
- Where medical management fails.
- Medical management cannot be instituted.
- Patients who have failed to ovulate after 7-8 cycles of all dose regimes of clomiphene citrate (Kistner).[13]
- Patient is unwilling to use gonadotropins due to the high cost of these drugs.
- Patient is unsuitable for use of gonadotropins due to high risk of OHSS.
- Patient is undergoing laparoscopy/laparotomy for other indications.

TECHNIQUES

Wedge Resection

Wedge resection requires that approximately 50 percent of ovarian substance is removed. As much of the cortex is preserved as possible. This procedure is associated with a loss of a lot of ovarian tissue and adhesion formation. Therefore it has been given up, to be replaced by less invasive laparoscopic follicular puncture, electrocautery, or laser diathermy.

Operative Laparoscopy

The development of operative laparoscopy has resulted in the introduction of minimally invasive method designed to replace bilateral ovarian wedge resection. The arguments that favor laparoscopic ovulation induction include,

Multiple ovulatory cycles after single treatment and virtually no cyclic monitoring of ovulation induction is required.[9] There is no risk of multiple gestation or ovarian hyperstimulation. Spontaneous abortion rate is less than that compared with medical ovulation induction. Laparoscopic procedure is less expensive and less cumbersome than gonadotropins. Hence, it is argued that after CC failure, the next best option is to select laparoscopic ovarian follicular diathermy.

Currently employed is the four-point laparoscopy technique. A 10 mm scope is employed as the visual axis, the operating axis is one of the portals with a 5 mm sheath placed on one side at the lateral border of the rectus muscles. The suprapubic portal is employed for suction irrigation and retraction, whereas the lateral portals are employed for alternate grasper and monopolar needle cautery applications. Continuous flow of CO_2 helps to keep the intestine away from the operative field. At the outset the uterus, the tubes, the ovaries and the peritoneal folds are examined for any pathology and tubal patency confirmed by hydropertubation. By grasping the ovarian ligament, the ovary could be lifted and rotated to a more convenient position for puncture. The needle is held perpendicular to the ovarian surface and the follicles are punctured with simultaneous application of current for approximately one second. Attempt is made to puncture almost all the prominent follicles, which amounts to 10 punctures on each ovary. The fluid mixed with the irrigating solution is completely aspirated out through the suction cannula.

EVALUATION OF VARIOUS LAPAROSCOPIC APPROACHES

Needle Puncture

Simple needle puncture was carried out in some cases with the thought that it will lead to minimal stromal damage. This proceedure was associated with bleeding and the chance of periovarian adhesions. At the same time the results in term of fertility rates is poor as compared to the other procedures. The use of transvaginal ultrasound guided follicular aspiration, using a technique similar to that of IVF programmes, and the ovulation rate was 87.5 percent and the fertilization rate was 50 percent. The procedure remains the same that the ovary is stabilized and the follicles are punctured with the help of a simple needle. Ferraretti et al[14] reported a fertilization rate of 66 percent and pregnancy rate of 72 percent after transvaginal ovarian drilling and Cibula[15] reported an ovulation rate of only 27 percent (3 out of 11 women) in a trial with multiple ovarian biopsy.

Electrocauterization

By grasping the ovarian ligament, the ovary could be lifted and rotated to a more convenient position for puncture. Monopolar cautery is used by holding the needle perpendicular to the ovarian surface. The follicles are punctured with simultaneous application of current for approximately one second. Power setting is 20-30 watts in cutting mode. Cortex is usually penetrated at 10-15 sites for a depth of 3-5 mm. Attempt is made to puncture almost all the prominent follicles, which amounts to 10 punctures on each ovary. The fluid mixed with the irrigating solution is completely aspirated out through the suction cannula. The ovaries are lavaged with Ringer's solution containing hydrocortisone and heparin. The bleeding is usually self-limiting and is arrested by diathermy if required. The electrocautery causes thermal damage and necrosis of the "excess" ovarian stroma. As no tissue is removed, less raw bleeding from the surface would be anticipated. Various authors have reported an ovulation rate of 70 to 90 percent with pregnancy rates of 53 to 72 percent in various studies. Kriplani et al[16], Tulandi et al[17], Radwan et al[18], Ligouri et al[19] etc are some of these authors. Saleh[20]et al have reported that beneficial effects were found after electrocauterization, whereas Amer et al[21] have reported that there was an improvement in hirsutism in 25 percent of patients and 40 percent in acne in cases treated with electrocauterization. Lemieux[22] has reported that there was a fall in the serum levels of androstenidione by 43 percent, testosterone by 48 percent, free testosterone by 48 percent and these might be reflected as the reduction in the acne and hirsutism. Felembam[23] has reported a post-operative adhesion rate of 27 percent.

Laser

When laser the KTP and CO_2 Laser[9] is used, The technique is similar to that of electrocautery, namely the ovarian cortex is vaporized over follicles. Because KTP and CO_2 laser focus their energy more precisely than electrocautery less peripheral thermal damage is inflicted. Either an ultra pulse CO_2 laser (40-80 watts, 25-200 mj) or the super pulse CO_2 laser (25-40 watts) is used. All visible subcapsular follicles are vaporized and a 2-4 mm crater is made in the ovarian stroma. It is recommended that the number of punctures be more, approximately 30 or so, or that all visible follicles be drained. With Nd: YAG laser the technique is a somewhat different. There is much more thermal diffusion in the non-contact mode with this laser. Also, the laser is divergent once it passes the sapphire tip of the delivery system. As a result, the coagulation of the tissue is achieved. A wedge shaped area of 4 to 10 mm is thus coagulated without opening the cortex. This laser has also been used in the contact mode to cut out a wedge shaped portion of the ovary not unlike the bilateral ovarian resection. The laser is now regarded to produce more excessive ovarian surface trauma, leading to adhesion formation. This is in relation to the stromal damage, which is thought to hamper ovulation. As a result, attention is now shifting towards the use of monopolar needle electrodes, that are insulated where they contact the ovarian surface. The needle punctures the ovarian surface to the depth of the insulated hub and the deeper stroma can be cauterized with minimal surface damage. Various authors like Muenstermann et al,[24] Heylen,[25] Daniell,[26] Verhelst,[27] Fukaya[28] and Huber[29] have reported an ovulation rate of 71 to 82 percent in various series with use of laser, with a pregnancy rate ranging from 41 to 75 percent. Keckstein et al[30] have reported a reduction in serum levels of Androstenidione by 63 percent and Verhelst[27] has reported no significant fall in SHBG, Prolactin, DHEA, LH levels after laser surgery. Fukaya et al[28] have, however, recorded a significant fall in LH, Testosterone and androstenidione levels with a rise in the FSH levels.

Heylen[25] et al have reported a postoperative adhesion rate of 10 percent and Osterzenski[31] has reported a rate of 8 percent.

RESULTS OF LAPAROSCOPIC TREATMENT

The summary of outcome analyzed from the aggregation of statistics by Donesky and Adashi (1995)[32] state that the results of ovarian laparoscopic surgery compare favorably with that of medical ovulation induction. The observation of lower miscarriage rate, with no risk of ovarian hyperstimulation and multiple gestation and the fact that the conception rate in subjects who failed to conceive with clomiphene was 27.59 percent after laparoscopic diathermy, all point to the fact that laparoscopic treatment indeed offers a real benefit to PCOD subjects who are attempting to conceive.

SUMMARY

What modality to choose, laser or electrocautery? From the data available to us till date, it can be concluded that ovarian follicular puncture by electrocautery and laser have similar results, with ovulation rates of 70-90 percent for electrocautery and 71-84 percent with laser. Though not many authors have studied the effects of follicular puncture by simple needle it is not thought to be equally effective. The pregnancy rates, when compared are 53-72 percent for electrocautery and 41-75 percent for laser.

The effects on the endocrine milleu are also comparable.

As far as the postoperative adhesion rates are considered the studies done so far have reported an adhesion rate of 27 percent for electrocautery and 8-10 percent for laser. The potential risk involved in the form of post operative adhesions, eventhough usually minimal and mild, is a fact to be borne in mind when operating on infertile subjects, least we convert the ovarian factor to a tubal factor. This data is, however, inadequate and more studies are required in this regard.

The cost factor and the unwieldy apparatus with the inherent hazards of laser to the operating personnel make laser surgery difficult. This is countered by the easy availability of electrocautery and the much lower cost to the health care provider gives electrocautery an edge over laser at present.

Thus, we could anticipate that, in the future we would understand the pathophysiological basis of PCOS in a better way and make the use of surgery for ovulation induction a rare event. Till then laparoscopic surgery for ovulation induction deserves an important place in the therapeutic armamentarium for anovulatory infertility.

REFERENCES

1. Stein JF, Levinthal ML. Amenorrhea associated with bilateral polycystic ovaries. Am J Obstet Gynecol 1935;29:181-91.
2. Polson DW, Wadsworth J, Adams J, Franks S. Polycystic ovaries: A common finding in normal women. Lancet 1988;1:870-2.
3. Adams J, Polson DW, et al. Multifollicular ovaries: Clinical and endocrine features and response to gonadotropin releasing hormone. Lancet 1985;2,1375-8.
4. Carey AH, Chan KL, Short F, White D, Williamson R, Franks S. Evidence for a single gene effect causing polycystic ovaries and male pattern baldness. Clin Endocrinol (Oxf) 1993;38(6):653-8.

5. Balen A, Conway GS, Kaltsas G, et al. Polycystic ovary syndrome: The spectrum of disorder in 1741 patients. Human Reprod 1995;10:2107-11.
6. Fox R, Corrigan E, Thomas PA, Hull MG. The diagnosis of polycystic ovaries in women with oligo-amenorrhoea: predictive power of endocrine tests. Clin Endocrinol (Oxf). 1991;34(2):127-31.
7. Bridges NA, Cooke A, Healy MJ, Hindmarsh PC, Brook CG. Standards for ovarian volume in childhood and puberty. Fertil Steril 1993;60(3):456-60.
8. Malkawi HY, Qublan HS, Hamaideh AH. Medical vs. surgical treatment for clomiphene citrate-resistant women with polycystic ovary syndrome. J Obstet Gynaecol 2003;23(3):289-93.
9. Vandermolen DT, Ratts VS, Evans WS, Stovall DW, Kauma SW, Nestler JE. Metformin increases the ovulatory rate and pregnancy rate from clomiphene citrate in patients with polycystic ovary syndrome who are resistant to clomiphene citrate alone. Fertil Steril 2001;75(2):310-5.
10. Kocak M, Caliskan E, Simsir C, Haberal A. Metformin therapy improves ovulatory rates, cervical scores, and pregnancy rates in clomiphene citrate-resistant women with polycystic ovary syndrome. Fertil Steril 2002;77(1): 101-6.
11. Parsanezhad ME, Alborzi S, Motazedian S, Omrani G. Use of dexamethasone and clomiphene citrate in the treatment of clomiphene citrate-resistant patients with polycystic ovary syndrome and normal dehydroepiandrosterone sulfate levels: A prospective, double-blind, placebo-controlled trial. Fertil Steril 2003;80(1):230-1; author reply 231.
12. Rajan R. Hyperinsulinemia and polycystic ovary syndrome J Obstet Gynaecol India 2001;51(4):126-8.
13. Kistner RW. The use of clomiphene citrate in the treatment of anovulation. Semin Drug Treat 1973 Autumn;3(2):159-76.
14. Ferraretti AP. Transvaginal ovarian drilling: A new surgical treatment for improving the clinical outcome of assisted reproductive technologies in patients with polycystic ovary syndrome. Fertil Steril 2001;76(4):812-6.
15. Cibula D, Cifkova R, Fanta M, et al. Increased risk of non-insulin dependant diabetes mellitus, arterial hypertension, coronary heart disease in perimenopausal women with history of the polycystic ovary syndrome. Hum Reprod 2000;15:785-9.
16. Kriplani A. Laparoscopic ovarian drilling in clomiphene citrate-resistant women with polycystic ovary syndrome. J Am Assoc Gynecol Laparosc 2001;8(4):511-8.
17. Tulandi T. Effects of laparoscopic ovarian drilling on serum vascular endothelial growth factor and on insulin responses to the oral glucose tolerance test in women with polycystic ovary syndrome. Fertil Steril 2000;74(3):585-8.
18. Radwan J. The effects of micro-laparoscopic ovarian electrocautery as a method of polycystic ovary syndrome treatment] Ginekol Pol 2001;72(8):642-6. Polish.
19. Ligouri G. Laparoscopic ovarian treatment in infertile patients with polycystic ovarian syndrome (PCOS): Endocrine changes and clinical outcome. Gynecol Endocrinol 1996;10(4):257-64.
20. Saleh A. Effects of laparoscopic ovarian drilling on adrenal steroids in polycystic ovary syndrome patients with and without hyperinsulinemia. Fertil Steril 2001;75(3):501-4.
21. Amer S A. Long-term follow-up of patients with polycystic ovarian syndrome after laparoscopic ovarian drilling: Clinical outcome. Hum Reprod 2002;17(8):2035-42.
22. Lemieux S, Lewis GF, Ben-Chetrit A, et al. Correction of hyperandrogenaemia by laparoscopic ovarian cautery in women with PCOS is not accompanied by improved insulin sensitivity or lipid lipoprotein levels. J Clin Endocrinol Metab 1999;84:4278-82.
23. Felembam A. Laparoscopic treatment of polycystic ovaries with insulated needle cautery: A reappraisal. Fertil Steril 2000;73(2):266-9.
24. Muenstermann U. Long-term GnRH analogue treatment is equivalent to laparoscopic laser diathermy in polycystic ovarian syndrome patients with severe ovarian dysfunction. Hum Reprod 2000;15(12):2526-30.
25. Heylen SM. Polycystic ovarian disease treated by laparoscopic argon laser capsule drilling: Comparison of vaporization versus perforation technique. Hum Reprod 1994;9(6):1038-42.
26. Daniell JF. Polycystic ovaries treated by laparoscopic laser vaporization. Fertil Steril 1989;51(2):232-6.
27. Verhelst J. Clinical and endocrine effects of laser vaporization in patients with polycystic ovarian disease. Gynecol Endocrinol 1993;7(1):49-55.
28. Fukaya T. Laser vaporization of the ovarian surface in polycystic ovary disease results in reduced ovarian hyperstimulation and improved pregnancy rates.Am J Obstet Gynecol 1995;173(1):119-25.
29. Huber J. Polycystic ovarian syndrome treated by laser through the laparoscope. Lancet. 1988 Jul 23;2(8604):215.
30. Keckstein G; The effect of laparoscopic treatment of polycystic ovarian disease by CO_2-laser or Nd:YAG laser. Surg Endosc 1990;4(2):103-7.
31. Osterzenski A. Endoscopic carbon dioxide laser ovarian wedge resection in resistant polycystic ovarian disease. Int J Fertil 1992;37(5):295-9.
32. Donesky BW, Adashi EY. Surgically induced ovulation in PCOS, wedge resection revisited in the age of laparoscopy. Fertil Steril 1995;63:439-63.

23 Laparoscopic Management of Benign Ovarian Mass

Pravin Patel, Manish Banker, Manish Shah

INTRODUCTION

Ovarian masses occur in all stages of a woman's life, from childhood to menopause. During childhood germ cell tumors are most common accounting for one half to two-third of cases.[1] Functional cysts of ovary mainly predominate during reproductive ages while almost 30 percent of the ovarian masses during menopause are borderline or malignant. Majority of ovarian tumors are benign (80-85%) and most of them (66%) of them are occurring in female of reproductive age group (Table 23.1).[2]

Advent of new techniques and gadgets has widened the scope of operative laparoscopy. Advantages of laparoscopy compared with laparotomy are well known. These advantages have been demonstrated in operations for benign ovarian cysts by laparoscopy by Mais et al in 1996.[3] Whether treatment is conservative (intra or transparietal cystectomy) or radical (salpingo-oophorectomy), several series have established that operative laparoscopy offers efficient surgical management of benign ovarian cysts, even in the case of dermoid cysts and endometriomas. Laparoscopic removal of benign ovarian cysts is an effective technique, involving little risk of complications.[4] However, thorough preoperative evaluation of the patient considering the risk of possible malignancy is the most important thing, as inappropriately carried out laparoscopy in patients with malignancy may hamper future prognosis (Figure 23.1).

Preoperative Screening

Preoperative screening consists of clinical history, bimanual pelvic examination, ultrasound preferably vaginal, color Doppler study of ovarian mass and tumor markers such as CA 125 and CEA.

Bimanual pelvic examination establishes the nature of the mass and its relationship to the adjacent organs. An ipsilateral mass smaller than 7-8 cm in size, unilocular with smooth surface, freely mobile mostly favors the diagnosis of benign ovarian cyst.[5]

High frequency vaginal ultrasound produces greater image resolution (sensitivity 100% and specificity 83%)

Table 23.1. Classification of benign ovarian mass

Functional cysts	Follicular cysts (Figures 23.2 and 23.3) Corpus luteum cysts Theca lutein cysts
Inflammatory	Tubo-ovarian abscess or complex
Neoplastic	Germ cell tumor Benign cystic teratoma Epithelial tumors Serous cystadenoma Mucinous cystadenoma Fibroma Cystadenofibroma Brenner tumor Mixed tumor
Others	Endometrioma

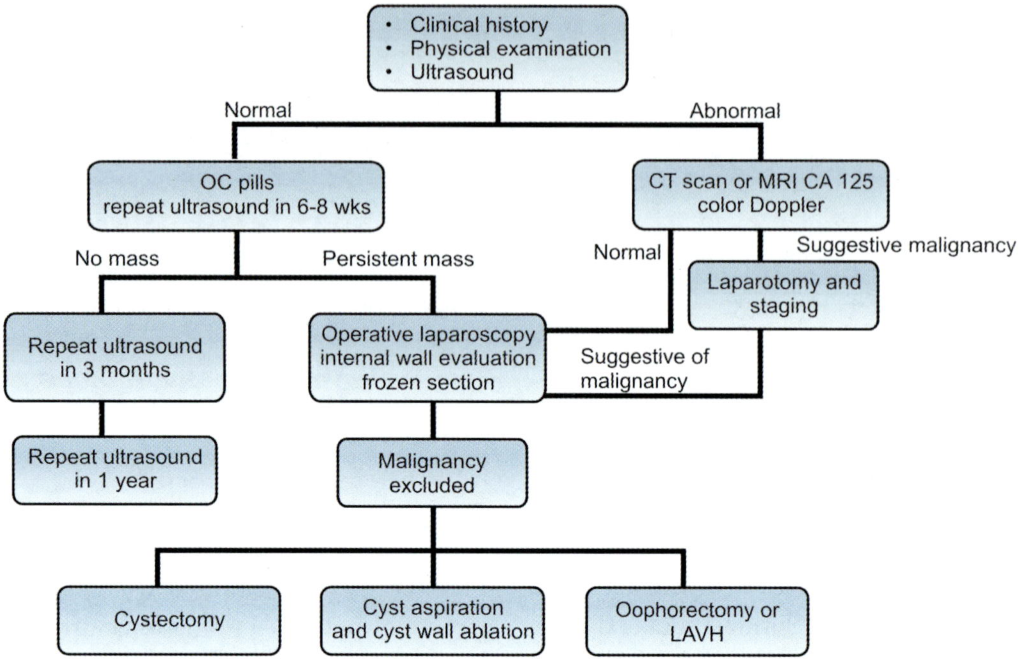

Figure 23.1. Laparoscopic management of benign ovarian masses: An overview

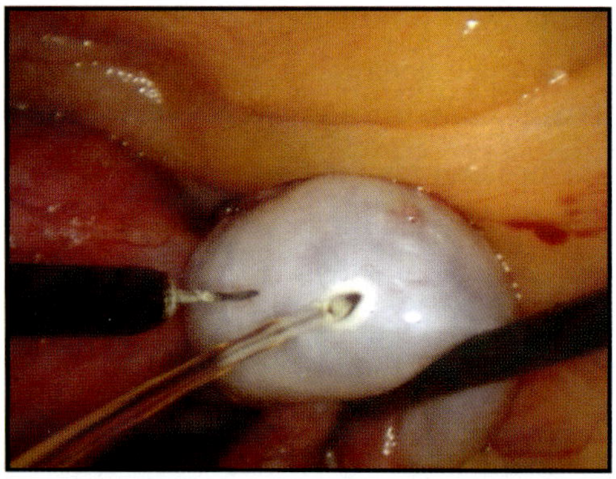

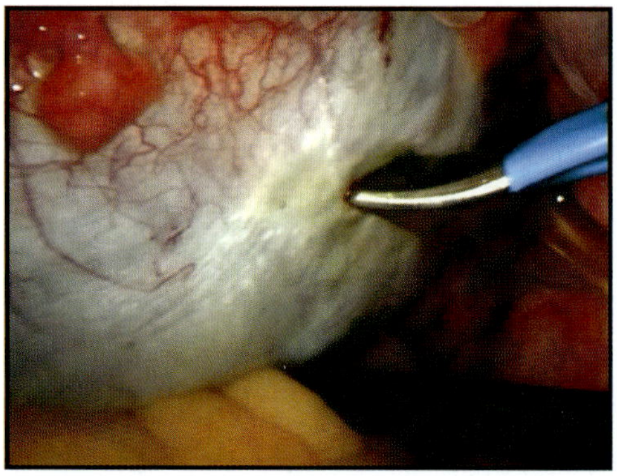

Figures 23.2 and 23.3. Puncture of simple follicular ovarian cyst at its most dependant part using scissors or monopolar needle

than the abdominal, thus allowing more detailed morphological assessment of ovarian masses and thus helps in ruling out ovarian malignancy.[6] Maggino et al[7] has proposed the following criteria for classification of ovarian masses.

Class I: Probable Benign Mass

- Dimensions < 5 cm
- Clear thin wall
- Non-echogenous content
- No septa or up to three thin septa
- No free fluid in pouch of Douglas.

Class II: Borderline Malignant Mass

- Dimensions from 5 to 10 cm and/or
- Clear, smooth, thick wall and/or
- Hypoechogenic liquid content or solid homogenous content and/or
- More than three thin septa and/or
- Thick but regular septa and/or

- Absence of endocystic projections and/or
- Absence of free peritoneal fluid.

Class III: Malignant Mass

- None of the above features are observed.

Transvaginal color Doppler ultrasound further classifies the mass by studying its vascularization. It allows the positioning of the probe closer to the mass and visually reflects the state of blood flow of the ovarian tumor; it permits the detection of low resistance intramural blood vessels, characteristic of malignant tumors. Bourne and co-workers[8] reported that low impedance (pulsatility index PI <1) was associated with malignant ovarian tumors. Based on these measurements, Fleischer[9] et al has proposed following parameters for differentiating benign and malignant mass.

Benign tumors

- PI > 1 (high impedance flow)
- Peripheral blood flow
- Diastolic end

Malignant tumors

- PI < 1 (low impedance flow)
- Central blood flow
- No diastolic end.

Preoperative evaluation of serum CA 125 level especially in patients of perimenopausal age in excess of 65 IU/ml distinguishes malignant from benign disease with a specificity of 92 percent and sensitivity of 75 percent.[10]

Ultrasound guided aspiration of ovarian cysts followed by cytological examination has a diagnostic reliability of 85-95 percent. However, this method is not sufficient to rule out malignancy.

High-resolution CT scan and MRI provide high quality images of the ovaries and are equally sensitive as sonography.

Intraoperative assessment ovarian mass based on the visual characteristics of ovarian surface such as vascularization, papillary or vesicular projections, and adhesions to other organs helps in deciding the future course of surgery. It is important to differentiate between organic and functional cysts also; 10-20 percent of functional cysts do not disappear after 3 months of treatment with combination oral pills. In retrospective study of 226 patients, Mage and colleagues[11] reported that the diagnosis of malignant tumors by laparoscopy was 100 percent accurate. They have laid down five laparoscopic criteria to differentiate between functional and organic cysts (Table 23.2).

Table 23.2. Laparoscopic criteria for differentiation between functional and organic ovarian cysts

Criterion	*Organic cysts*	*Functional cysts*
Utero-ovarian ligament	Lengthened	Normal
Cyst wall	Thick	Thin
Ovarian vessels	Numerous and regular starting from mesovarium	More scanty, coral like
Cyst fluid	Clear, dark, brown, or dermoid	Saffron yellow
Internal cyst wall appearance	Smooth or fibrotic with areas of hyper-vascularization	Retina like aspect

SURGICAL PROCEDURES

Ovarian cystectomy is choice of surgery for women of reproductive age with a purpose of preserving the fertility. All the benign ovarian pathologies can be managed by this method in three ways:

- Intact cyst removal (Figures 23.4 to 23.6).
- Aspiration and excision of cyst wall (Figures 23.7 and 23.8).
- Aspiration and ablation of cyst wall (Figure 23.9)

Complete ovarian cyst removal with minimal trauma to the residual ovarian tissue provides specimen for histology and minimizes the chances of recurrence. Canis et al[12] and Childers et al[13] both have individually advocated enucleation of ovarian cyst and possibly saving the ovarian tissue. Aspiration and ablation of cyst wall (Figure 23.9) does not destroy the entire cyst wall and increases chances of recurrence and damages the underlying cortex by heat. Therefore, excision is preferred but intact excision of larger cysts of more than

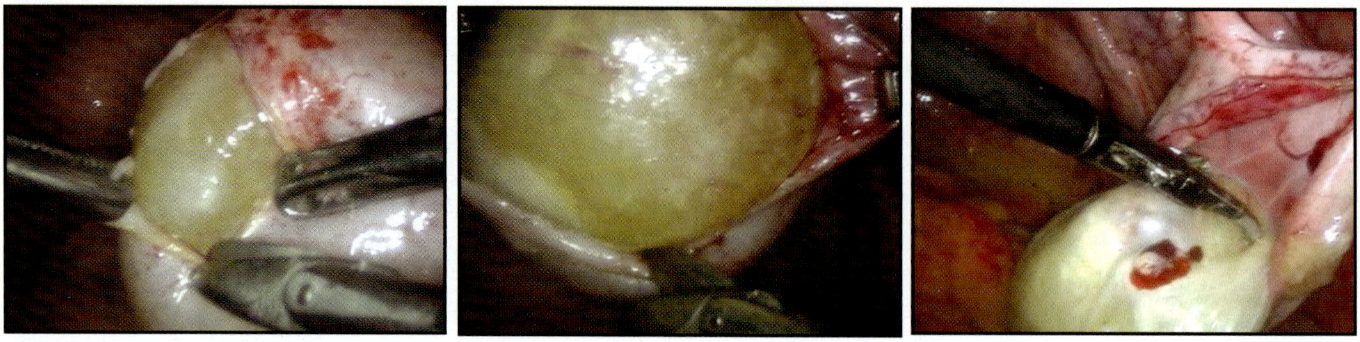

Figures 23.4 to 23.6. Ovarian cortex incision with scissors: Removal of dermoid cyst en mass

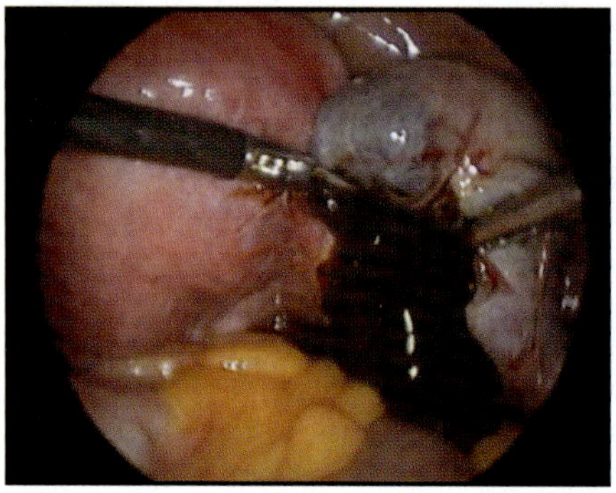

Figure 23.7. Puncture of chocolate cyst and drainage of fluid

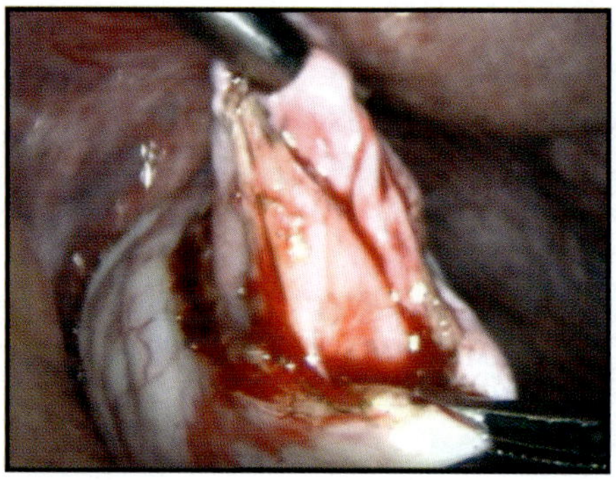

Figure 23.8. Chocolate cyst wall enucleation

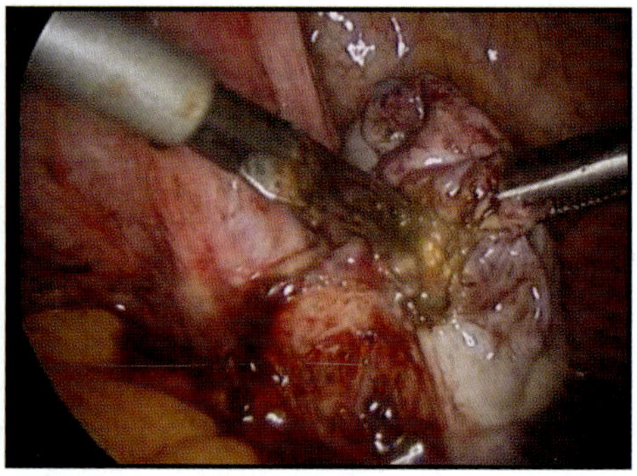

Figure 23.9. Chocolate cyst wall ablation

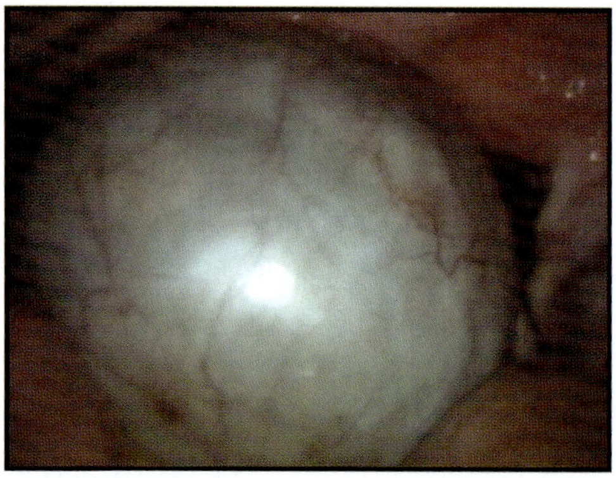

Figure 23.10. Large ovarian cyst

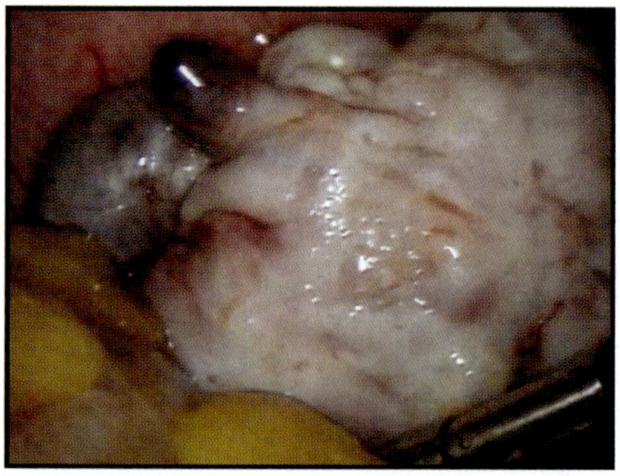

Figure 23.11. Large chocolate cyst

10 cm in diameter (Figures 23.10 and 23.11) may sometime be difficult. It may rupture during manipulation. A large cyst is first punctured with an 18-gauze needle or by direct trocar insertion in to the cyst and aspiration of contents (Figures 23.12 and 23.13). Interior of the cyst wall is then checked for any intracystic vegetation (Figure 23.14). If they are found then, a biopsy with frozen section is carried out before a decision is made whether to perform cystectomy or oophorectomy.

Complete separation of cyst wall from the surrounding ovarian cortex is carried out using atraumatic forceps (Figure 23.8). By traction and counter-traction, the dissection is carried out and the cyst is removed. Injection of 3-5 ml of dilute vasopressin or only normal

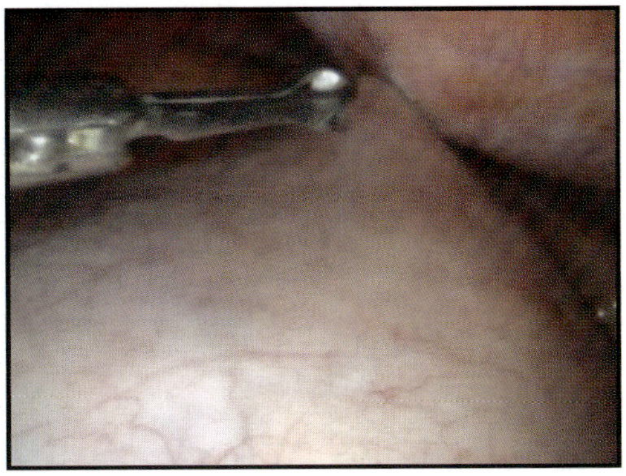
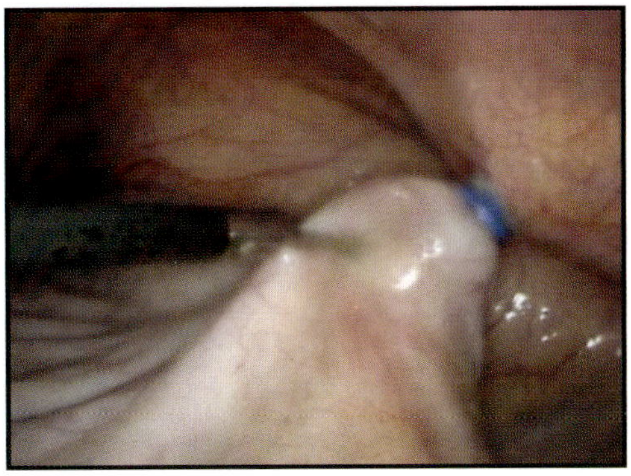

Figures 23.12 and 23.13. Decompression of large chocolate cyst by direct insertion of trocar into the cyst and suction of the cyst contents. This avoids spillage of contents into the peritoneal cavity

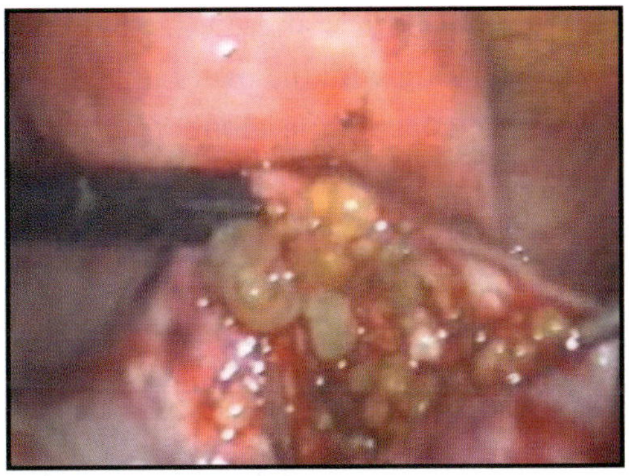

Figure 23.14. Borderline ovarian tumor having papillary excrescences

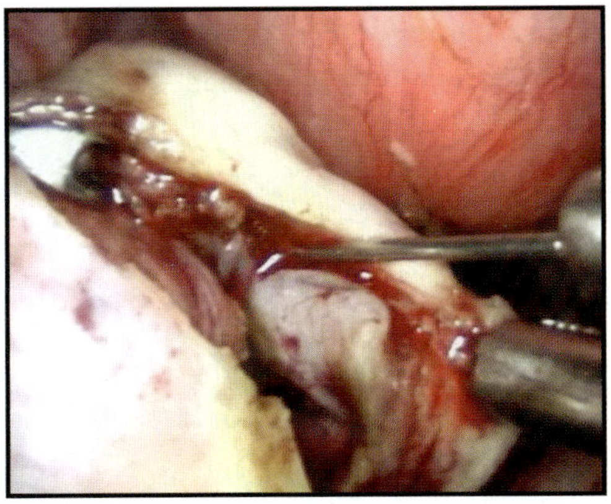

Figure 23.15. Hydrodissection using saline injection for cyst wall enucleation; this facilitates easy plane of cleavage for complete cyst wall removal

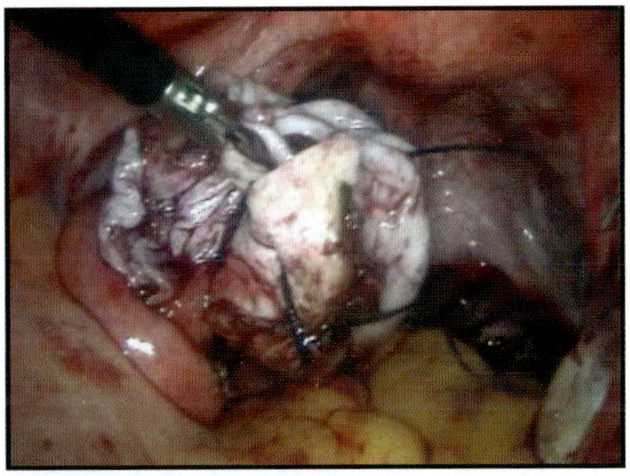

Figure 23.16. Ovarian suturing

saline between the capsule and ovarian cortex creates tissue plane (Hydrodissection) and reduces bleeding (Figure 23.15).[14] After the cyst is excised, the base is coagulated with the help of bipolar forceps. However, aggressive electrocoagulation can be the cause of ovarian destruction and premature ovarian failure. Generally, the bleeding is self-limiting and the ovary heals without the need for suturing. Ovarian edges approximate spontaneously. In cases of large cysts where approximation is problem, suturing is preferred option using 2-0 delayed absorbable materials (Figure 23.16). Use of titanium clips or fibrin sealant[15] is useful in controlling microvascular or capillary bleeding and closing the ovarian cortex after cystectomy.

In cases of endometrioma, Donnez proposed only opening the cyst, coagulating the borders and letting the endometrioma dry out.[16] This practice is based on the theory of how an endometrioma is formed. However, enucleation of cyst wall is the preferred method (Figure 23.8) and when it is not possible, bipolar coagulation of cyst lining is done (Figure 23.9).

In cases of dermoid cysts, complete enucleation of dermoid cyst without spillage of the contents in young patients is preferred (Figures 23.4 to 23.6). Oophorectomy or salpingo-oophorectomy is performed only in postmenopausal women. Postoperative lavage with 5 to 7 liters of saline decreases the chances of adhesions and patient morbidity.[17]

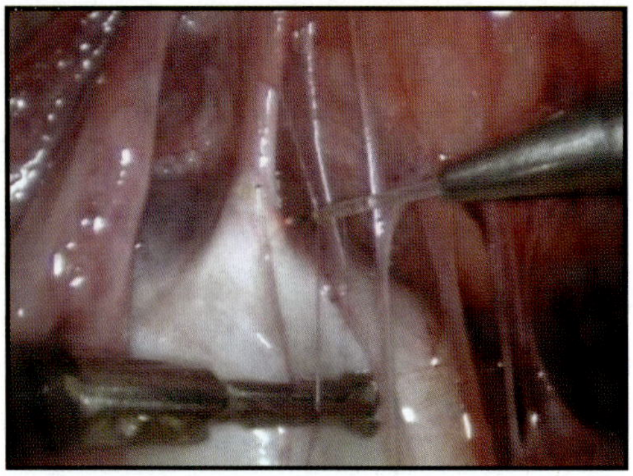

Figure 23.19. Adhesiolysis using Nd: YAG laser exposing the ovarian mass

Laparoscopic Oophorectomy (Figures 23.17 and 23.18) is usually indicated in perimenopausal women with an ovarian mass who have finished childbearing or in cases of severe damage to the ovarian tissue or when there is no viable tissue left after cystectomy. Tubes are usually removed along with the ovary unless previously removed. Bipolar coagulation along with excision has completely replaced the earlier method of applying pre-tied loop ligatures and cutting the ovary. One of the recent technique for laparoscopic oophorectomy is automatic stapling device which reduces the operating time but more expensive than bipolar coagulation. In certain cases of ovarian adhesions, aquadissection, blunt probing, scissors, and judicious use of bipolar coagulation are necessary to mobilize the ovary for laparoscopic removal (Figure 23.19). Aggressive ovariolysis increases the risk of ureteral or bowel injury, or severe bleeding. Extensive ovarian adhesiolysis to avoid incomplete removal of all functional ovarian tissue is necessary to avoid possible chances of persistent ovarian remnant syndrome in some cases.[18]

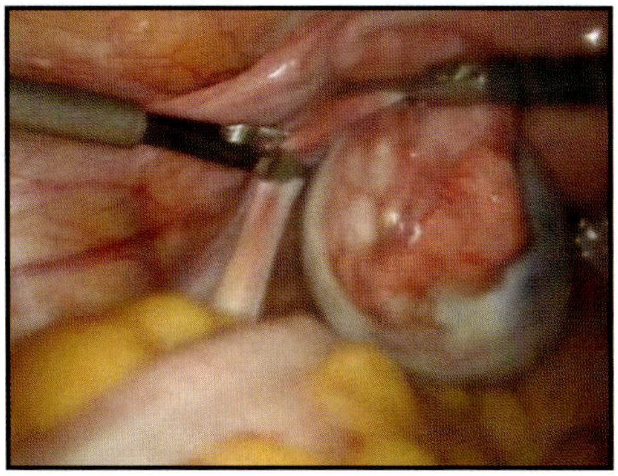

Figure 23.17. Salpingo-oophorectomy: Infundibulopelvic ligament being grasped and coagulated

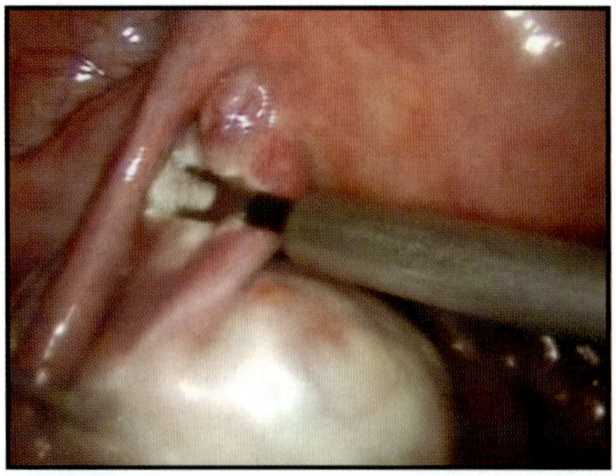

Figure 23.18. Salpingo-oophorectomy: Utero-ovarian ligament being grasped and coagulated

TISSUE RETRIEVAL METHODS

Removal in Endobag (Figures 23.20 and 23.21)

After enucleation of cyst wall or oophorectomy, the tissue is grasped with forceps and removed from the abdominal cavity. However, this type of removal is possible only when there is a small ovarian cyst. Larger tissue mass is usually removed by placing it into a specially designed Endobag introduced inside the abdominal cavity through a 10 mm trocar. The bag is then removed by applying

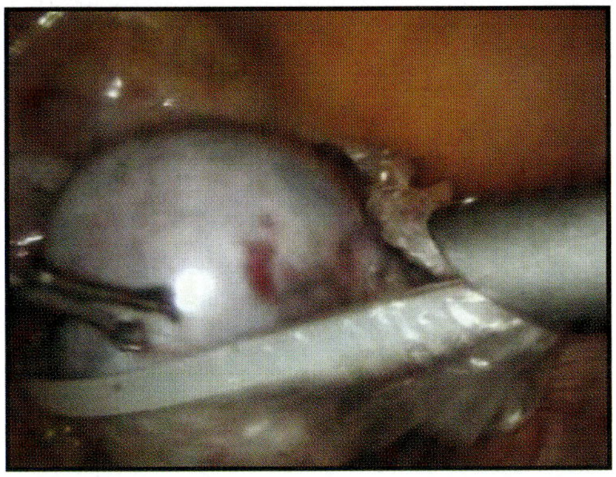

Figure 23.20. Removal of intact dermoid cyst using Endobag: As cyst is decompressed inside the bag, this avoids spillage of contents into the abdomen

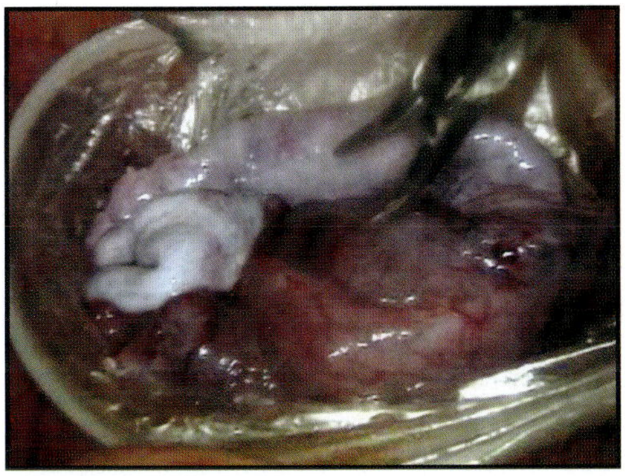

Figure 23.21. Cyst wall retrieval using Endobag

traction to the bag and pulling it through a trocar incision by removing the port. Aspirating the cyst contents deflates the cyst and cyst is then pulled out of abdomen. Bigger tissue mass is morcellated inside the bag only and then removed piecemeal. This method of tissue retrieval is most widely accepted as it nullifies chances of possible spillage in cases of undiagnosed ovarian malignancy.[18,19]

Direct Tissue Removal through Abdominal Incision

In confirmed benign pathologies, the tissue is removed directly with an instrument introduced through a suprapubic incision without using a bag. However, there are some reports of developing ovarian remnant or induced endometriosis at the site of trocar insertion.[21] Nezhat and co-workers have not observed this phenomenon in their 1-3 year follow-up in the patients who underwent this technique of cyst wall removal.[22]

Culdotomy

In cases of large tissue mass such as dermoid cyst, the mass is placed in the cul-de-sac and colpotomy is carried out and cyst is removed intact or aspirated through vagina. Directing a needle through the vagina usually decompresses cyst. Thick contents of cysts are removed by introducing a suction cannula through the incision followed by copious intraperitoneal irrigation.

Ovarian Torsion (Figure 23.22)

As it is a surgical emergency, diagnosis of this condition has to be prompt. Clinical correlation along with color Doppler ultrasound or in rare cases MRI, CT scan diagnoses the condition. If it remains undetected, the cyst becomes hemorrhagic, necrotic and ischemic. Too much delay causes gangrenous changes, which are irreversible, and adnexectomy is the final treatment. Ovarian torsion can occur in all types of ovarian cysts. However, large ovarian mass, dermoid cysts, ovarian hyperstimulation, and cysts associated with adhesions are commonest conditions associated with it. Immediate untwisting of the pedicle using atraumatic forceps and simultaneous

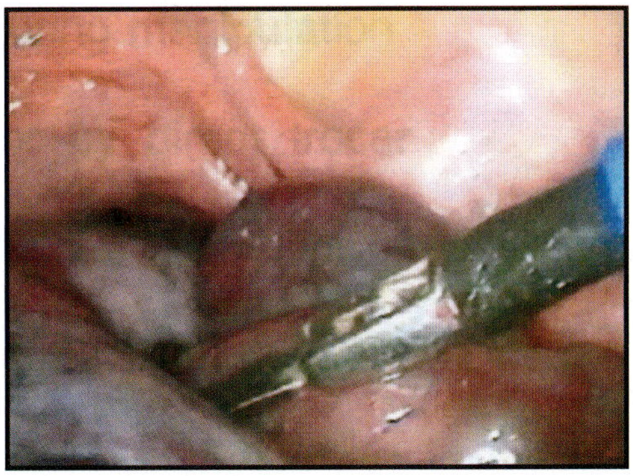

Figure 23.22. Ovarian torsion resulting in hemorrhagic ovarian mass

correction of underlying cause is the treatment of choice. Rarely stay sutures to prevent recurrence is necessary.

CONCLUSION

Most of the ovarian pathologies can be treated by laparoscopy. However, careful preoperative and perioperative examination is required to eliminate the possibility of malignancy and worsening the prognosis for the patient. Laparoscopic operations have changed postoperative morbidity, length of hospitalization, blood loss and quality of life. Though, advantages outweigh the risk in cases of benign ovarian mass, surgeon should be prepared to proceed with staging laparotomy if suspicious malignant lesion found unexpectedly so as to give optimum benefit to the patient.

REFERENCES

1. Granberg S, Norstorm A, Wikland M. Tumors in lower pelvis as imaged by vaginal ultrasound. Gynecol Oncol 1989;37:224.
2. Goldstein SR, Subramanyam B, Snyder JR, Beller U, Raghavendra N, Beckman EM. The postmenopausal cystic adnexal mass: The potential role of ultrasound in conservative management. Obstet Gynecol 1988;73:80.
3. Mais V, Ajossa S, Piras B. Treatment of non-endometriotic benign adnexal cysts: A randomized comparison of laparoscopy and laparotomy. Obstet Gynecol 1996;86: 770-4.
4. Bruhat MA, Mage G, Chapron C, et al. Present day endoscopic surgery in gynecology. Eur J Obstet Gynecol Reprod Biol 1991;41:4-13.
5. DiSaia, Creasman WT. The adnexal mass and ovarian cancer. Clinical Gynecologic Oncology. Fourth edition, Mosby-Year Book Inc 1993;295.
6. Sassone AM, Timor-Tritsch IE, Artner A, Westhff C, Warren WB. Transvaginal sonographic characterization of ovarian disease: Evaluation of a new scoring system to predict ovarian malignancy. Obstet Gynecol 1991; 78:70-6.
7. Maggino T, Gadducci A, D'Addario V, Percorelli S, Lissoni A, Stella M, et al. Prospective multicenter study on CA 125 in postmenopausal pelvic masses. Gynecol Oncol 1994;54:117-23.
8. Bourne T, Campbell S, Steer C, et al. Transvaginal color flow imaging: A possible new screening technique for ovarian cancer. Br Med J 1989;299:1367-70.
9. Fleischer AC, Rodgers W, Kepple D, Williams L. Color Doppler sonography of ovarian Masses: A multicenter analysis. J Ultrasound Med 1993;I:41-8.
10. Malkasian GD, Knapp RC, Lavin PT, et al. preoperative evaluation of serum CA-125 levels in premenopausal and postmenopausal patients with pelvic masses: Discrimination of benign from malignant disease. Am J Obstet Gynecol 1988;159:341-6.
11. Mage G, Canis M, Manhes G, et al. Kystes ovariens et coelioscopie. A propos de 226 observation. J Gynecol Obstet Biol Reprod 1987;16:1053-61.
12. Canis M, Pouly JI, Wattiez A, Mage G, Manhes H, Bruhat MA. Laparoscopic management of adnexal masses suspicious at ultrasound. Obstet Gynecol 1997;5(1):679-83.
13. Childers JM, Nasseri A, Surwit EA. Laparoscopic management of suspicious adnexal masses. Am J Obstet Gynecol 175(6):1451-57; discussion 1996;1457-59s
14. Nezhat C, Winer WK, Nezhat F. Laparoscopic removal of dermoid cyst. Obstet Gynecol 1989;73:278-80.
15. Donnez J, Nisolle M. Laparoscopic management of large ovarian endometrial cysts: Use of fibrin sealant. J Gynecol Surg 1991;7:163-7.
16. Donnez J, Nisolle M, Smoes P. Peritoneal endometriosis and endometriotic nodules of the rectovaginal septum are two different entities. Fertil Steril 1996;66:362-8.
17. Lin P, Falcone T, Tulandi T. Excision of ovarian dermoid cyst by laparoscopy and by laparotomy. Am J Obstet Gynecol 1995;173(3 Pt 1):769-71.
18. Campo S, Garcea N. Laparoscopic conservative excision of ovarian dermoid cysts with and without an Endobag. J Am Assoc Gynecol Laparosc 1998;5(2):165-70.
19. Teng FY, Muzsnai D, Perez R, et al. A comparative study of laparoscopy and colpotomy for the removal of ovarian dermoid cysts. Obstet Gynecol 1996;87(6):1009-13.
20. Hsiu JG, Given FT, Kemp GM. Tumor implantation after diagnostic laparoscopic biopsy of serous ovarian tumors of low malignant potential. Obstet Gynecol 1986;68:91-3.

24 Laparoscopic Management of Adnexal Masses

M Ramesh

INTRODUCTION

At the outset I wish to state that I am not a Gynecologist by profession, but have been associated with several of my colleagues including three members in my family, who are all gynecologists. Having pioneered laparoscopic surgery in my region I have been involved in performing several types of laparoscopies including GI, Endocrine, Thoracic, Gynecological and Urological surgeries. Having performed a few thousands of gynecological laparoscopies and having trained over a hundred gynecologists to perform laparoscopic surgeries. I take it as my prerogative to write this article.

Over the last 30-40 years ever since laparoscopic tubal ligation was started there has been a total revolution by which today almost all adnexal masses are being managed by laparoscopy.[7,8] The distinct advantage of laparoscopy over open surgery, apart from decreased morbidity[10] has been a significantly improved vision of adnexa which are situated deep inside the pelvis behind the broad ligaments. A magnified vision has also given us an opportunity to manage most pathologies surgically with more precision.[5,9] Besides, laparoscopic adnexectomy can be performed during pregnancy also.[25]

Most women with an adnexal mass do not have any symptoms. The mass is detected either during a routine physical examination or more commonly during ultrasonological examination of the pelvis. Because ovarian malignancy is always a possibility these masses deserve due respect. Coming to the diagnosis of these masses several factors need to be considered:

Age

In girls younger than 9 years 80 percent of ovarian masses are malignant and are generally germ cell tumors. During adolescence 50 percent of adnexal tumors are adult cystic teratomas.[18] Women with gonades that contain Y chromosome have a 25 percent chance of developing a malignant neoplasm. Endometriosis is present in almost 50 percent of those who present with a painful mass. In sexually active adolescents tubo-ovarian abscess may be a common cause.

Pain

Pain that recurs periodically may be associated with torsion which may eventually lead to infarction. Once infarction has set in, pain is continuous and progressively worsens. Peritoneal signs may be present in these cases. Pain related to menstrual cycles suggest endometriosis. Acute pain of short duration particularly after exertion or intercourse may be due to rupture of a cyst. Intraperitoneal bleeding should be considered if such a pain becomes progressively worse. If pain is preceded by amenorrhea or pregnancy symptoms ectopic pregnancy should be strongly suspected.

Clinical Findings

Adnexal masses that are fixed, irregular or solid are suspicious of malignancy. The presence of ascites or upper abdominal mass should be considered malignant unless proved otherwise.

ULTRASOUND

It is the hallmark of diagnosis of adnexal masses. Ovarian ultrasound requires special expertise and best results are obtained by using high-resolution equipment. The test helps to localize the lesion (e.g. ovarian, uterine, etc.) Scoring systems such as that suggested by DePriest and associates[20] can than be used to determine the likelihood of a malignant component.[29,30] Suspicious findings of malignancy include a mass with irregular borders, papillations, solid areas, thick septae, ascites or matted bowel. Transvaginal sonography has proved to be of good value for screening and detection of early ovarian cancer.[17,19,20]

Hysterosonography may be used to help distinguish between uterine masses and those arising from other pelvic structures.

Color Doppler ultrasonography can evaluate the resistive index of the mass vessels, which when low, is indicative of malignancy.[17]

CT SCAN

This helps to identify the size of the mass and its relation to other organs. It is less effective than ultrasonography for determining the internal architecture of these masses. CT angiograms have been useful for evaluating the vasculature of the masses. This is particularly useful in sarcomas.

MRI SCANS

MR imaging has been used for those who do not tolerate contrast material necessary for CT scanning. Gadolinium-enhanced MR imaging is highly accurate in the detection and characterization of complex adnexal masses.[23]

OTHER INVESTIGATIONS

A barium enema or colonoscopy is required to rule out large bowel neoplasms in older women. Intravenous pyelography is reserved for cases that need to exclude congenital anomalies of the urologic system, especially pelvic kidney.

The hormonal assays do not generally have much value in adnexal masses. However, estrogen and progesterone estimation may be helpful in cases suspected to have germ cell tumors and in girls younger than 12 years presenting with a mass. Beta hCG estimation is important in gestational trophoblastic tumors.

CA-125 value greater than 35 U/ml in a post-menopausal patient is not conclusive, but leads to suspicion of malignancy.

GENERAL CONSIDERATIONS OF LAPAROSCOPIC SURGERY FOR ADNEXAL MASSES

Patient is examined under general anesthesia to assess the adnexal mass under total relaxation. Pneumoperitoneum is created either by Veress needle technique or Hasson's technique through a subumbilical incision. The author prefers the latter as the present meta-analysis indicates that injuries are about 15 percent less with open technique. A general survey of the whole of the abdomen is done. A secondary port is introduced in the left iliac fossa avoiding the subcutaneous and the inferior epigastric vessels. A similar port is introduced on the opposite side. A third secondary port is introduced in the midline in the suprapubic region, above the urinary bladder. On many occasions surgery can be performed with only two ports, and if it is so, then either the right or the midline port is omitted. The patient is placed in the Trendelenburg position and the bowel is lifted off from the pelvis. Uterine manipulation is done to antevert and lift the uterus. Careful inspection of the pelvis is done methodically starting from the urinary bladder, UV fossa, anterior surface of the uterus, fundus, round ligaments, tubes, ovaries, infundibulo-pelvic ligaments, posterior surface of the uterus, uterosacral ligaments and the pouch of Douglas.

This can be done by simultaneous uterine manipulation which helps in visualization of the various uterine surfaces and also stretch the adnexa, along with manipulation of the adnexa with instruments. A blunt tipped instrument or a palpation probe is inserted between the lateral border of the uterus and the ovarian ligament as far as the cervix and abutting against the broad ligament, is slowly swept laterally. This movement stretches the ovarian ligament, then pushes the ovary out of the pelvis and rotates the ovary so that the anterior surface of the ovary can be visualized. Besides the tube is also pushed laterally and cranially so that the lateral part of the tube and fimbria are seen. Sometimes this maneuver may be difficult on the left side as the sigmoid colon may be adherent to parts of the left pelvic wall and broad ligament, and in such cases we need to use another instrument to keep the colon away or pull up the ovary as the instrument is being moved laterally. Then the ovary and tube move medial to the sigmoid colon and can be seen.

The specific steps of surgery for various pathologies are considered individually.

POLYCYSTIC OVARY AND ANOVULATION

Anovulation is the key factor for polycystic ovarian syndrome. 50 percent of women are amenorrheic; there is dysfunctional uterine bleeding in 30 percent. Hirsutism is found in 70 percent of them. Obesity is the common factor, present in 35-60 percent in women with PCO. Approximately 20-40 percent may have normal LH : FSH ratio.

CLINICAL RECOMMENDATIONS

It is advisable to perform endometrial biopsy to rule out hyperplasia. The duration of unopposed estrogen should determine who should undergo biopsy. If the treatment is not for infertility Medroxy Progesterone acetate 10 mg, cycle days 1-10 per month is adequate for protection.[28] In patients with increased cardiovascular risk, abnormal lipids, hirsutism, no desire for pregnancy, but who have a need for contraception, oral contraceptives are appropriate. Treatment of hirsutism with glucocorticoids should be done with caution in women with insulin sensitivity. Spirinolactone and Frusemide do not affect insulin sensitivity, weight loss should be recommended to all patients above ideal body weight.

The surgical treatment of polycystic ovaries is by performing ovarian drilling. The advantages of this procedure is that it is cheaper and easier than the hormonal approach which requires an ongoing monitoring by repeated hormonal assays and ultrasound scanning. It also decreases the risk of multiple pregnancy. Laparoscopic ovarian drilling has been found to carry less risk of adhesion formation than after laparotomy and wedge resection.

TECHNIQUE OF OVARIAN DRILLING

The following ports are introduced:

A primary 5 mm port at the umbilicus, two 5 mm secondary ports, one in each iliac fossa. If the patient is very obese and reaching out to the other iliac fossa is difficult, then a midline suprapubic port may be preferred to the right iliac fossa port.

- Uterus is anteverted using a uterine manipulator.
- A preliminary inspection of the uterus and adnexa is done.
- An atraumatic grasper is introduced through the left iliac fossa port and the right ovarian ligament is grasped. The ovary is lifted and rotated to bring it out of the pelvis and move it away from the right fallopian tube. A needle is introduced through the right iliac fossa or midline port and brought in contact with one of the cysts on the right ovary. Holding the needle in this position, monopolar diathermy is applied with cutting mode of energy, to cause a puncture in the cyst opposed to the needle. Now the needle is brought in contact to another cyst and diathermy is applied similarly for a very short spurt. Care is taken not to penetrate the needle tip deep into the ovary so that the ovarian stroma is not damaged by the thermal effect of diathermy. This is repeated in about 10 sites

where cysts are seen. Soon after the drilling is completed, saline irrigation is carried out, to cool the ovary. Hemostasis is achieved by bringing needle in contact to any of the puncture sites that is bleeding and applying coagulation mode of diathermy.

- The grasper is now introduced through the right sided port to grasp the left ovarian ligament and the needle is introduced from the left side. The same procedure is repeated on the left ovary.
- All the fluid collected in the pouch of Douglas is aspirated as this fluid is rich in LH and is prone to cause adhesions in the pelvis.

PROBLEMS

If uterus is acutely retroverted or uterine manipulation is difficult an extra port can be introduced to retract bowel, lift the uterus and anteverted introduce the grasper between the lateral border of the uterus and ovarian ligament, apply a lateral sweep on the ovary and tube and this maneuver should bring the ovary up and laterally.

If the ovaries are very large manipulation and rotation is difficult. If manipulating the ovarian ligament is not able to bring all the cysts in access to the needle then the ovary can be lightly grasped with a large atraumatic grasper and moved. An extra port can also be introduced to either manipulate the ovary or puncture the cysts from a different direction or to retract other organs.

There can be bleeding either from the sites of ovarian puncture or due to a tear of the ovarian ligament during ovarian manipulation. If bleeding persists applying pressure for some time helps. Use of bipolar diathermy with a microbipolar forceps can control bleeding without much damage to neighboring tissue.

Care should be taken to isolate all organs and tissues away from the needle, especially while using diathermy.

Other complications of ovarian drilling include formation of pelvic adhesions, ovarian atrophy and premature menopause. The risk of adhesions should be minimized by careful hemostasis, good peritoneal lavage and suction of all the fluid as well as by leaving either Ringer's lactate solution or normal saline at the end of procedure.

OVARIAN CYSTECTOMY

Simple cysts bigger than 7 cm are considered pathological and are taken up for surgical removal. Post-menopausal women with simple cysts more than 3 cm need to be excised.[21]

Small cyst of the ovary can be treated by aspiration. The ovary is steadied with a grasper holding either ovarian ligament or pushing the ovary against the pelvic wall or broad ligament, a needle is introduced into the cyst and all the fluid is aspirated.

They can also be treated by partially excising the cyst wall. The ovary is steadied with a grasper either holding the ovarian ligament or the ovary itself. Using monopolar needle or scissors, the cyst wall along with the overlying capsule of the ovary is excised partially. The rest of the cyst is inspected. The remaining cyst wall is destroyed by superficial diathermy or laser.

Thin walled cysts of the ovary can be excised by two methods:[2,3,7]

Open Technique

The ovary is steadied with a grasper holding either ovarian ligament or pushing the ovary against the pelvic wall or broad ligament. A needle is introduced into the cyst and all the fluid is aspirated. Alternatively if the cyst is large the trocar is directly pierced into the cysts and a 5 mm suction cannula is used through the cannula to aspirate the cyst contents (Figures 24.1 to 24.4). The puncture site is incised further till the ovarian capsule and cyst wall are separately seen. These two structures are held separately with graspers and peeled apart till the inner cyst wall is extracted everting the ovarian capsule. There may be a small part of the ovarian cyst densely adherent to the ovarian stroma. This part is separated using bipolar diathermy and short dissection. The inside of the ovary is inspected for any oozing (Figure 24.5). Hemostasis is ensured using bipolar diathermy (Figure 24.6). Irrigation

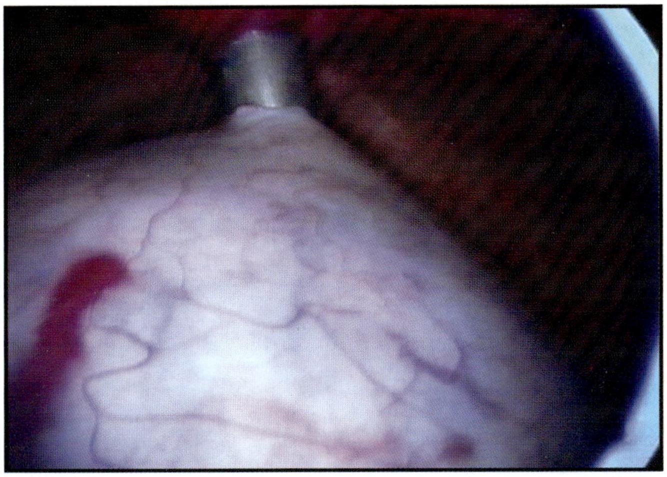

Figure 24.1. Trocar insertion into cyst

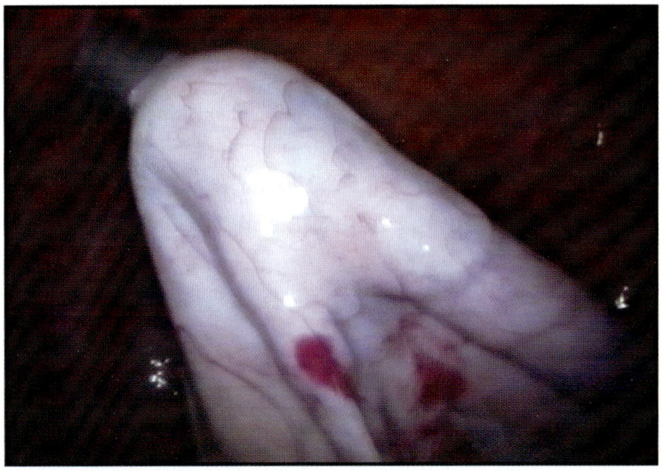

Figure 24.2. Aspiration of contents without spill

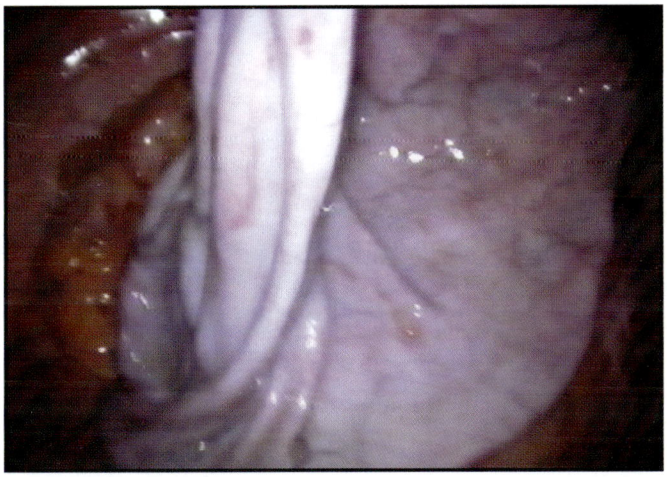

Figure 24.3. Large ovarian cyst emptied

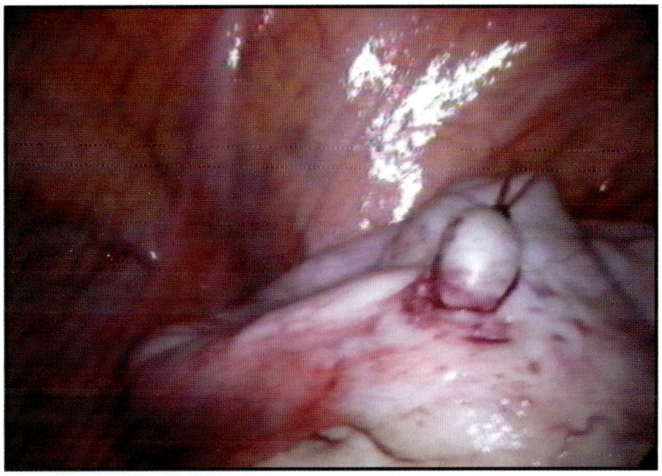

Figure 24.4. Ligation of cyst puncture site

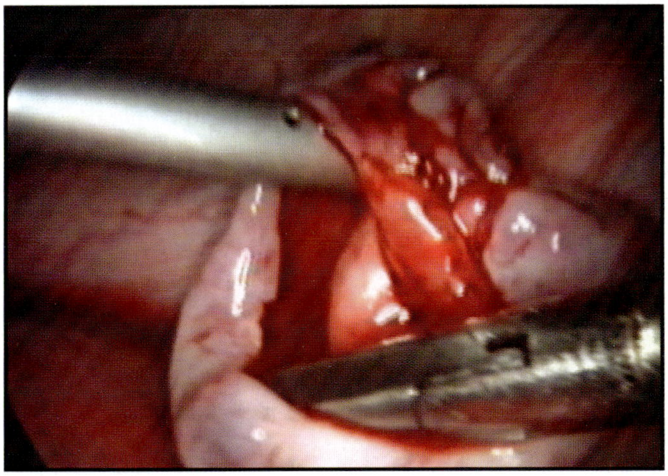

Figure 24.5. Normal ovary after cyst removal

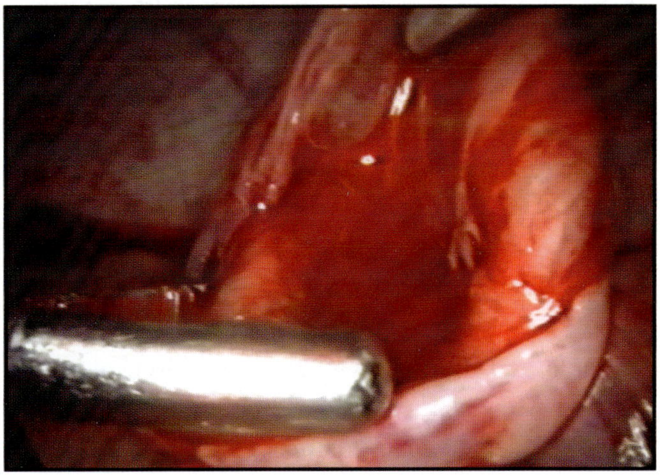

Figure 24.6. Irrigation of ovary after cyst wall excision

is used appropriately for visualization of the bleeding spots. This method can be performed with only two secondary ports of 5 mm. The cyst is extracted through the 10 mm port using a 5 mm telescope through one of the secondary ports. Alternatively the cyst can be held with a grasper introduced through one of the 5 mm ports and pushed out through the 10 mm port by rail-roading technique. The advantages of this method is that it requires a smaller incision on the ovary and is faster to perform and cyst extraction is easier. This method can also be used for very large cysts. The disadvantage of this method is that spillage of cyst fluid content occurs.

Closed Technique

Bipolar diathermy is applied on a small part of the ovarian capsule overlying the cyst. This part of the capsule is incised using a scissors. Two graspers are used to hold the cut edges and peel of the capsule slowly from the cyst wall. Diathermy is applied along the capsule and a scissors is used to cut on the line of coagulation. The two graspers are used to hold the ovary and the cyst in a suitable position and diathermy is applied between the cyst and the ovarian tissue. This part is cut to dissect the cyst from the rest of the ovary. As the cyst is being peeled off, an area where the cyst is adherent to the ovarian stroma is approached. Small spurt of diathermy is applied between the cyst wall and the ovary and the coagulated area is cut in very small increments each time. Suction and irrigation can be used whenever there is oozing from the dissected area. It is very important to keep the dissecting area clear in order to identify the line of demarcation between the cyst and rest of the ovary accurately. This method will help to excise the cyst in toto without the risk of cyst fluid leak into the peritoneal cavity. The cyst is introduced into an endobag. The opening of the endobag is brought out, the cyst is then aspirated and the cyst wall removed along with the endobag. Morcellation of the cyst wall is required if it is large. This method is ideal for mucinous cyst and dermoid cyst. The advantage of this method is that there is no fluid spillage, but the disadvantages include a larger ovarian incision that needs to be taken to excise the cyst, the longer duration required to perform the surgery, the risk of the cyst rupturing at any point during surgery, inability to excise very large cyst and the difficulty in extracting such a cyst. Large adnexal masses can also be removed by posterior calpotomy. Using a CCL extractor, the ball is pushed against the posterior vaginal fornix. Using monopolar diathermy electrode an incision is made against the ball, strong gasper is introduced through the cannula and cystic mass is brought close to the incision. This can be drained and morcellated before being extracted through the vagina. The culdotomy incision is sutured through the vaginal route.

Problems

Sometimes the cyst wall will be very thin and densely adherent to the ovary. In such cases, the part of the cyst attached to the ovarian stroma is left *in situ*. The cyst wall lining can be fulgurized if necessary.

There can be severe bleeding while separating the cyst wall. This is normally controlled by pressure usage of hemostatic agents and use of energy sources.

Excessive use of diathermy can damage the adjacent ovarian tissue. This can further go on to premature ovarian failure.

The fallopian tube can get stretched over the ovarian cyst and, hence, normal anatomy is disturbed. The stretched out tube is difficult to identify at times and is prone to damage during dissection of the cysts. The blood supply to distal part of the fallopian tube needs to be preserved by careful dissection as this may be damaged due to change in the anatomy.

ENDOMETRIOSIS

There are two verieties–Genital and extra genital. Genital endometriosis occurs in the uterine musculature, cervix, tubes, ovaries, lower pelvis, doom of the bladder, vagina and in the rectovaginal septum. Extragenital endometriosis may be seen in intestines, bladder, ureter, lungs, pleura and skin. Laparoscopy helps in diagnosis and also initiates all treatment of option of genital endometriosis. Often the diagnosis of endometriosis is made during treatment of the infertility. Endometriosis can affect fertility by impairment of ovulation, interference with conduction of ovum and fertilization and disturbances in nidation. Endometriotic cysts in the ovary can interfere with normal follicular growth. Endometriosis can cause pain due to compression and invasion of neighbouring organs as well as deep infiltration in the rectum.

Operative treatment of endometriosis is indicated when there is significant genital endometriosis and when there is formation of ovarian cysts. Presence of severe pain also warrants operative management.

LAPAROSCOPIC MANAGEMENT

All adhesions to the uterus and adnexa are released. Adhesiolysis is started from the periphery to progress towards the ovarian cyst. Adhesions are normally dense and would require use of energy sources; either lasers or bipolar diathermy can be used for this purpose. Among lasers used for photovaporization either carbon dioxide laser or the Potassium Titanyl Phosphate (KTP / 532) laser or argon beam can be used. Deeply penetrating lasers like Nd:YAG are not preferred. Bipolar diathermy is widely used and is found to be very effective. The thermal damage of diathermy is minimized by constant irrigation by either normal saline or ringers lactate solution using a irrigation cannula over the diathermised areas. One of the most common areas of endometriosis is over the uterosacral ligaments and between the ovary and broad ligament, lateral to the uterosacral ligaments. Adhesions tend to be progressively dense and in these cases combination of diathermy, blunt, hydro and sharp dissections are used. Both ovaries trend to be pulled medially and in many cases will be in contact are densely adherents to each other. Adhesiolysis of the adnexal mass is carried out over the posterior uterine surface and the ovary is released from the broad ligament to which it is normally attached. Chocolate material is frequently seen between the ovary and broad ligament. As the invagination of the ovarian capsule progresses, the chocolate cysts are formed. The ovary is released of all around it. A wide opening is made over the invagination site in cases of chocolate cysts and the fibrotic ring at the site of invagination is resected. The cyst is excised as far as possible. Small cysts which cannot be excised are laid open, the lining of the cyst is destroyed by bipolar coagulation or laser photocoagulation or vaporization. The chocolate cyst wall is much thicker than a simple serous cysts and needs to be peeled from the normal ovarian tissue with much larger force and use of diathermy or laser wherever adhesions are very dense. Stripping of the cyst wall is associated with fewer recurrences but this removes more follicles than does laser oblation of the cyst capsule inside the ovary. When the cysts are very large, the operative procedure is carried out in two steps with an interval of 2 - 3 months between the two. It is found that cystic structures regressed and the ovary resumes almost regular size. Further adhesiolysis, superficial coagulation of residual endometriotic tissue and restoration of normal anatomy is carried out in the second stage. Special precaution is taken while retrieving endometriotic tissue from the abdomen to make sure it does not come in contact with the abdominal wall. As this could lead to scar endometriosis. Rectovaginal septum is different pathological entity among the types of endometriosis this may also need a two stage procedure, the second stage being carried out after a period of medical treatment.

ADNEXAL TORSION

This is normally seen as an emergency with severe pain, vomiting and sometimes hemodynamic disturbance. Doppler scan would be useful in picking up lack of blood flow to the affected viscera. More commonly this is seen in cases of fimbrial, para-ovarian and ovarian cysts.

Operative Technique

Normally two secondary ports are sufficient, but sometimes the third may also be necessary. Initially the uterus and adnexa along with pouch of Douglas and the tissues beyond the twists are carefully inspected. If it is found to be frankly gangrenous, then the tissue is excised this can be done in 2 ways:

1. **Using energy sources**: Normally a bipolar coagulation for cysts is introduced. The viable tissues just beyond the twist is coagulated and then cut with the scissors (Figures 24.7 to 24.12). Alternatively ultracision, ligasure or other sources like carbon dioxide laser can be used for the dissection.
2. **Using ligature**: Loop knot can be tied just proximal to the twisted tissues, then the twisted tissue is excised. It is also possible to suture-ligate the pedicles on both sides and then excise it (Figures 24.13 to 24.16).

The necrosed tissue is brought out in an endobag. Morcellation is done if required, taking care to prevent spillage of any tissue.

If the tissues are only dusky, then de-rotation helps in restoring blood supply.[15] This is done by using 2 instruments gently holding the rotated tissue and twisting it in the opposite direction. Even if the ovary is slightly dusky it can be left alone.

TUBO-OVARIAN ABSCESS

This is normally seen in adolescent and young women who are sexually active.[27] This can be managed by draining the abscess by a culdotomy. In cases presenting early there may only be a mass without liquifaction. Adhesions to the neighboring bowel is common.

Operative Technique

2 secondary ports are introduced in the lower abdomen if adhesions are present, it is released either by blunt hydro or diathermy dissection. Use of bipolar diathermy only is strongly recommended (Figures 24.17 to 24.21). Care needs to be taken to avoid damage, to bowel or ureter. After initial inspection the adnexal abscess is dissected. Mild inflammatory changes can be accepted and in these conditions conservative line of treatment is followed, presence of any pus is removed. A drain is left *in situ*. Grossly infected or damaged adnexa need to be removed. This is done either by diathermy dissection or suture ligation of pedicles. Excised tissue is removed through an endobag.

BROAD LIGAMENT FIBROID

This can easily be confused to a malignant adnexal mass. It is removed surgically, if found to be symptomatic or causing pressure effects.

Operative Technique

The broad ligament is incised after injecting diluted vasopressin solution or copious amount of normal saline, till blanching of the local area is seen. Using spatula an incision is made in the leaf of broad ligament over the fibroid (Figures 24.22). Using blunt dissection the fibroid is further dissected. If necessary a myoma screw is applied to the fibroid and traction is applied (Figure 24.23). Simultaneously the sites of the fibroid are dissected with 2 instruments (Figures 24.24 and 24.25). Bipolar diathermy is used wherever necessary in larger fibroids. Care has to be taken to avoid damage to bowel, bladder, ureter and uterine vessels. The fibroid can be removed either by morcellation or enlarging the port. The residual defect after removal of the fibroid is closed by either intracorporeal suturing or by assisted surgery wherein the suprapubic port site is enlarged to use conventional open surgical suturing (Figures 24.26 to 24.28).

ADNEXAL MASSES

If adnexal masses are fixed, irregular or solid, malignancy is suspected.[13,14,32] The presence of ascites or upper abdominal mass strongly raises the suspicion of malignancy. The following staging procedure is important in patients with suspicion of malignancy. Ascitic fluid is collected from the pouch of Douglas at the out set. Washings are obtained. The whole abdomen is inspected with special attention to the following sites: Right and left diaphragm, surface of the liver, Gallbladder, Stomach, Spleen, Right and Left kidney, Right and left paracolic gutter, small bowel, mesentery, appendix, ascending

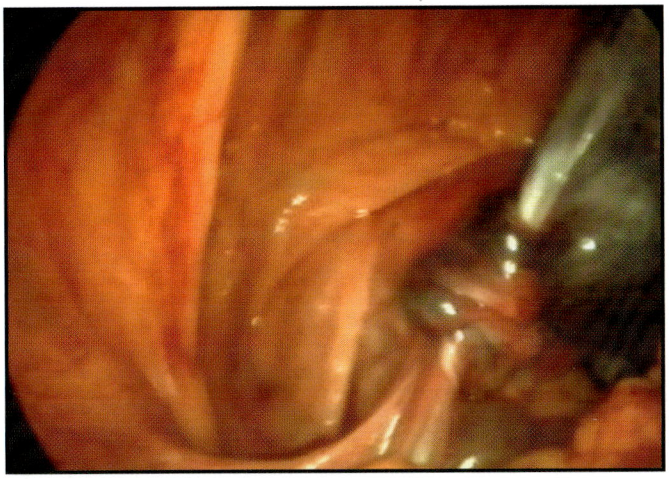

Figure 24.7. Left twisted ovarian cyst

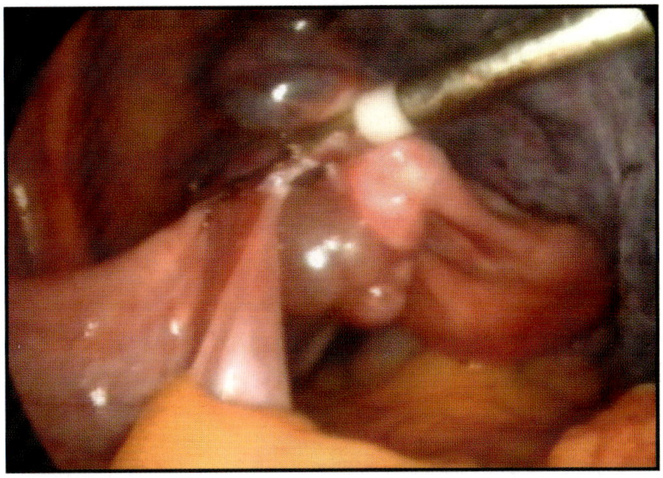

Figure 24.8. Salpingo-oopherectomy using bipolar diathermy

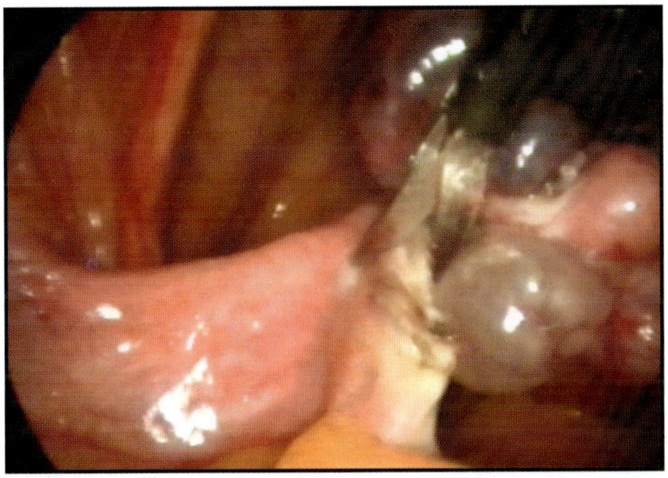

Figure 24.9. Salpingo-oopherectomy scissor use

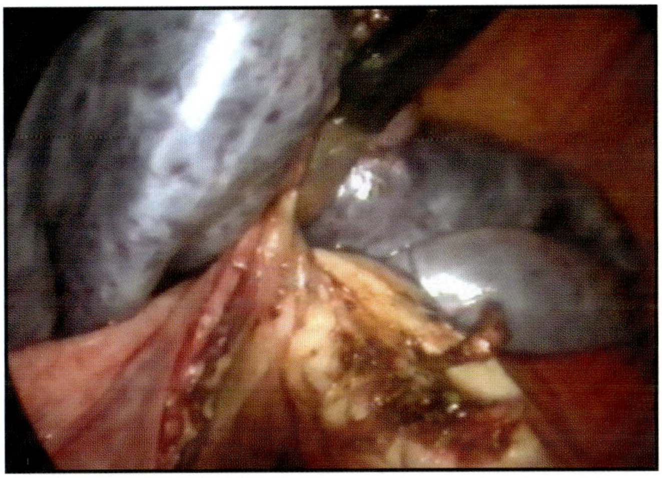

Figure 24.10. Salpingo-oopherectomy bipolar scissor

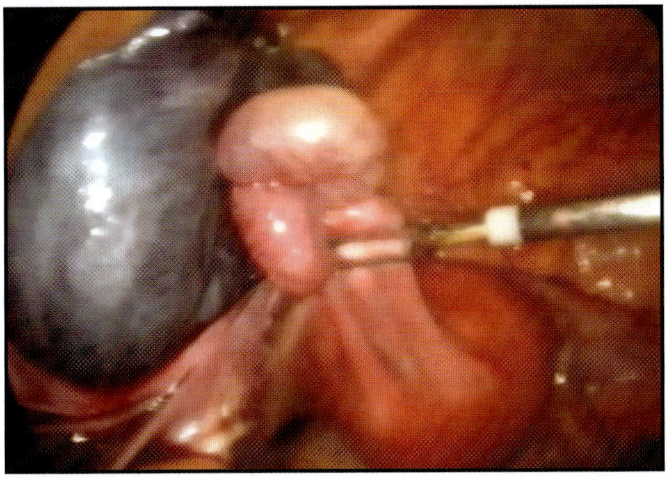

Figure 24.11. Bipolar diathermy of infundibulopelvic diathermy

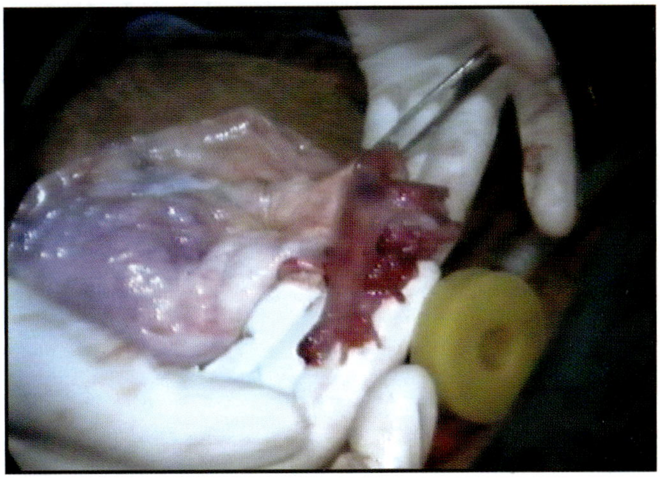

Figure 24.12. External view of excised adnexa

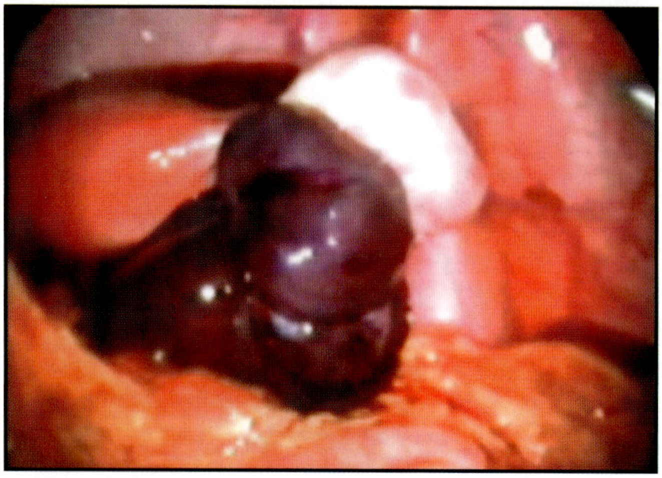

Figure 24.13. Gangrenous twisted tube

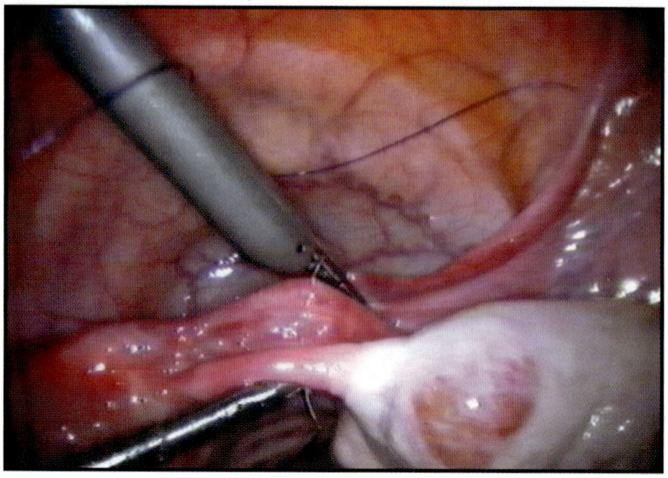

Figure 24.14. Suturing of adnexa

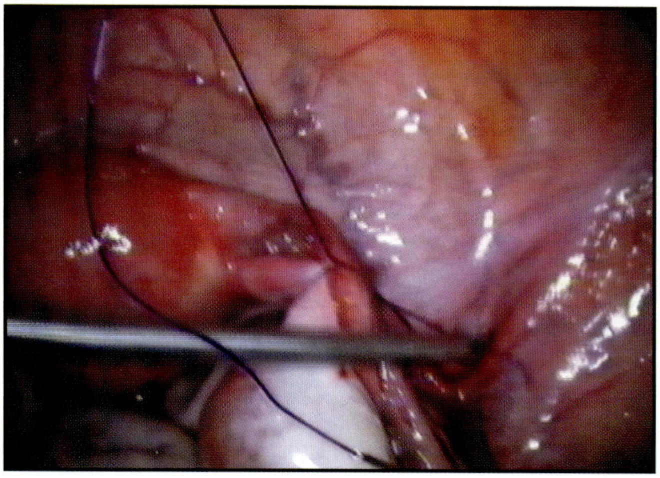

Figure 24.15. Ligation of adnexal mass

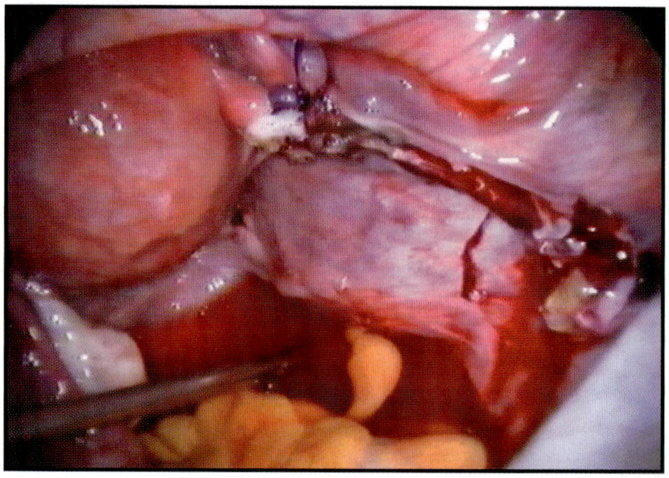

Figure 24.16. After adnexectomy

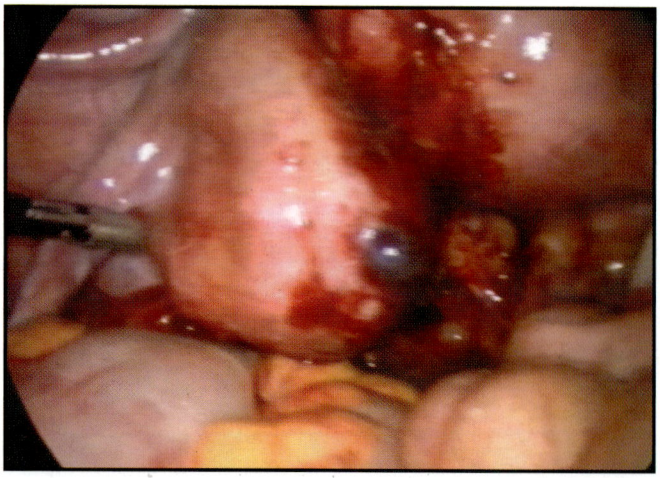

Figure 24.17. Left pyosalpinx

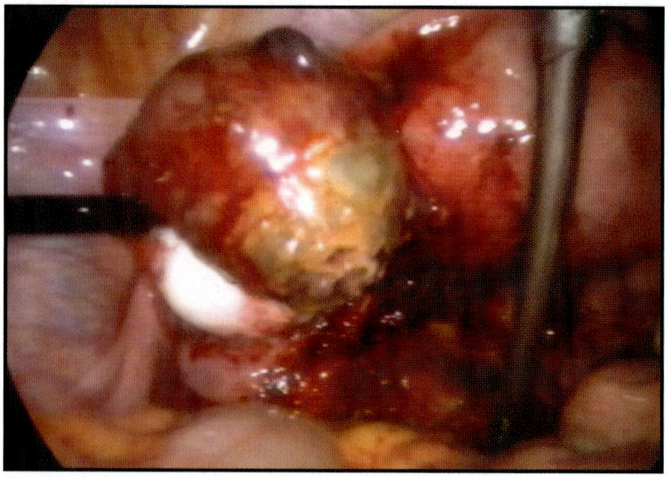

Figure 24.18. Pointing of left pyosalpinx

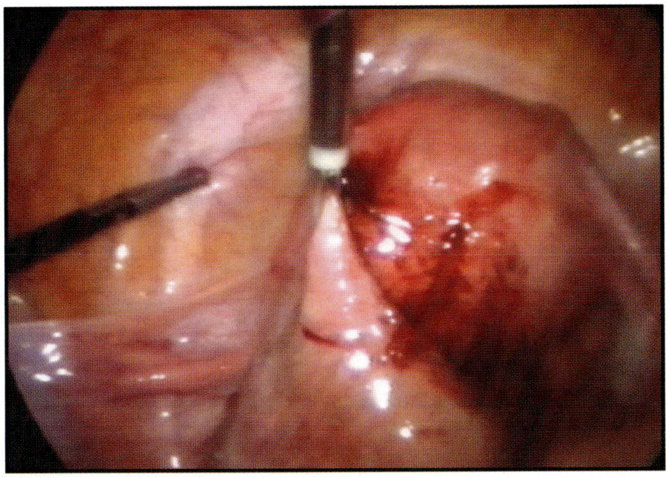

Figure 24.19. Use of bipolar diathermy

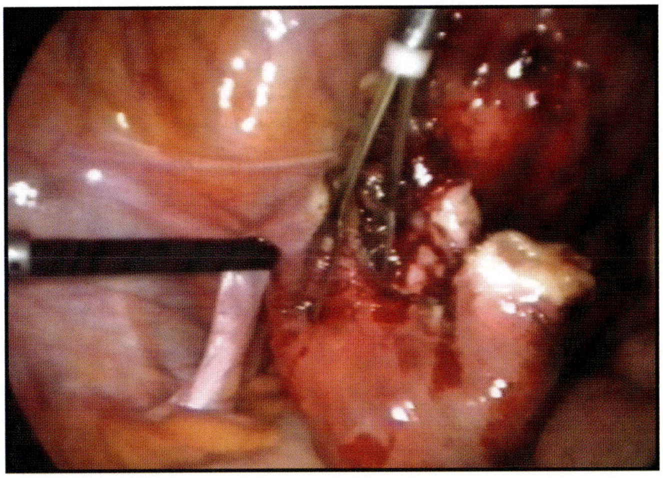

Figure 24.20. Use of bipolar diathermy

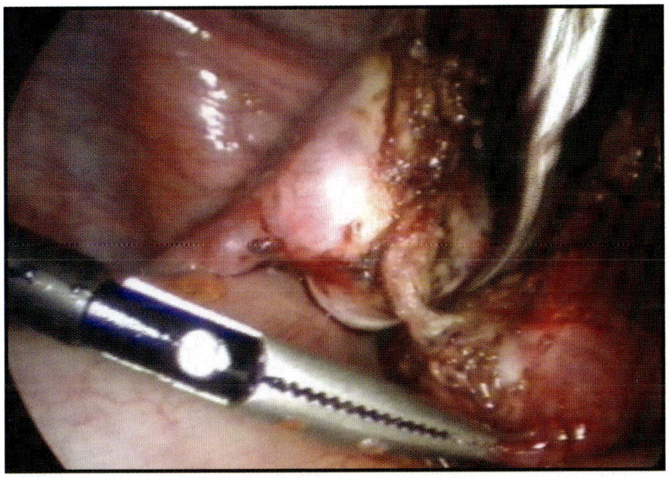

Figure 24.21. Sharp dissection with cautery

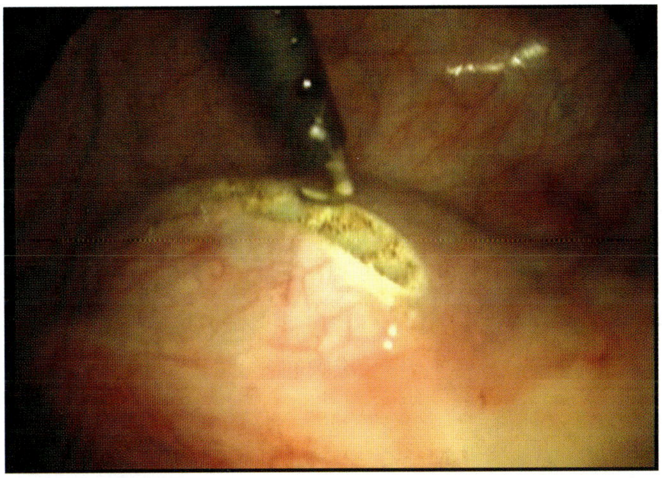

Figure 24.22. Broad ligament myoma-monopolar diathermy

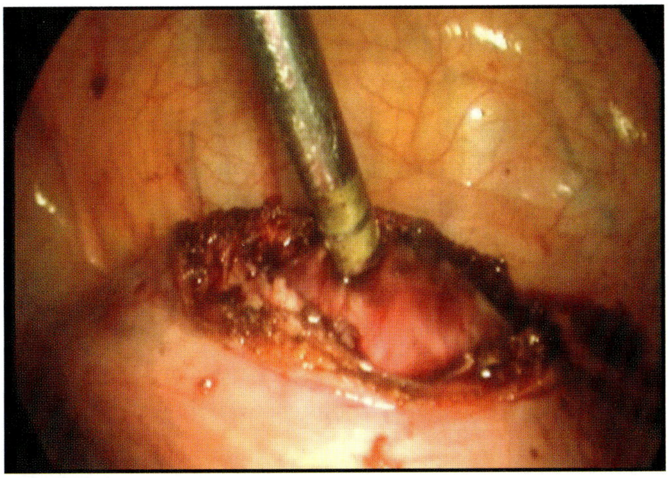

Figure 24.23. Entry of myoma screw into the myoma

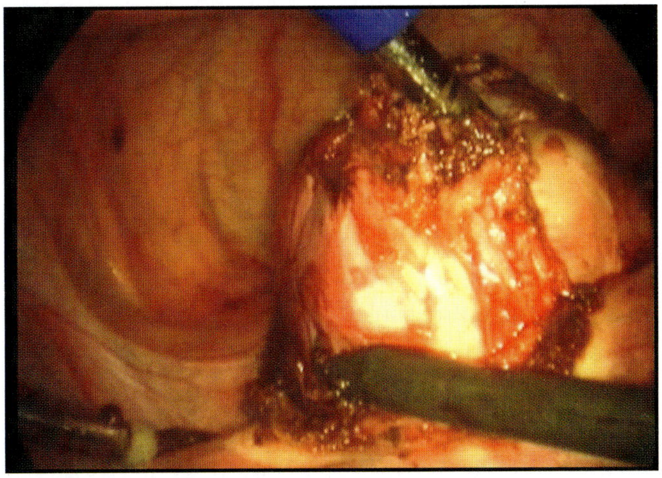

Figure 24.24. Enucleation of the myoma

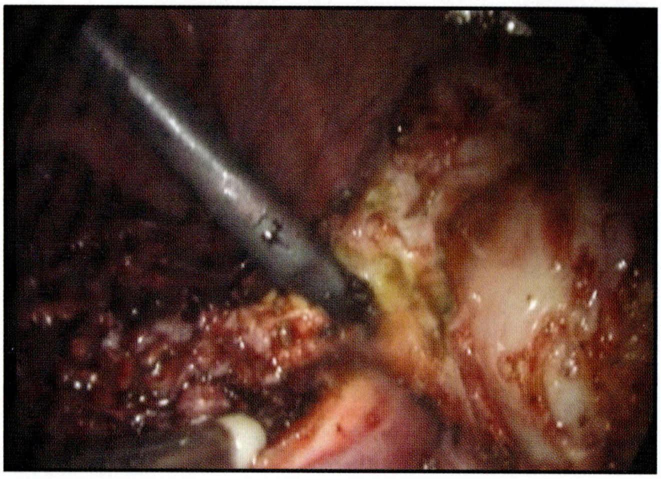

Figure 24.25. Coagulation of the base of the myoma

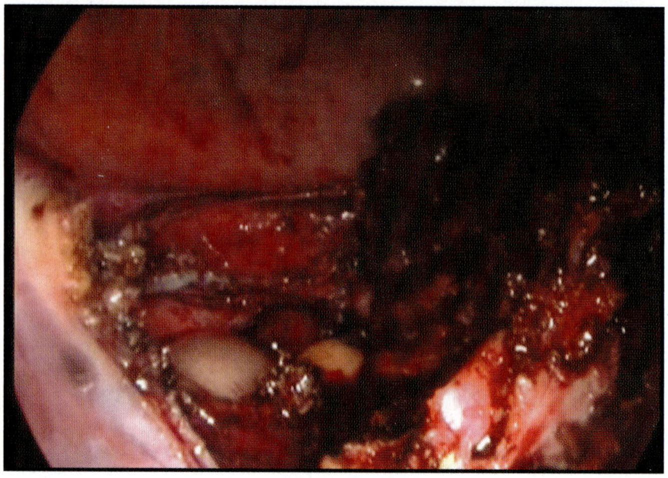

Figure 24.26. Myoma bed hemostasis check

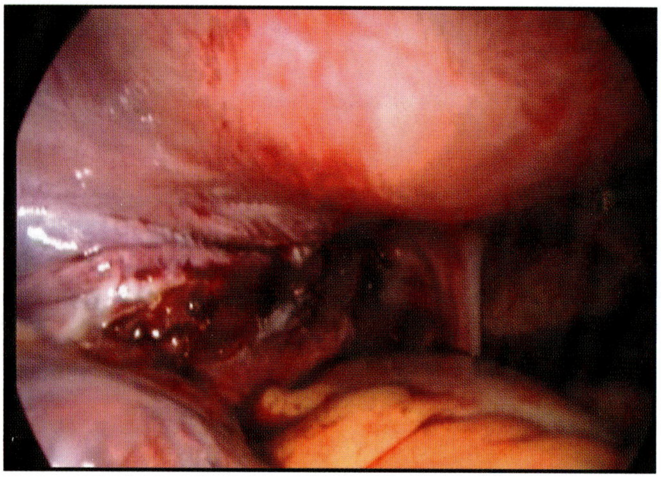

Figure 24.27. Approximation of the myoma bed

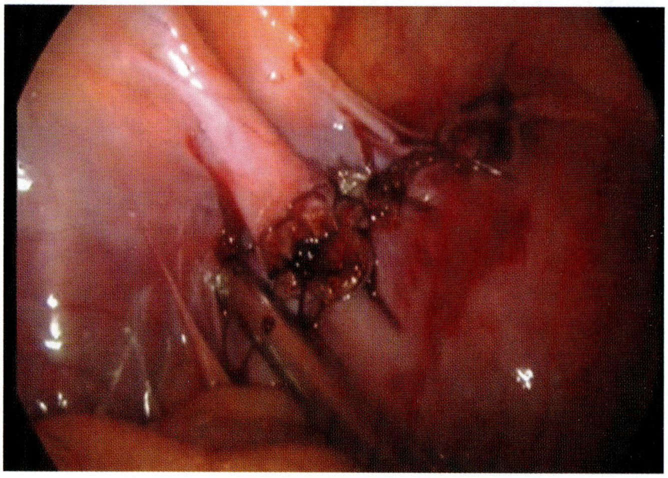

Figure 24.28. Approximation of the myoma bed by suturing

transverse, descending and rectosigmoid colon, omentum, lesser sac, para-aortic and pelvic nodes, uterus and adnexa and bladder peritoneal.[1]

Whenever there is suspected malignant ovarian lesion which is confined to the ovary, Diagnostic Ovariectomy can be performed using laparoscopy, but in such cases the ovary has to be removed without spillage of contents or rupture of the capsule.[4,16,31] The intact cyst can be removed in an endobag'. Obvious benign masses can be removed without damage to the rest of the adnexa.[6] The dissection must take into consideration the women's desire regarding future fertility.[12,26] Any possible technical factors that would come in way of future reproductive abilities should be considered as far as possible.[7]

When disseminated malignancy is evident a complete staging protocol must be performed. The abdomen is explored by laparotomy, the uterus both adnexae, omentum, pelvic and para-aortic lymphnodes are removed, biopsies are taken from the undersurface of the right and left diaphragms, paracolic gutters and bladder wall.[22,24,37-40] Resection needs to be as maximal as possible and may have to include parts of bowel warranting the need for colostomy in some occasions.[33-36]

REFERENCES

1. Chapron C, Dubuisson JB, Samouh N, Foulot H, Aubriot FX, Ansquer Y, et al. Treatment of ovarian dermoid cysts. Place and modalities of operative laparoscopy. Surg Endosc 1994;8:1092-5.
2. Canis M, Mage G, Pouly JL, Wattiez A, Manhes H, Bruhat MA. Laparoscopic diagnosis of adnexal cystic masses: A 12-year experience with long term follow-up. Obstet Gynecol 1994;83:707-12.
3. Mettler L, Caesar G, Neunzling S, Semm K. Stellenwert der endoskopischen ovar-chirurgie, Kritische analyse von 626 pelviskopish operierten ovarialyzsten an der Universitäts- Fraenklinik Kiel 1990-1991. Geburtsh u Frauenheilk 1993;53:253-7.
4. Nezhat F, Nezhat C, Welander CE, Benigno B. Four ovarian cancers diagnosed during laparoscopic management of 1011 women with adnexal masses. Am J Obstet Gynecol 1992;167:790-6.
5. Semm K, Mettler L. Technical progress in pelvic surgery via operative laparoscopy. Am J Obstet Gynecol 1980; 138:121-7.
6. Reich H. Laparoscopic oophorectomy and salpingo-oophorectomy in the treatment of benign tubo-ovarian disease. Int J Fertil 1987;32:233-6.
7. Nezhat C, Nczhat F, Silfen SL. Videolaseroscopy for oophorectomy. Obstet Gynecol 1991;165:1323-30.
8. Perry CP, Upchurch JC. Pelviscopic adnexectomy. Am J Obstet Gynecol 1990;162:79-81.
9. Pittaway DE, Takacs P, Bauguess P. Laparoscopic adnexectomy: A comparison with laparotomy. Am J Obstet Gynecol 1994;171:385-95.
10. Tintara H, Leetanaporn R. Cost-benefit analysis of laparoscopic adnexectomy. Int J Gynecol Obstet 1995;50:21-5.
11. Daniell JF, Kurtz BR, Lee JY. Laparoscopic oophorectomy: comparative study of ligatures, bipolar coagulation and automatic stapling devices. Obste Gynecol 1992;80:325-8.
12. Leng JH, et al. Role of laparoscopy in the diagnosis and treatment of adnexal masses. Chin Med J (Engl) 2006;119(3):202-6.
13. Chapron C, Dubuisson JB, Fritel X, Morice P, Aubriot FX, Foulot H. Techniques et indications de l'utilisation du sac endoscopique dans la prise en charge des kystes ovariens. Contracept Fertil Sex 1994;22:682-4.
14. Chapron C, Dubuisson JB, Capella-Allouc S. Salpingo-oophorectomy for adnexal masses. Place and results for operative laparoscopy. Eur J Obste Gynecol Reprod Biol (In press).
15. Chapron C, Capella-Allouc S, Dubuisson JB. Treatment of adnexal torsion using operative laparoscopy. Hum Reprod 1996;11:998-1003.
16. Chapron C, Dubuisson JB, Fritel X, Rambaud D. Management of organic ovarian cysts: Place and modalities for laparoscopy. Hum Reprod Update, (In press).
17. Alcazar JL, Ruiz-Perez ML, Errasti T. Transvaginal color Doppler sonography in adnexal masses: Which parameter performs best? Obstet Gynecol Surv 1973;28(5):suppl:357-81.
18. Barber HR, Graber EA.Gynaecological tumors in childhood and adolescence. Obstet Gynecol. 1997;89(5 Pt 1):679-83.
19. Canis M, Pouly JL, Wattiez A, Mage G, Manhes H, Bruhat MA. Laparoscopic management of adnexal masses suspicious at ultrasound Gynecol Oncol 1997;65(3):408-14.
20. DePriest PD, Gallion HH, Pavlik EJ, Kryscio RJ, van Nagell JR Jr. Transvaginal sonography as a screening method for the detection of early ovarian cancer. Am Fam Physician 1998;57(10):2471-6, 2479-80.
21. Drake J. Diagnosis and management of the adnexal mass South Med J 1997;90(10):972-81.
22. Gallup DG, Talledo E. Management of the adnexal mass in the 1990s Radiology 2000;214(1):39-46.
23. Hricak H, Chen M, Coakley FV, Kinkel K, Yu KK, Sica G, Bacchetti P, Powell CB. Complex adnexal masses: detection and characterization with MR imaging–multivariate analysis Obstet Gynecol 1991;77(4):563-5.
24. Maiman M, Seltzer V, Boyce J. Laparoscopic excision of ovarian neoplasms subsequently found to be malignant JSLS 1997;1(1):17-27.
25. Nezhat FR, Tazuke S, Nezhat CH, Seidman DS, Phillips DR, Nezhat CR. 1: Laparoscopy during pregnancy: A literature reivew Pediatr Clin North Am 1999;46(3):573-92.
26. Pfeifer SM, Gosman GG. Evaluation of adnexal masses in adolescents. J Adolesc Health. 1996;18(6):397-403.
27. Slap GB, Forke CM, Cnaan A, Bellah RD, Kreider ME, Hanissian JA, Gallagher PR, Driscoll DA. Recognition of tubo-ovarian abscess in adolescents with pelvic inflammatory disease. Am J Obstet Gynecol 1973;116(4): 551-6.
28. Spanos WJ. Preoperative hormonal therapy of cystic adnexal masses. Am J Obstet Gynecol 1999;181(1):57-65.
29. Timmerman D, Bourne TH, Tailor A, Collins WP, Verrelst H, Vandenberghe K, Vergote I. A comparison of methods for preoperative discrimination between malignant and

benign adnexal masses: The development of a new logistic regression model. Cancer 1999;86(11):2280-90.
30. Twickler DM, Forte TB, Santos-Ramos R, McIntire D, Harris P, Scott D. Charles Chapron, Jean-Bernard Dubuisson, Sylvie Capella-Allouc and Xavier Fritel The ovarian Tumor Index predicts risk for malignancy Service de chirurgie Gynécologique, Clinique Universitaire Baudelocque, CHU Cochin Port-Royal, 123, Boulevard Port-Royal, 75014, Paris, France Policy and Practice Guidelines Committee of the Society of Obstetricians and Gynaecologists of Canada No. 97, 2000.
31. SOGC/GOC/SCC POLICY AND PRACTICE Policy and Practice Guidelines Committee of the Society of Obstetricians and Gynaecologists of Canada No. 97, November 2000.
32. Dubuc-Lissoir J, Drouin P, Ehlen T, et al. Guidelines for the laparoscopic management of the adnexal mass. J Soc Obstet Gynaecol Can 1998;20(10):983-9.
33. Allen DG, Baak J, Belpomme D, et al. Advanced epithelial ovarian cancer: 1993 consensus statements.Ann Onc 1993;4:S83-8.
34. Trimbos JB, Bolis G. Guidelines for surgical staging of ovarian cancer. Obstet Gynaecol Survey 1994;49:814-6.
35. Morgan RJ, Copeland L, Gershenson D, et al. NCCN ovarian cancer practice guidelines. Onc 1996;10:293-310.
36. NIH Consensus Development Panel on Ovarian Cancer. Ovarian cancer: Screening, treatment, and follow-up. J Amer Med Assoc 1995;273:491-7.
37. Hoskins W, Rice L, Rubin S. Ovarian cancer surgical practice guidelines. Onc 1997;11:896-904.
38. Hoskins WJ, Bundy BN,Thigpen JT,Omura GA.The influence of cytoreductive surgery on recurrence-free interval and survival in small volume stage III epithelial ovarian cancer: A gynecologic oncology group study. Gynaecol Onc 1992;47:159-66.
39. Junor EJ, Hole DJ, McNulty L, Mason M,Young J. Specialist gynaecologists and survival outcome in ovarian cancer: A Scottish national study of 1866 patients. Brit J Obstet Gynecol 1999;106:1130-6.
40. Scarabelli C, Gallo A, Zarrelli A,Visentin C, Campagnutta E. Systematic pelvic and pata-aortic lymphadenectomy during cytoreductive surgery in advanced ovarian cancer: Potential benefit on survival. Gynecol Onc 1995;56:328-37.

Index

A

Adhesiolysis 20
  laparoscopic management 23
Adnexal mass 215, 222
  clinical findings
    CT scan 216
    MRI scans 216
    ultrasound 216
  factors
    age 215
    pain 215
  laparoscopic surgery 216
    bipolar diathermy 220
    laparoscopic management 221
    ovarian cystectomy 218
    polycystic ovary and anovulation 217
    technique of ovarian drilling 217
Adnexal torsion 221

B

Benign ovarian mass
  classification 207
  preoperative screening 207
    borderline malignant mass 208
    malignant mass 209
    probable benign mass 208
  surgical procedures 209
    laparoscopic oophorectomy 212
    ovarian cystectomy 209
  tissue retrieval methods 212
    culdotomy 213
    direct tissue removal 213
    ovarian torsion 213
    removal in endobag 212
Broad ligament fibroid 222

C

Cardiac arrhythmias 75
Complications at laparoscopy 3, 46
  anesthesia related 3
  bladder and ureteric injuries 5, 56
  electrosurgical injuries 8
  gastrointestinal injuries 7
  injuries from energy sources 54
  morcellator related injuries 8
  nerve injuries 3
  patient positioning 3, 48
  pelvic inflammatory disease 57
  postoperative wound infections 57
  prevention of anesthesia complications 46
  safety at creating pneumoperitoneum 47
  safety at use of operative instruments 55
  safety involving trocar or veress needle related injuries 4, 48
    bladder injury with veress and trocar 53
    bowel injury 48
    incisional hernia 53
    injury to great vessles 52
    injury to omental or mesenteric vessels 52
    injury to vessels in abdominal wall 52
    specific procedures and bowel injury 51
  tumor seedings 57
Culdoscopy 10

D

Distal tubal occlusion 161
  classification
    hydrosalpinx follicularis 162
    hydrosalpinx simplex 162
    hydrosalpinx with pachysalpinx 162
  operative techniques
    adhesiolysis 163
    cuff salpingostomy 165
    everting the mucosa 165
    fimbrioplasty 164
    laparoscopic salpingostomy 164
    opening the tube 165
    salpingectomy 166
    stabilizing the eversion 165
  pathology 161
  preoperative evaluation
    couple fertility 162
    hysterosalpingography 163
    hysteroscopy 163
    salpingoscopy 163
  surgical anatomy 161

E

Ectopic pregnancy
  diagnosis 168
  surgical management 170
    laparoscopic approach 170
    laparotomy or laparoscopy 170
    salpingectomy 171
    salpingostomy 171
    segmental resection 171
  treatment 168
    chemotherapy 169
Electrosurgery or laser 54
Endometrioma 25
  clinical presentation 26
  diagnosis 26
  endometrioma and infertility 30
    pathogenesis 30
    treatment 30
  medical management 27
  pathogenesis 25
  surgical management 28
    aspiration of endometriomas 27, 32
    laparoscopic cyst wall ablation 33
    ovarian cyst excision 31
    role of adjunctive surgical procedures 30

Endometriosis 36, 220
classification 36
diagnosis 36
treatment 37
Endoscopic instrumentation
basic instruments 63
camera equipment 65
insufflator 63
light cables 65
light sources 64
telescopes 63
hand instruments 65
bipolar forceps 67
graspers/forceps 66
monopolar hook and needle 67
myoma screws 67
scissors 67
suction and irrigation apparatus 67
trocar 65
veress needle 65
maintenance and sterilization of instruments 70
newer developments 70
operating room set-up 70
specialized devices
electrocautery 67
harmonic scalpel 68
laser 68
ultrasound systems 68
specialized instruments
suturing instruments 68
uterine manipulators 69
tissue retrieval methods 69
endobag 70
morcellator 69

F

Falloposcopy 181
coaxial technique 182
complications 185
falloposcope 182
linear everting catheter system technique 182
management of fallopian tubal luminal disease 184
patient preparation 181
pitfalls of scoring system 184
potential therapeutic applications 185
results 183
Fertiloscopy
concept 10
contraindications 12
indications 10
procedure 11
Fibroids or leiomyomas 87

G

Gas embolism 74

H

Hysteroscopic myomectomy 87, 88, 130
precautions 132
prerequisites 130
role 130
Hysteroscopic surgery
metroplasty 156
polypectomy 155
synechiolysis 155
Hysteroscopy complications 57
dilation of the cervix 58
hazards of distension media 58
CO2 and other gases 58
high-viscosity fluids 58
liquid distension media 58
low-viscosity fluids 58
mechanical complications 59
instrumental and electrosurgical injuries 59
perforation 59
postoperative complications 60
preoperative preparation 58
safety at anesthesia 57

I

Indications for tubal endoscopy 180
ectopic pregnancy 181
endometriosis 181
pelvic inflammatory disease 181
prior to assisted fertilization 181
proximal tubal disease 180
unexplained infertility 181
Infertility 148
diagnostic hysteroscopy 150
endometrial hyperplasia 150
evaluation of cervical canal 150
evaluation of endometrial cavity 150
intrauterine adhesions 150
intrauterine pathology 150
uterine malformation 150
diagnostic modalities 148
hysterosalpingography 149
hysteroscopy before ART 149
sonohysterography 148
ultrasonography 148
instrumentation
conventional diagnostic hysteroscopy 149
microcolpohysteroscope 149
office hysteroscopy 149
management
hysteroscopic myomectomy 152
hysteroscopic surgery 152
preoperative endometrial reduction 153
pregnancy rates after hysteroscopic myomectomy 155
Intrauterine adhesions 137
classification 139
clinical manifestations 138
contributing factors 137
diagnosis 139, 150
hysterosalpingography 139
hysteroscopy 140
magnetic resonance imaging 140
ultrasonography 140
etiology 137
hysteroscopic adhesiolysis 141
adjunctive procedures 142
management of perforations 143
procedure related complications 143
surgical modalities and techniques 142
technical nuances 141
outcomes and prognosis 143
pathogenic processes 138
treatment options 141

L

Laparascopy surgery 78
anesthesia techniques 80
choice of anesthetic drugs 80
epidural, spinal anesthesia 81
monitoring 80
intraoperative complications 82
location of surgery 79
pain management 82
physiologic changes associated with 79
preoperative evaluation 80
selection of patient 79
Laparoscopic assisted myomectomy 95
complications 105
difficulties 103
indications 95
laparoscopic procedure 98, 99
preoperative evaluation 96
Laparoscopic myolysis 128
Laparoscopic myomectomy 90, 112
clinical study 91
complications 125
breakage of myoma screw 125
endometrial serosal fistula 126
indications 127
patient selection and preparation 90
place of laparoscopic assisted myomectomy 127